DIGESTIVE WELLNESS FOR CHILDREN

DIGESTIVE WELLNESS FOR CHILDREN

How to Strengthen the Immune System &
Prevent Disease Through Healthy Digestion

ELIZABETH LIPSKI, PH.D., C.C.N.

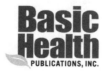

Basic
Health
PUBLICATIONS, INC.

The information contained in this book is based upon the research and personal and professional experiences of the author. It is not intended as a substitute for consulting with your physician or other healthcare provider. Any attempt to diagnose and treat an illness should be done under the direction of a healthcare professional.

The publisher does not advocate the use of any particular healthcare protocol but believes the information in this book should be available to the public. The publisher and author are not responsible for any adverse effects or consequences resulting from the use of the suggestions, preparations, or procedures discussed in this book. Should the reader have any questions concerning the appropriateness of any procedures or preparation mentioned, the author and the publisher strongly suggest consulting a professional healthcare advisor.

Basic Health Publications, Inc.
28812 Top of the World Drive
Laguna Beach, CA 92651
949-715-7327

Library of Congress Cataloging-in-Publication Data

Lipski, Elizabeth.
    Digestive wellness for children : how to strengthen the immune system
& prevent disease through healthy digestion / Elizabeth Lipski.
        p. cm.
    Includes bibliographical references.
    ISBN-13: 978-1-59120-151-9
    ISBN-10: 1-59120-151-9
    1. Nutrition disorders in children. 2. Diet therapy for children.
3. Children—Nutrition. I. Title. 010a 2006001689

    RJ399.N8.L37   2006
    618.92'39—dc22

                                        2006001689

Editor: Kate Johnson
Typesetting/Book design: Gary A. Rosenberg
Cover design: Mike Stromberg

Printed in the United States of America

10   9   8   7   6   5   4   3   2   1

Contents

This book is dedicated to my children:

*Aron, who so generously offers his time and expertise,
and for his love of learning;*

*Kyle, my friend, whose mature insights amaze me,
and whose wit keeps me laughing;*

Arthur, curious, bright, and capable, who shares my heart;

*and Cora, who inspires me to reflect on
independence, privacy, and style.*

Foreword

I have long been greatly concerned about all the parents out there who feel helpless when their children have health problems. They feel alone and inadequate in dealing with problems that impact their children's health and well-being. The truth is that every day, parents make choices that affect their family's ability to be healthy. Each choice is like a droplet of water in an upward or downward stream of health. When added together, these choices have an enormous collective effect, taking us either towards or away from health. In terms of diet, we are often guided by what's convenient, fast, and affordable. Computers, electronic games, and television have replaced playing outdoors, sports, and family conversation. We treat our children with antibiotics and medications that help in the short run, but depress our children's overall ability to bounce back on their own. So what's a parent to do?

Thankfully, the complex issues related to our children's health are made simpler in *Digestive Wellness for Children* by Elizabeth Lipski, Ph.D., C.C.N. As both Dr. Lipski and I have been aware for nearly two decades, digestion plays a key role in the overall health of our children. Dr. Lipski offers many important concepts and breakthroughs that lead us to rethink common children's health issues. Such far-reaching issues as asthma, irritable bowel syndrome, chronic abdominal pain, attention deficit disorder, headaches, juvenile arthritis, and many more health concerns can be resolved by changes in lifestyle and diet. When digestion is improved, immune function improves and comes back into balance. Your child's energy, behavior, and sense of well-being improve on all levels.

This book is a must-read for every parent who is interested in being proactive about their child's health and wellness. Dr. Lipski artfully weaves the scientific information into an easy-to-read and extremely usable guide for parents. *Digestive Wellness for Children* will give you the confidence to try new options, because they are based upon current scientific research.

You will become more fully informed about the increase in children's illnesses in our country and how our busy lifestyles contribute to the problem. You'll find practical ideas about creating healthy family meals, making the transition to a healthier diet, and shopping. You'll also find specific information about how digestion works and why probiotic bacteria are so critical to gut health. You'll begin to understand why your child is so sensitive to his/her environment and what you can do to reduce food and environmental sensitivities. Finally, you'll find specific information and recommendations on more than thirty-five specific health conditions—from infancy through adolescence.

For many years, I have been impressed by the way that Elizabeth Lipski has kept abreast of the latest knowledge and information in the nutritional sciences, and how it applies to health conditions that can challenge your children. Her first book, *Digestive Wellness,* has become a classic in the field. *Digestive Wellness for Children* is a companion to that earlier work. We now recognize that the digestive tract plays an important role in determining our health. We are not "what we eat" but rather "what we absorb from what we eat," "what wastes we can eliminate," and "how well our gut ecology is balanced." Many of our children have long-standing health issues that can be resolved when these issues are addressed.

This book makes an important contribution to people's understanding of the important relationships between gastrointestinal physiology, diet, and health. For parents who are not familiar with this exciting and important topic, this book will provide an introduction and a guide to how they can gain better control over digestive function and its relationship to their children's health.

Dr. Lipski's book helps the reader to understand how to approach this objective with precision. Enjoy.

—Ann Louise Gittleman, Ph.D., C.N.S.
New York Times award-winning author of more than twenty-five books
including *The Fat Flush Plan, Before the Change,* and
The Fast Track ONE-DAY Detox Diet

Our Children's Health

All ancient systems of healing, however much they differ among themselves, share with one another a common skein that divides them from modern clinical medicine. They all approach sickness as a problem of balance and relationship, the result of disharmony between the sick person and his environment rather than the product of specific diseases. To the traditional healer, disease itself has no reality independent of the person who is sick and the web of relationships of which he is part. By understanding how this universal wisdom was displaced from the conceptual basis of modern Western medicine, we can learn how to restore it.

—LEO GALLAND, *THE FOUR PILLARS OF HEALING*

OUR CHILDREN ARE NOT WELL

Our kids are in trouble. Consider the following statistics on childhood disease in the United States:

- About 300,000 of our children have arthritis. Rheumatoid arthritis, the most devastating type, affects 70,000–75,000 children.

- According to the U.S. Centers for Disease Control and Prevention, asthma prevalence among children and teenagers increased approximately 5 percent *each year* during the period of 1980–1995. Asthma now afflicts 4.8 million of our children (15 percent of boys and 10 percent of girls) under the age of eighteen, and 600 die from the disease each year.

- 12 percent of our children suffer from respiratory allergies or hay fever.

- Over 8 million of our children get migraine headaches, resulting in over a million lost days of school each year.

1

- Approximately 10 percent of our infants and young children develop eczema, and 60 percent of these children will continue to have problems with eczema into their adult years.

- It is estimated that irritable bowel syndrome affects 17 percent of our high-school students and 8 percent of our middle-school students.

Learning, behavioral, developmental, and mental health challenges have increased as well, afflicting an estimated 17 percent of our children—that's 12 million kids:

- Eight percent of our children (10 percent of boys and 5 percent of girls) have a learning disability.

- Three to 6 percent have an attention deficit disorder.

- The diagnosis of autism and pervasive developmental disorder is skyrocketing, with at least a tenfold increase in the United States in the last twenty years.

According to the U.S. Surgeon General, 10 percent of our children and adolescents suffer from mental illness that is severe enough to warrant medical attention. For example:

- Between 2 and 6 percent of our children and adolescents are depressed.

- Suicide is the third leading cause of death in children aged ten to nineteen years old.

- In 2002, 11 million prescriptions for antidepressants were written for children—but recent studies indicate that the use of antidepressants in children doubles their risk of suicide.

- In the past twenty years, the average age of onset of bipolar disorder (also known as manic depression) has fallen from the early thirties to the late teens.

Overall, between 5 and 30 percent of American children have a chronic illness. And "adult" illnesses such as type II diabetes and heart disease, formerly rare in childhood, are now appearing in children at alarming rates.

Baby Blues

Despite all of the advantages of the American lifestyle, many of our children get off to a rough start. How many of us have spent long nights pacing with an unhappy baby? Sixteen to 26 percent of infants experience colic in their first few months, and as many as 10 percent of infants experience eczema, diaper rash, and/or cradle cap.

Food allergies affect 2 to 8 percent of infants, and allergy to milk is the most common; in infants, cow's milk intake is also strongly associated with spitting up and vomiting. Spitting up and an unusual amount of vomiting occurs in half of all newborns and two-thirds of infants aged up to four months old. It's normal for babies to spit up from time to time, but 0.3 to 8 percent of infants have more serious gastroesophageal reflux disease that may be associated with poor weight gain, fussiness, hiatal hernia, cystic fibrosis, or other health problems.

Bigger Children, Bigger Problems

Simple, natural strategies can solve some of the health problems of infancy, and many others are quickly outgrown. But as our children grow, they can develop other digestive health issues. Constipation, for example, accounts for 3 percent of all visits to pediatricians and 25 percent of children's visits to gastroenterologists. Encopresis (fecal soiling or unplanned bowel movements in children older than four years) affects 1 to 3 percent of our children. Celiac disease, which limits the body's tolerance of gluten-containing grains, affects 1 in 300 American children.

Our Kids Are Fat

Young people in our culture have unhealthful eating patterns, and television, computers, and video games contribute to their lack of physical activity. Forty-three percent of adolescents, for example, watch more than two hours of TV daily. (*Author's note:* As one of my sons commented, "You don't break bones while playing Nintendo.") Obesity in our children has become a grave concern. In 1999, 13 percent of children aged six to eleven years, and 14 percent of adolescents and teenagers, were overweight. According to the Surgeon General's 2003 report, the percentage of overweight children and adolescents has more than tripled in the last twenty years!

CHRONIC ILLNESS IN CHILDREN: THE DIGESTION CONNECTION

What is the common denominator here? If your child's digestion isn't working well, his/her overall health will suffer. The purpose of eating is to provide healthful nutrients to each cell of the body; if this is interrupted, or if proper nutrients aren't taken in, children begin to show mental, behavioral, and medical symptoms.

Many children's health problems actually stem from poor food choices, unhealthful lifestyles, and faulty digestion. It may also surprise you to learn that digestive problems are directly linked to a slew of seemingly unrelated juvenile illnesses including arthritis, attention deficit disorders, autism, migraines, asthma, depression, diabetes, and more. And much of this illness is preventable, controllable, or curable! You can learn to recognize the digestive factors in your child's health and behavioral issues, how to find solutions, and how to encourage a healthier diet for your entire family. There is something you can do.

Digestive Wellness for Children provides parents with a step-by-step plan for making healthful changes in their family's lifestyle. The approach is from a biological rather than a medical viewpoint. The standard medical approach is to diagnose and provide "appropriate" treatment, either drugs or surgery. The biological approach involves cleansing, feeding, and nurturing the child's entire being—using simple but effective tools to improve the way he/she feels. By understanding the functions of the gastrointestinal tract and looking for the underlying causes of disease rather than settling for mere treatment of symptoms, we can begin to correct our children's problems in a lasting way.

It is recommended that you start by reading the first two sections of this book. Then, in the second two sections, you can go directly to the specific chapters that apply to your child's health needs.

The first chapters of the book explore the causes of digestive illness that are related to the American lifestyle. Then we take a trip through the digestive tract, where we find a beautifully orchestrated system of integrated harmony. We look at the microbes that populate our internal world, and at the effects we feel when they are out of balance. We move on to discuss dysbiosis and leaky gut syndrome, which often underlie digestive illness and many other health problems. These chapters provide the groundwork to really understand the causes and effects of poor lifestyle choices and medical therapies on your child.

Then we focus on health improvement and problem solving, with information and practical tips on how to develop a wellness lifestyle. The biological approach is based on the concept of "biochemical individuality"; just as each of us has a unique face, body, and personality, so too do we each have a unique biochemistry and unique needs. One child's need for a specific nutrient can be thirtyfold higher or lower than another's. When it comes to food, one person's pleasure is another's poison. Although you may believe that it's important to eat certain foods like bread, eggs, meat, milk, oranges, and tomatoes, these may or may not be healthful for your child (or for you). It depends on how well that specific person can use them.

The last two sections of the book discuss strategies for dealing with digestive and digestion-related health problems, including information about the latest research on nutritional and herbal therapies. Certain digestive issues characteristically occur at various stages of childhood, from infancy through the teen years. Other health issues like arthritic conditions, migraine headaches, and skin problems may actually be the consequence of faulty digestion. The goal is to help your child's body reach its own natural balance, which will allow it to heal. Day in and day out, cell by cell, the body continually replenishes itself. With the correct balance of nutrients and activity, your child can become healthier and more resilient each year.

The book contains some exercises and questionnaires designed to help you shop and cook more wisely, and to increase your awareness of your child's body and mind so you can help him/her breathe more deeply, relax more fully, and live more freely. Finally, the Resources section lists professional organizations that can refer you to nutritionally oriented physicians and health professionals, and the Appendices provide detailed information on laboratory tests and natural treatments.

Functional medicine, which is concerned with early intervention in health problems and improving the chances of a return to full health, is an integral part of the biological approach. Much of the information in the field of functional medicine is new, and most physicians will be unfamiliar with many of the laboratory tests recommended herein. Take this book to your pediatrician's office, and ask the doctor to work with you in this new way.

Although we may not be aware of it, we all practice medical self-care. When we get a headache, we take an aspirin or go for a walk. If we have indigestion, we take an antacid or drink ginger tea. We know when we're too sick to go to work. Most of the time, we make our own assessment and treatment plan, expecting that the problem will pass with time; when these plans fail, we seek professional help. This book will expose you to new plans, ideas, and tools so you can be your own family's health expert. Just as one tool won't work for every job, not all of these tools will work for you, but some will, and even your failures may yield information that you can apply toward the goal of your child's best health.

PART ONE

An Overview of Children's Health Issues and Digestion

CHAPTER 1

Our Kids: Overfed and Undernourished

It's appalling that here in this land of plenty, with access to a wide variety of foods, that we still have a significant proportion of the population selecting foods that lead to inadequate intakes of critical nutrients.

—JANET KING, CHILDREN'S HOSPITAL OAKLAND RESEARCH INSTITUTE, CHAIRPERSON OF DIETARY GUIDELINES, SCIENTIFIC ADVISORY COMMITTEE

Grocery store shelves are filled with high-profit, tasty foods that ultimately make us sick. Packaged foods can be healthful, or not; there are some high-quality packaged foods, but the vast majority are stripped of most nutrients and loaded with antinutrient chemicals. Fresh is always best—and yet despite the abundance of fresh produce available to us all year, we turn to frozen vegetables and canned fruits. We eat microwaved and/or genetically modified foods. We feed our children processed Lunchables because it's convenient. The producers of all of these "foods" reap the profits, while our overall health as a nation declines.

THE NEW "NORMAL"

Our culture offers an enormous amount of choice and options—but much of what we consider "normal" is killing us. We think it's normal to eat packaged foods on the run or to skip meals entirely, to immunize our children with chemical-laden vaccines, to stare at computer screens all day, to eat dinner in front of the television, and to drive around a parking lot looking for the "perfect space" rather than walking half a block. We think it's normal for our kids to spend their days hooked into an electronic lifestyle and snacking on sweets and junk foods.

We are, essentially, three or four generations into an enormous, uncontrolled experiment, and we are already seeing the problems that can result. The air we breathe, the water we drink, the foods we eat, the cleaning products we use, and the personal-care products we use expose us to chemicals that simply weren't present in our environment a hundred years ago. Each day, for example, the average person is exposed to over 100 different chemicals. If we get enough antioxidants (substances like vitamins C and E that protect cells against oxidative damage) from our foods, we can easily slough off most chemical toxins. But what happens when we eat poorly or are exposed to more chemicals than our bodies can handle? What will occur as generation after generation of Americans grows up on highly processed, nutrient-depleted foods that are filled with pesticide residues, colorings, man-made fats, and fake sugars?

The purpose of this chapter is to look at some of what our culture overlooks as normal and to confront some of the lifestyle challenges that we face as parents today. Our children's world is vastly different from when we were children. If we simply accept the normal, we will surely do ourselves and our families a huge disservice.

MODERN-DAY EATING: TOO MUCH, AND YET TOO LITTLE

We are the most overfed and undernourished people in the world. Nearly half of our daily caloric intake comes from high-calorie, nutrient-poor foods. Although current studies report that we are consuming more nutrients than ever before, this is due to an alarming increase in our total daily calories. And it is clear that not only what we eat but also the way we eat has changed—for the worse. We often eat the same way we put gas in our cars: stop, fuel, and go. Forty-five percent of our meals are eaten away from home (that's up from 39 percent in 1980). Many of us skip breakfast, and others skip both breakfast and lunch.

The Standard American Diet Is "SAD"

Even if you are trying to feed your children well, foods just aren't what they used to be. According to the food tables published by the U.S. Department of Agriculture (USDA) over the past fifty years, we've lost half of the calcium in broccoli, 88 percent of the iron in watercress, and 40 percent of the vitamin C in cauliflower. Partly because of such nutritional changes in food and mainly due to poor food choices, we are eating more calories but not getting the nutrients we need. Today, 20 percent of women and children do not meet the recommended daily allowances for vitamin E and zinc. A study of high-school runners found that 45 percent of girls and 17 percent of boys were deficient in iron; 31 percent of female college athletes were also found to be iron-deficient.

The average American gets 18.6 percent of his/her calories each day from sugar, 21.4 percent from fats and oils, and 5 percent from sweetened soft drinks, versus only 4.5 percent from vegetables and 3 percent from fruits. It's worse for the average teenager, who gets 20 percent of his/her daily calories from refined sugar: an average of 34 teaspoons (544 calories) for boys and 24 teaspoons (384 calories) for girls. Such calories are called "empty calories" because their utilization by the body requires magnesium, B-complex vitamins, and chromium—all essential to energy production, bone health, nerve and muscle functions, and mood regulation—but the refined sugar itself contains none of these nutrients.

In the 1950s, Coca-Cola sold only a 6.5-ounce bottle, but today, some stores market a 64-ounce, 600-calorie version! Soft drinks are our biggest dietary source of refined sugar, accounting for about a third of our sugar intake. We're now consuming twice as many soft drinks as in 1974, and children consume a disproportionate amount; they drink more soft drinks than fruit juice by the age of five years, and more soft drinks than milk, fruit juices, or fruit drinks by the age of thirteen.

The teen years are a prime time to build bone and help prevent future osteoporosis. Instead, teenagers put themselves at greater risk of broken bones because soft drinks deplete bones of strengthening minerals without contributing any. A boy aged twelve to nineteen years drinks an average of 24 ounces of soda per day (that's 868 cans per year), and a girl in that age range drinks 18 ounces daily (651 cans annually). Unfortunately, girls get only about 60 percent of their recommended calcium on average, and girls who drink soft drinks get only about 48 percent. Calcium is critical to healthy bones, teeth, and proper nerve, brain, and muscle function. We also use it in nearly every cell in the body.

The Real Cost of Eating Out

Now that we're eating on the run and on the road, our "food dollar" has much more to do with convenience and taste temptation than with nutritional value:

- In 1997, almost half of all money spent on food was for food and drinks outside the home.

- Also in 1997, one-third of our food dollars was spent on fast foods.

- Older children eat a higher percentage of meals away from home (26 percent) than preschoolers do (18 percent).

- Restaurant and fast-food consumption in children increased nearly 300 percent between 1977 and 1996.

- Children who drink soft drinks take in an average of 188 more calories per day than children who drink other types of drinks.

- In 1977–1978, we ate 18 percent of our total calories from food prepared outside of the home. By 1996, this had increased to 32 percent.

- Compared to home-cooked meals, meals prepared outside the home were higher in calories and fat, yet lower in fiber, calcium, and iron.

What Do We Eat per Person per Year?

These USDA statistics on what we ate per person in 2001 might surprise you!

- 142 pounds of caloric sweeteners (nearly 6.3 ounces per day): cane and beet sugar consumption was down to a mere 61 pounds, consumption of hidden corn sweeteners rose substantially to 79.2 pounds per person, and we each ate 0.3 pounds of syrups and 1.1 pounds of honey (percentage-wise, children eat more sweeteners than adults do)

- 24.3 gallons (388.8 cups) of coffee

- 87.9 pounds of added fats and oils, including 32.5 pounds of hydrogenated vegetable shortening

- 26.7 quarts of ice cream, sherbet, frozen yogurt, and ice-milk

- 25.1 gallons of alcohol: beer 21.6, wine 2.2, distilled liquor 1.3

- 46.4 gallons of carbonated soft drinks: diet soda 11.1, caloric soft drinks 35.3

- 4.2 pounds of potato chips

- 22 pounds of candy

- 38 donuts

—*source: Economic Research Service, USDA, Food Consumption Data 2001, www.ers.usda.gov/data/ foodconsumption/FoodAvailSpreadsheets.htm*

- Only 34 percent of dinner entrées are completely "homemade," and nearly 7 percent of those are sandwiches.

- The average American purchased carry-out meals 118 times in 2002.

- Americans get a full quarter of their vegetables from eating potato chips or French fries.

- Fast-food chains and restaurants have "supersized" foods so we eat more and spend more, and they have higher profits. (Rent the movie *Supersize Me!*)

- We spend $110 billion on fast foods today, in comparison to $6 billion in 1970.

Given the facts above, it is perhaps not surprising that 16 percent of children aged six to eleven years, and 14 percent of teenagers, are overweight or obese—rates that have tripled in the past twenty years. Our thinness-oriented culture, however, encourages our young people to combat this excess weight with a variety of methods. When surveyed, 43 percent of students reported trying to lose weight, most through exercise, and many combining exercise with eating less food or less fat, which are all healthful ways to shed unwanted pounds. But 13 percent of the students who had tried to lose weight said that they fasted for twenty-four hours or more; 8 percent said they took diet pills, powders, or liquids; and 7 percent of girls and 2 percent of boys reported using laxatives or vomiting to assist with weight loss. Obviously, we have a serious problem here!

THE WILL TO CHANGE

Our physical bodies are composed of the foods we eat, and if we don't get the nutrients we need, our bodies first begin to show the deficiencies as irritability, lack of attention, and other mood changes. Is it a coincidence, then, that 20 percent of our children have learning and behavior problems?

It's time to focus on health rather than convenience and to develop better habits. Instead of asking, "Does this look and taste good?" we should ask, "Is this healthful, will it contribute to my biochemical balance and help me feel better, and will it taste good?" We need to exercise regularly and think positive thoughts. We need to relax by ourselves and with friends. We need to create balance in our lives. And we need to impart this lifestyle to our children by modeling healthful behavior for them.

Take breakfast, for example: Studies show that eating breakfast enhances school-aged children's ability to learn and behave in a classroom setting, and that's why many public schools offer breakfast to students. Although school breakfast and lunch programs may not offer the most exciting foods, children who partake of them have higher nutrient status than children who don't. Small, frequent meals keep children's energy levels even and their minds alert. Snacking also reduces the incidence of children's tantrums!

Think of the body as a woodstove: You light the stove in the morning so it will warm the house while you work; throughout the day, you put in small amounts of wood; and at night, you fuel the stove and then let it die down before you go to sleep. Similarly, if we give our children small meals and nutritious snacks throughout the day, they are utilized and burned efficiently. Although we eat primarily to nourish our bodies, we mustn't forget that meals are also a time for relaxation, rest, and renewal. Numerous studies show that we digest food better if we are relaxed, and many people seem to know this intuitively, as indicated by the global customs of saying grace or taking a couple of moments to "center ourselves" before a meal.

CHAPTER 2

Chemicals and Convenience: Consumer Be Aware!

Today, not a single child is born free of synthetic chemicals.
—BILL MOYERS, PBS DOCUMENTARY *TRADE SECRETS*

Research now confirms what many parents and teachers have long suspected: that some children experience behavior, learning, or respiratory problems when they eat foods containing petroleum-based additives like dyes, synthetic flavorings, and certain preservatives.
—JANE HERSEY, DIRECTOR, FEINGOLD ASSOCIATION

Eighty-nine (89) percent of 10,500 ingredients used in personal-care products have not been evaluated for safety by the CIR, the FDA, nor any other publicly accountable institution.
—COSMETIC INGREDIENT REVIEW PANEL, FDA OFFICE OF COSMETICS AND COLORS

Thousands of years ago, nomadic people foraged and hunted for food. When populations increased, farming and animal husbandry enabled more people to be fed with regularity. Foods were grown nearby and eaten fresh and primarily in season. Nowadays, however, a global economy supplies our food, and it seems perfectly normal to buy Granny Smith apples imported from New Zealand, apricots from Turkey, salmon from Norway, and mineral water and wine from France. We have grown accustomed to nectarines in winter and oranges in summer.

Are foods shipped from far away just as nutritious as foods grown locally? A ripe, juicy tomato from your backyard has about the same measurable nutritional value as those pale hothouse tomatoes sold in winter. But even though these foods share some of the same scientific measurements, our intuitive measurement tells us they are different in some important ways. This chapter will give you a "heads up" on what lurks in your foods and personal-care items. You'll also get some insight into microwaved, irradiated, and genetically modified foods.

FOOD ADDITIVES—AND SUBTRACTIONS

Americans love the convenience of frozen foods—but most frozen foods contain additives that make them less perishable. Aseptic packaging to lengthen food's shelf-life kills much of the bacteria that cause spoilage and food poisoning—but simultaneously kills the beneficial bacteria that actually help maintain our health. Today's food production, transportation, and processing methods destroy or extract valuable nutrients, add preservatives and other chemicals, and even change the very genetic makeup of foods to "enhance" them.

Preservatives and Other Problems

From earliest times, meats and other foods were salted and "cured" to preserve them. Later, foods were jarred and canned with sugar, salt, and vinegar to keep them from perishing. Pickling foods like cabbages and cucumbers is a way to preserve them while retaining their original character and much of their nutrient value; pickling actually adds enzymes and beneficial bacteria that support health. But because so much of today's food is shipped from afar and packaged to last months or years, chemicals are added to stabilize and preserve it. In the United States alone, more than 3,000 food additives (dyes, artificial flavorings, dough conditioners, texturing agents, anticaking agents, and so on) are used to extend shelf-life and enhance flavor, appearance, and consistency. The average American eats an alarming 14 pounds of additives each year!

It is well documented that a class of common preservatives called sulfites causes asthma and respiratory problems in certain individuals. (*Author's note:* Current research indicates that only a tiny percentage of the population is sensitive to preservatives and other food additives, but in my practice as a clinical nutritionist, I have seen many people with these sensitivities. One fifteen-year-old told me that eating a single drop of food coloring would put her in anaphylactic shock, a severe, possibly life-threatening allergic reaction, within ten minutes. Another client can no longer eat in restaurants because of her severe reactions to monosodium glutamate.)

Children consume more of these potentially harmful substances per body weight than adults do. Ben Feingold, M.D., a pioneer in the field of food sensitivity and child behavior, found that many food additives caused significant behavior and learning problems. The long-term effects of additives on developing children are of special concern—but no one really knows what those effects are. And although additives have been tested singly, they have never been tested in combinations, so we have no idea of their synergistic effects either. (*Author's note:* This ongoing dietary experiment reminds me of my favorite experiment with a childhood chemistry set; I used to mix two chemicals together and then watch the test-tube explode.)

"Just Like Sugar"

Splenda, also called sucralose, is one of our newest eating experiments. This sweetener is manufactured from real but nutritionally depleted sugar through a five-step process in which three hydroxyl groups in each molecule are replaced by

Splenda Symptoms?

People who use Splenda are starting to report allergic reactions such as hives; others say eating the sweetener causes them to be overly emotional and display symptoms of mental illness. Recently, I saw a client who began having intense stomach pains right after she began using Splenda. Consider the following list of possible symptoms resulting from Splenda consumption, adapted from Dr. Joseph Mercola's website at www.mercola.com:

- Flushing, redness, and/or burning feeling of the skin
- Rash and/or itching
- Swelling
- Blisters or welts
- Nausea
- Stomach cramps
- Dry heaves
- Feelings of food poisoning
- Bloated abdomen
- Diarrhea
- Vomiting
- Pain (body, chest)
- Headache
- Seeing spots
- Dulled senses
- Becoming withdrawn and/or losing interest in usual activities
- Feeling forgetful
- Moodiness
- Unexplained crying
- Feeling depressed
- Altered emotional state such as feeling irate, impatient, hypersensitive
- Trouble concentrating/staying in focus
- Seizures
- Shaking
- Feeling faint
- Anxiety
- A panicky or shaky feeling
- Panic attacks
- Mental or emotional breakdown

three chlorine atoms, converting the sugar (which, by the way, never had any chlorine in it before) to a chemical called 1,6-dichloro-1,6-dideoxy-BETA-D-fructofuranosyl-4-chloro-4-deoxy-alpha-D-galactopyranoside. This chemical is 600 times sweeter than sugar by weight.

Marketers, focusing on the fact that we eat too much sugar and running with the current low-carbohydrate craze, advertise Splenda as "just like sugar but without the calories," and the sweetener has already found its way into hundreds of food products. In response to consumer interest, General Mills is creating low-sugar versions of its three most popular cereals by reducing the amount of sugar by 75 percent and replacing it with small amounts of Splenda. This will potentially affect a *huge* number of children.

We want to believe that this chemical will let us eat our cake (or cereal) and still be thin, but we are letting ourselves be duped, as no scientific findings indicate that Splenda will help us lose weight or be healthier in any way. Surely long-term research has shown it to be harmless? No: there have been few studies at all, none in children, and no long-term studies in humans—except for the one we are now conducting by eating it! (See the inset "Splenda Symptoms?" on page 16.)

WAVES OF THE FUTURE

Modern food processing and preparation seriously deplete the average American diet of many nutrients. In making white flour from whole-wheat kernels, twenty-two vitamins and minerals are removed; when the bran and germ go, so do 98 percent of the vitamin B_6, 91 percent of the manganese, 84 percent of the magnesium, and 87 percent of the fiber. In making breakfast cereals (even many health-food brands) by extruding a slurry of grains through nozzles to create shapes, the high temperatures and pressures destroy vitamins, antioxidants, and essential fats. And now that 90 percent of American homes have a microwave oven, even the health benefits of a home-cooked meal are suspect.

Microwave Cooking

Microwaving has spread like brushfire over the last two decades. Despite the apparent public consensus that microwaving is safe, not much scientific literature has clarified either its safety or its danger. In 1991, Hans Ulrich Hertel and Bernard Blanc of the Swiss Federal Institute of Technology studied some of the effects of microwave usage by giving eight people specific foods that were prepared raw, cooked in a conventional oven, or cooked in a microwave oven. The researchers reported that microwave cooking lowered hemoglobin levels and cholesterol levels while elevating white blood cell counts. Hemoglobin carries oxygen to our cells, so low levels indicate anemia and fatigue. A rise in white blood cells indicates that the body's immune system is gearing up to defend against a challenge, most typically an infection. (*Author's note:* A current client of mine who has used microwave cooking exclusively for the past thirty years also has low hemoglobin and elevated white blood cell levels.)

The researchers also found structural changes in the microwaved food that were not seen in the conventionally cooked food. Dr. Hertel stated,

> There is extensive scientific literature concerning the hazardous effects of direct microwave radiation on living systems. It is astonishing, therefore, to realize how little effort has been taken to replace this detrimental technique of microwaves with technology more in accordance with nature. Technically produced microwaves are based on the principle of alternating current. Atoms, molecules, and cells hit by this hard electromagnetic radiation are forced to reverse polarity 1–100 billion times a second. There are no atoms, molecules, or cells of any organic system able to withstand such a violent, destructive power for any extended period of time, not even in the low energy range of milliwatts.

Another study showed that when breast milk was microwaved to 98.6°F, almost all its protective antibodies and lysozymes were destroyed and its vitamin C level was reduced. But a different study reported that if breast milk was heated to 140°F, there was no damage to its vitamin B_1, vitamin E, or essential fatty acids. Microwaving is too recent an innovation for us to know what the long-term effects are.

One Child's Journey into Health

At a conference many years ago, I heard a naturopathic physician speak about a child who would not eat and was nearing starvation. After questioning the parents in detail, the doctor discovered that all of the child's formula and cooked food had been heated in a microwave oven; that a computer was left running in each room of the home twenty-four hours a day; and that the child watched a great deal of television. The doctor believed that the child's difficulties may have been due to electromagnetic disruption. Within twenty minutes of being given a dose of a single homeopathic remedy, the child said he was hungry. The doctor instructed the parents to turn off computers and TV sets unless they were being used, and to cook all of their son's foods conventionally. With these simple changes, the child flourished.

Given the possible health concerns, does it really take that much longer to cook in a conventional oven or on the stovetop?

Irradiation

Another questionable modern technology used on our food supply is irradiation. Irradiation is a clever way of utilizing nuclear waste materials to keep food fresh longer and reduce the risk of food poisoning. It kills all bacteria (like *Salmonella*, a major problem in poultry, meat, and egg production) and leaves no radiation in the food itself, but the process may destroy more than we want it to; irradiated milk, for example, loses 70 percent of its vitamin A, thiamin, and riboflavin.

Irradiated foods contain molecules found nowhere in nature. The U.S. Food and Drug Administration (FDA) groups these "radiolytic by-products" in two categories: "known radiolytic products" such as formaldehyde and benzene, which are proven carcinogens, and "unique radiolytic products," which are new molecules that haven't been characterized. What's frightening is that no one knows the long-term effects of these "unique" molecules on our health. Studies in the 1950s, however, showed that animals eating irradiated foods had a wide variety of health problems including premature death, reproductive dysfunction, a rare form of cancer, chromosomal abnormalities, liver damage, low weight gain, and vitamin deficiencies.

Figure 2.1. This pretty little picture, called a Picowave Radura, indicates that a food has been irradiated. Most people, however, don't know what this symbol means.

The FDA has approved irradiation for use in beef, pork, chicken, other poultry, eggs in the shell, fruits and vegetables, wheat, wheat flour, juice, spices, dried-vegetable seasonings, and sprouting seeds. Seventy-five percent of our beef producers and 50 percent of our poultry producers have signed agreements to use this technology. Due to lingering health and safety concerns, however, the European Parliament limits the use of food irradiation to spices, dried herbs, and seasonings. Many researchers are opposed to such massive experimentation done at our risk, and worry about all the environmental problems associated with handling radioactive materials at small irradiating facilities throughout the country.

Irradiation Identification

Irradiated foods are labeled as such only when sold to the first buyer. The standard wording is "treated with radiation," "treated with irradiation," or "electronically pasteurized" and is allowed to be as small as the other smallest labeling on the package. Consumers are supposed to see irradiation labeling, if applicable, on the following foods:

- Plant foods sold in whole form in a package (for example, a label on a bag of beans or oranges)
- Fresh, whole fruits and vegetables (a label on a fruit or vegetable, box, or display)
- Whole meat and poultry in a package (a label on a package of chicken breasts)
- Unpackaged meat and poultry (a label on the butcher's display)
- Irradiated meat and poultry that are part of another packaged food (a label on a frozen chicken pot-pie showing that it contains irradiated chicken)

You won't see any such labeling, however, when irradiated ingredients are provided at salad bars or deli counters; served in school lunches, restaurants, hospitals, or nursing homes; or used in processed foods like soups or applesauce. There is also no labeling on irradiated spices or seeds. Whole cases of irradiated fruits and vegetables are marked with a symbol on the crates (see Figure 2.1), but consumers typically see only the unpacked contents.

Genetic Engineering

For more than a hundred years, most of our produce has been hybridized, meaning that two or more varieties of a particular plant have been cross-pollinated to create a new variety. Many hybridized foods often look or taste better than their "old" counterparts, but their nutritional value is often sacrificed for ease of transportation or resistance to pests, drought, heat, or cold. Corn, for instance, contains 14 percent less protein now than it did forty years ago. Today's technologists are taking hybridization a step further by splicing genes into dozens of foods to make foods bigger, sweeter, juicier, longer lasting, and more plentiful. Most of us eat genetically modified foods (GMFs)—also called genetically engineered (GE) foods—on a regular basis, and yet many people are completely unaware of the issues involved in their creation.

Agricultural genetic engineering generally involves changes to seeds. Many soy and corn varieties, for example, have been modified to be resistant to an herbicide called Round-Up so that a field can be sprayed with the herbicide and only the weeds, not the crop, will be killed. Other varieties have been given genes from the soil bacterium *Bacillus thuringiensis,* which makes the resulting "Bt" plant resistant to insects that go through a larval stage. Proponents of this biotechnology assert that it will reduce pesticide and herbicide use, make crops more resistant to frost damage and drought, increase food's nutritional value, and even help clean up environmental contaminants. Opposition, however, is based on the fact that little long-term testing has been performed on GMFs prior to their release into the food supply.

Although the outcry against GMFs has been large in Europe, Americans have been relatively quiet. Japan, the European Union, Russia, and many other countries require the labeling of GMFs. The FDA has refused thus far to require labeling of GMFs in the United States. In fact, up to 60 percent of the foods now on our supermarket shelves contain genetically modified (GM) ingredients. Many processed foods contain soy derivatives, corn syrup, or cornstarch, and if you eat foods containing soy or corn that has not been organically grown, you are probably consuming GMF products. This includes any food that contains corn syrup, soybean oil, soy protein, tofu, corn chips, popcorn, tortillas, and more. Despite some consumer protest, farming of genetically modified crops is increasing steadily in the United States:

- Soybean acreage was 17 percent GM in 1997, 68 percent by 2001, and 80 percent in 2003.

- Bt corn (introduced in 1996) was 8 percent of corn acreage in 1997, 26 percent in 1998, down to 19 percent in 2001, and then up to 30 percent by 2003.

- 10 percent of cotton was herbicide-resistant in 1997 versus 56 percent in 2001.

Because genetically engineered crops were first developed in the mid-1990s, their long-term costs and environmental consequences are yet to be determined. In an initial study of such issues, researchers at Cornell University dusted Bt corn pollen onto the leaves of milkweed plants, which are the sole food for the caterpillar stage of the endangered monarch butterfly. Nearly half of the monarch caterpillars that fed on those leaves died, and the remainder grew to only half their normal size. What other animal species may also be affected by genetically altered plants? Suffice it to say that more testing must be done before we can know the long-term effects that these crops may have on the environment—or, for that matter, on our health.

ENVIRONMENTAL EXPOSURES

Exposure to environmental toxins is a serious public health issue. According to the U.S. Environmental Protection Agency (EPA), 50,000 synthetic chemicals are dispersed into our environment, many of which are known to disrupt the normal functions of our body's systems. Children are especially vulnerable to the effects of these chemicals, beginning *in utero,* when fat-soluble metals and other toxins are pulled from the mother's body to the baby's during pregnancy. The Environmental Working Group and the Red Cross examined umbilical cords from ten newborns. They identified 287 industrial chemicals in the newborns' tissues with an average of 200 per umbilical cord. Compared to adults, children breathe more air, drink more water, and eat more food for their relative weight, and may also be less capable of eliminating some toxins; for example, children absorb about half of the lead they ingest, whereas adults absorb only one-tenth. Children also play close to the ground and have hand-to-mouth activity that increases their exposure to toxins.

Before Food Is Food

Farmers used to grow many different foods, rotate their crops, and use "natural" fertilizers. Today, most food grown in America comes from corporate agrifarms that produce monocrops, and our soils are being depleted as a result. Chemical fertilizers add only the nutrients necessary for healthy plants, not nutrient-rich foods. Worse, chemical pesticides can damage our nervous and immune systems and are especially harmful to children, who are exposed to more pesticide per unit of weight than adults are. Nearly three-quarters of the produce consumed by small children contains pesticide residue.

In 2003, the U.S. Centers for Disease Control (CDC) looked at pesticides in the blood of ordinary citizens. Of the thirty-four pesticides tested, the average person had thirteen in his/her bloodstream, and blood levels of chlorpyrifos (an organophosphate pesticide banned for residential use in 2001 because of its negative effects) were found to be twice as high in children as in adults. The CDC report showed that children and women of child-bearing age carried the heaviest pesticide burdens—which is alarming, because pesticide exposure in the womb and during the first three years of postnatal life has been found to lower birth weight, increase the incidence of birth defects, and hinder normal neurological development and reproduction.

In 1993–1997, pesticide residues were found on 19 to 24 percent of all produce in the United States. Pesticide residues on imported foods have increased in the last decade, and we currently import many foods grown with DDT and other pesticides that have been banned for use in the United States. As of January 2006, however, all imported foods are required to meet current United States standards for allowable pesticide types and residue level. And fortunately, organic farming and integrated pest management (combining natural insect-control methods to reduce the use of pesticides) are gaining momentum.

Tobacco

An emerging concern is second-hand smoke or environmental tobacco smoke

(ETS), which is the smoke that drifts into a room from a cigarette plus the exhaled smoke from a smoker. About a quarter of American adults smoke, half to a third of all children under the age of five years live in a household with a smoker, and children who live with smokers have more respiratory problems and more health problems in general. A 1992 study by the EPA reported that ETS causes 150,000–300,000 respiratory tract infections in infants and toddlers under the age of 18 months, resulting in as many as 15,000 hospitalizations. Children with asthma are especially at risk from ETS. ETS affects between 200,000 and 1 million asthmatic children each year.

Your child's risk of hospitalization from your smoke doubles with just half a pack a day. Mothers who smoke during pregnancy run a greater risk of having children with hyperactivity and/or lower intelligence. And of the over 4,000 chemicals that have been found in cigarette smoke, at least forty-three of them are known to cause cancer.

Cotinine, an easily measured metabolite of nicotine, is used to determine the health risks of people who are around smoke. High cotinine levels, which correlate with cancer risk, are commonly found in nonsmokers. Between CDC statistics gathered in 1991–1994 and 1999–2000, cotinine levels decreased by 58 percent for children and 55 percent for teenagers, indicating that children's exposure to cigarette smoke was dropping, but cotinine levels were still found to be twice as high in children as in adults. So if you smoke, it's not just your own health that you affect, but also the lifelong health of your children and other family members.

Heavy Metals

A child's nervous system begins forming long before birth, as embryonic neurons branch out and make the connections that transport information to and from the brain and body. The more branches and connections made, the larger the brain will be. The neural pathways formed in your child's first three years of life are the basis for his/her ability to learn and develop; during this time, exposure to heavy metals can have significant, detrimental consequences.

Lead

Lead is toxic even at extremely low levels. There is no known biological use for the element in the human body and no known safe level of lead in children. Early lead exposure is associated with cognitive deficits that persist into adolescence and adulthood; one study, for example, demonstrated that high-school students with high lead levels in early childhood had a sevenfold increase in failure to graduate. High levels of lead have also been found in children with autism, attention deficit disorders, and learning problems. High lead levels, whether in childhood or adulthood, can translate into problems with thinking and behavior later in life, and in extreme cases can correlate with criminal problems.

A major effort has been made in the United States since the 1970s to reduce lead in the environment. In 1991, former U.S. Secretary of the Department of Health and Human Services Louis Sullivan declared lead poisoning to be the most serious environmental disease of North American children. A recent CDC report shows that the number of American children with lead levels above 10 parts per million dropped from 4.4 percent in 1991–1994 to 2.2 percent in 1999–2000. This great improvement is due to an active public health campaign to remove lead from gasoline, paint, and other products, but lead toxicity continues to be a huge problem in America and worldwide.

Mercury

The exposure of children to mercury during pregnancy and breast-feeding and from fish, vaccinations, dental amalgams, and coal-powered fuel plants is of grave concern for neurological development. Mercury readily passes through the placenta to the fetus. In one study, mothers measured for mercury prior to pregnancy and after birth showed decreased mercury levels because the babies' bodies pulled mercury from the moms' during pregnancy, and the newborns showed higher mercury levels than the mothers did. Even at low levels of exposure in the womb, the effects of mercury on the fetal brain and nervous system can lead to later problems with memory, attention, language, and other skills.

Through regular vaccinations, our infants and children take in potentially toxic doses of mercury from the vaccine preservative thimerosol, which is 49 percent ethylmercury by weight. The number of recommended immunizations rose significantly in 1989, and until recently a typical child received a cumulative total of 237.5 milligrams of mercury from standard vaccinations. Parental outcry has resulted in the removal of thimerosol from many current vaccines, but not all. Although most children are able to rid their bodies of this toxin, at least 15 percent of children have poor detoxification capabilities. A controversial but growing body of evidence links increasing levels of mercury in immunizations to outcomes including autism, developmental delays, and other learning disabilities (visit the website www.vaccinesafety.edu/thi-table.htm). Immunization is of great personal and public benefit, but be sure to ask your physician to use only vaccines that do not contain thimerosol.

In 2001, the National Wildlife Federation documented that concentrations of mercury in New England rainfall were up to four times the safety limit established by the EPA. Sixty-three percent of this mercury comes from coal-fired power plants and from incinerated mercury-containing products. Each year, approximately 160 tons of mercury is released into the atmosphere over the United States, with only about fifty tons collected by "scrubbers." And China may seem far away, but its mercury emissions of about 1,000 tons per year drift and fall on our waters and land. Mercury from these sources pollutes our water, air, and land, and ultimately our food supply.

Fish consumption is the most common source of mercury exposure in the general population. Ninety percent of the mercury in food is absorbed and deposited into our tissues, with the highest concentrations residing in our kidneys, liver, red blood cells, bile, brains, testes, and nervous systems. The FDA and EPA advise pregnant, potentially pregnant, and lactating women, as well as children under the age of five years, not to eat swordfish, shark, king mackerel, or tilefish, and to limit intake of albacore tuna to once weekly. They also advise a 12-ounce weekly limit on intake of low-mercury fish such as light tuna, shrimp, salmon, pollock, and catfish. Although I'm no longer of childbearing age, I follow the same recommendations to be on the safe side.

PERSONAL-CARE AND HOUSEHOLD PRODUCTS

Personal-care items can be a source of many "hidden" chemicals and allergens. A 2004 report from a nongovernmental "watchdog" called the Environmental Working Group (EWG) states that 99.6 percent of the 7,500 products analyzed contained one or more ingredients never studied for safety by the Cosmetics Ingredient Review (CIR, the cosmetic industry's self-regulating panel): "One of every 120 products on the market contains ingredients certified by government authorities as known or probable human carcinogens, including shampoos, lotions, make-up foundations, and lip balms manufactured by Almay, Neutrogena, Grecian Formula, and others. An astonishing one-third of all products contain one or more ingredients classified as possible human carcinogens."

What Lurks in Your Toiletries and Household Cleaning Products?

It's important to consider what's in your house-cleaning products as well. An innocuous dishwashing detergent usually contains several dangerous chemicals such as naptha (a central nervous system depressant), diethanolamine (a possible liver poison), and chlorophenylphenol (considered a toxin). And this is only one of many household items! Just think: air freshener, window cleaner, scouring powder, bleach, laundry detergent, all-purpose spray cleaner, toilet cleaner, oven cleaner, tub and tile cleaner, furniture polish.... Luckily, many cleaning products without these harsh chemicals can be found at health food stores and even in regular supermarkets.

As consumers, we naively assume that somewhere, some regulatory agency is looking out for our best interests, but apparently that isn't always the case; of the

75,000 chemicals registered with the EPA, only a fraction has undergone complete testing to determine its potential contribution to health problems. As with environmental toxins, children are more susceptible than adults are to the negative effects of household chemicals. Please take the time to examine the products you use in your home. For information on ingredients in common toiletries and cleaning products, visit the EWG's website at www.ewg.org/reports/skindeep.

What's in Baby Shampoo?

The other day, a mom proudly told me that she uses Johnson & Johnson Baby Shampoo on her baby every night. She probably feels safe using such a prominent product—but the EWG has identified several "red flags" among the shampoo's ingredients:

- Five ingredients (acrylates copolymer, cocamidopropyl betaine, PEG-14M, PEG-80 sorbitan laurate, and quaternium-15) may contain harmful impurities linked to cancer or other health problems.

- Two ingredients (PEG-14M and PEG-80 sorbitan laurate) may contain impurities linked to breast cancer.

- One ingredient (tetrasodium EDTA) may increase exposures to carcinogens and other ingredients of concern.

- One ingredient (fragrance) is an allergen.

- Nine ingredients (sodium hydroxide, glycerin, fragrance, sodium hydroxide, sodium trideceth sulfate, guar hydroxypropyltrimonium chloride, hydrolyzed silk, PEG 150 distearate, and amodimethicone) are unstudied for use by the CIR or have insufficient data.

Using Johnson & Johnson's Baby Shampoo probably won't harm your baby, but how can you know the cumulative effect of all the chemicals and cosmetics in your home? On the other hand, the ingredients of Tom's Baby Shampoo, a more natural product, are all foods or found in foods, and the possibility that these ingredients may be harmful is slim:

- One ingredient (fragrance) is an allergen.

- Six ingredients (fragrance, chamomile extract, citric acid, herbal tea [chamomile], glycerin [vegetable], and cocobetaine [coconut oil]) are unstudied or have insufficient data.

—source: www.ewg.org/reports/skindeep

The Hygiene Hypothesis: Too Clean!

Marketers make us believe that adding protective antibacterial substances to sponges, cleansers, soaps, and other personal-care and home-care products makes us safer. But many scientists believe that constant exposure to microbes in infancy and early childhood contributes to the health and responsiveness of the adult immune system. The hygiene hypothesis, a theory that our environment is actually too clean, suggests that our culture doesn't sufficiently challenge our immune system. We have improved sanitation, low bacterial availability in food, fewer childhood infections, increased use of antibiotics, and routine vaccinations. Children who have little challenge by microbes may be at increased risk for developing ongoing conditions such as allergies, eczema, and asthma.

OUR FOOD HAS CHANGED

The life in food gives us life. Once a plant is picked or an animal killed, a grain split or milk homogenized, it begins to lose its enzymatic activity. Transporting foods over long distances diminishes their life-giving capacity. Canned, frozen, and packaged foods often contain adequate nutrients, but we know instinctively that these foods are different from fresh or homemade foods. In fact, processed foods are enzyme-deficient; they don't contain the enzymes that are critical aids in digestion and metabolism. Fresh fruits, vegetables, local fish and game, grains, beans, nuts, and seeds give us these essential enzymes. A body that doesn't have to work overtime making enzymes has more energy for other processes.

Whole foods are in balance with themselves and with nature. When we eat them, we benefit from their balance. Later chapters in this book will show you how to bring the health-supporting benefits of whole foods to your family.

CHAPTER 3

A Journey Through the Digestive System

The surface area of the digestive mucosae, measuring up and down and around all the folds, rugae, villi, and microvilli, is about the size of a tennis court.

—SIDNEY BAKER, M.D.

For simplicity's sake, visualize the digestive tract as a 25- to 35-foot hose running from mouth to anus. From the time you swallow, whatever you eat is squeezed through that "hose" by peristalsis, which is the involuntary, rhythmic contraction of sets of smooth muscles that pushes your food from your throat on downward. (*Author's note:* When my son Arthur was seven years old, he demonstrated that peristalsis works even if you eat while standing on your head—yes, the food went down, or rather, up, as usual!)

Another analogy is an irrigation system in which a large water conduit gets narrower and narrower, finally trickling water into each tiny portion of a field. If that water supply becomes blocked upstream, the plants downstream from the blockage wither and die. Similarly, food passing through the digestive tract is broken down into basic components for absorption through the mucosa (the folded lining of the tract) and carried by the bloodstream to all the cells of the body. As with water in a field of plants, an unblocked flow of nutrients into the body is critical for optimal health and function of each organ and cell.

From birth to death, we continually create and recreate ourselves from the food we put into our bodies. The fundamental function of digestion is to turn foods into microscopic particles that our cells can use for energy, maintenance, growth, and repair. If digestive wellness is compromised (for example, by drug use, enzyme deficiency, "dead" foods, stress, or other factors), the body tries to find ways to make things work, but eventually our cells lose their capacity to function fully and we become unhealthy.

YOU AREN'T ONLY WHAT YOU EAT

The digestive process is considerably more complicated than the hose and irrigation analogies indicate. To digest, you must be able to take in foods and grind them into a mash if necessary, break the mash into tiny particles, absorb the particles into the bloodstream, transport nutrients and calories into the cells for use, and remove waste products from the body.

There are several digestive phases, involving numerous organs and functions:

- Eating occurs when food is chewed and swallowed. The mind makes food choices related to lifestyle, personal values, and cultural customs. The mouth serves as the portal for nutrients and other materials to enter the body.

- Digestion, or the actual breakdown of food into its components, begins with saliva in the mouth and movement through the esophagus, but mainly occurs in the stomach and small intestine. It requires cooperation from the liver, gallbladder, and pancreas, and proper levels of stomach acid and intestinal bacteria are critical.

- Through this stage, food is essentially "outside" the body, though in a tube going through it. Absorption occurs when nutrients are taken through the lining of the small and large intestines into the bloodstream for transport to the cells. It also entails the passage of some food components through the portal vein to the liver for filtration. (See Figure 3.1 on page 30.)

- Assimilation occurs when nutrients enter the cells for use as fuel and raw materials.

- Elimination occurs when cellular waste products (transported again by the bloodstream) and undigested food materials are excreted from the body through the kidneys, colon, lungs, lymphatic system, and skin.

Health can, and does, break down at any of these digestive phases. The old saying "You are what you eat" is primarily true, but it leaves out something important: You are also *how* you eat, or how well you digest. Although nutritious food is the right place to start on the path to digestive wellness, many people eat all the "right" foods and still have digestive problems. For example, absorption problems can lead to food sensitivities, fatigue, skin conditions, and migraine headaches. Diabetics have a problem assimilating glucose into their cells. Constipation and diarrhea are problems of elimination.

A GUIDED TOUR

The digestive system is beautiful, intricate, self-running, and self-healing. Because

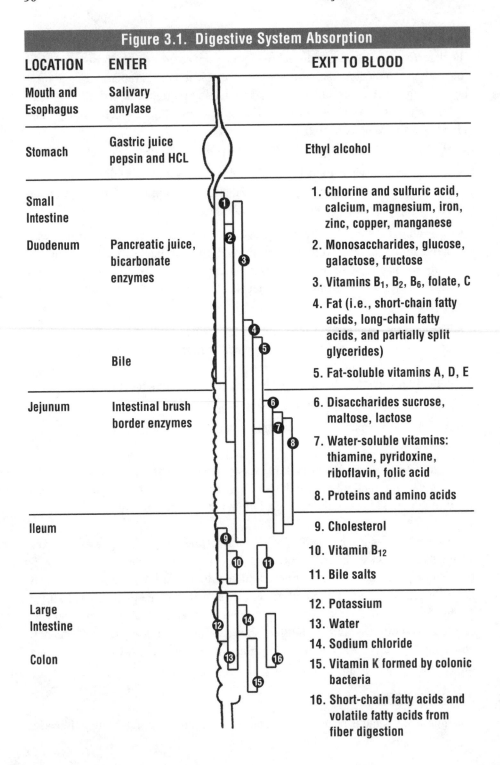

Figure 3.1. Digestive System Absorption

LOCATION	ENTER	EXIT TO BLOOD
Mouth and Esophagus	Salivary amylase	
Stomach	Gastric juice pepsin and HCL	Ethyl alcohol
Small Intestine		1. Chlorine and sulfuric acid, calcium, magnesium, iron, zinc, copper, manganese
Duodenum	Pancreatic juice, bicarbonate enzymes	2. Monosaccharides, glucose, galactose, fructose
		3. Vitamins B_1, B_2, B_6, folate, C
		4. Fat (i.e., short-chain fatty acids, long-chain fatty acids, and partially split glycerides)
	Bile	5. Fat-soluble vitamins A, D, E
Jejunum	Intestinal brush border enzymes	6. Disaccharides sucrose, maltose, lactose
		7. Water-soluble vitamins: thiamine, pyridoxine, riboflavin, folic acid
		8. Proteins and amino acids
Ileum		9. Cholesterol
		10. Vitamin B_{12}
		11. Bile salts
Large Intestine		12. Potassium
		13. Water
		14. Sodium chloride
Colon		15. Vitamin K formed by colonic bacteria
		16. Short-chain fatty acids and volatile fatty acids from fiber digestion

it works automatically, the average person knows very little about it. To gain a more thorough understanding, let's take a guided tour of the digestive system from brain to colon.

The Brain: Where Digestion Actually Begins

Digestion begins before we even put food into our mouths! Any sight, sound, odor, taste, or texture associated with food can trigger the body to prepare for the food to come. Digestive juices, enzymes, and hormones begin to flow in anticipation of eating. As the body "revs up" for the impending work of digestion, heart rate and blood flow can change.

One way to use the brain purposely to prepare the gastrointestinal (GI) tract is to say grace before a meal. This expression of gratitude promotes a relaxed attitude and gives you time to appreciate and welcome the food into your body. Although there isn't any published research on the health benefits of saying grace, I believe it augments the body's ability to digest and utilize food more fully.

The Mouth: Gateway to the Gut

The main function of the mouth is to chew and liquefy food. The salivary glands under the tongue produce saliva that softens food, begins dissolving soluble components, and helps keep the mouth and teeth clean. Saliva contains amylase, an enzyme that breaks down carbohydrates. Only a small percentage of starches are digested by amylase, but a piece of bread kept in your mouth for a long time will begin to taste sweet as the starch is split into simple sugars.

Chewing also stimulates the parotid glands (located behind the ears in the jaw), to release hormones that stimulate the thymus to produce T cells, which are critical to the normal functioning of the immune system. The immune and digestive systems are very closely associated, anatomically and otherwise, as you will learn in the section on gut-associated lymphatic tissue (page 34).

Many people eat so fast that they barely chew their food at all and then wash it down with liquids, so the stomach receives chunks of food instead of mush (these people, not coincidentally, often complain of indigestion or gas). This sidesteps the function of the teeth, which is to increase the food's surface area for more efficient breakdown by digestive enzymes in the GI tract. In *May All Be Fed* by John Robbins, this point is dramatically illustrated in an account of three men who survived a World War II concentration camp by chewing their food very, very well, while their compatriots starved and perished. Many digestive problems, in fact, can be solved just by chewing food completely.

Healthy teeth and gums are critical for proper digestion. The most common health problems in the mouth are sores on the lips or tongue—usually canker or cold sores—and tooth and gum disease. Babies, of course, experience teething, an irritation in the gums prior to tooth eruption.

The Esophagus: Down the Hatch

Peristalsis can push well-chewed food through this tube from the mouth to the stomach in about six seconds, but dry food can get stuck and take minutes to reach the cardiac or esophageal sphincter (ring of muscle) at the bottom. This little "door" separates the esophagus from the stomach and remains closed most of the time to keep stomach acid and food from coming back up; it opens when a peristaltic wave, triggered by swallowing, relaxes the sphincter.

The most common esophageal problems are gastric reflux or spitting up, gastroesophageal reflux disease, hiatal hernia, and eosinophilia esophagitis.

The Stomach: Your Body's Blender

Under the ribcage and just below the heart, the stomach's muscles contract vigorously, mixing and mashing our food into a liquid called chyme. Although most foods are digested and absorbed farther down the gastrointestinal tract, alcohol, water, and certain salts are absorbed directly from the stomach into the bloodstream (that's why we feel the effects of alcohol so quickly). Protein and fat digestion are initiated in the stomach as well.

Hydrochloric acid (HCl), produced by millions of parietal cells in the stomach lining, starts to break apart protein molecules, which are composed of up to 200 amino acids strung together. The enzyme pepsin, also made in the stomach, cuts the bonds between specific amino acids to split protein chains into short segments of just four to twelve. In addition, the stomach produces small amounts of lipase, a fat-digesting enzyme.

Stomach HCl kills some of the microbes that can cause food poisoning. This acid is strong enough to burn our skin and clothing, but the stomach lining is protected by a thick layer of mucus. If the mucus layer breaks down, however, HCl can burn a hole in the stomach lining and cause a gastric ulcer.

When the stomach has finished its job, food has been reduced to chyme, which is the consistency of split-pea soup. This generally takes two to four hours—less if it's a low-fat meal, more if it's a high-fat or high-fiber meal—before the chyme is passed in small amounts through the pyloric valve into the small intestine. Chronic stress lengthens the amount of time that food stays in the stomach, whereas short-term stress usually shortens the emptying time.

The most common problems associated with the stomach are gastric ulcers and underproduction of HCl in adults, and stomach-aches in children.

Vitamin B_12 and Intrinsic Factor

Early nutritionists knew that a certain unidentified nutrient in food, then dubbed "extrinsic factor," needed to join with a certain substance in the stomach, called "intrinsic factor," in order to be absorbed by the body. Eventually, extrinsic factor was found to be vitamin B_{12}, which is essential for blood formation, energy, growth, and cell division and function. Intrinsic factor binds vitamin B_{12} for transport through the intestinal wall.

With age, parietal cells become less efficient and their production of both HCl and intrinsic factor decreases. As a result, elderly people often have a vitamin B_{12} deficiency, which affects the body's ability to bring oxygen into the cells. The main symptoms are dementia, depression, nervous system problems, muscle weakness, and fatigue.

Vegan (completely vegetarian) children are often deficient in vitamin B_{12}, and some other children simply have difficulty absorbing vitamin B_{12} from their food; this can lead to megaloblastic anemia, impaired growth, speech and fine motor skill delays, failure to thrive, and other neurological problems. I worked with a B_{12}-deficient toddler whose seizures stopped once her B_{12} level was normalized. Physicians began experimenting with B_{12} injections in asthmatic children as early as the 1930s, and one study achieved a 50-percent cure rate with a daily 1-milligram injection for thirty days.

Many people benefit from prescribed B_{12} injections or sublingual B_{12} supplements, even if they do not yet have low serum B_{12} levels or pernicious anemia; by the time serum levels of the vitamin are low, the tissues are quite depleted.

The Small Intestine: Absorption and Protection

The small intestine would average 15–20 feet long if stretched. Here, food is completely digested and most nutrients are absorbed through the intestinal wall. The wall is lined with hundreds of tiny, fingerlike folds called villi, covered in turn by millions of microvilli. (Think of the loops on a terry-cloth towel, with even smaller threads projecting from the loops.)

The villi and microvilli are only one cell layer thick but perform multiple functions: producing digestive enzymes, absorbing nutrients, and simultaneously blocking absorption of foreign substances that aren't useful to the body, such as chemicals, bacterial products, and other large molecules found in food. The intestinal lining repairs and replaces itself every three to five days; enzymes and fluids in the sloughed material are recycled by the body to aid in digestion.

The small intestine has three parts: the duodenum (the first 12 inches), jejunum (the next 40 percent), and ileum (the last segment). Specific nutrients are absorbed at specific parts of the small intestine. The duodenum's environment, for instance, is acidic because of stomach HCl, facilitating absorption of calcium, copper, iron, folic acid, thiamin, manganese, vitamins A and B_2, and zinc; people with low HCl levels may therefore become deficient in one or more of these nutrients. The duodenum is also the site of further protein digestion and fat digestion by bile from the liver and gallbladder. In the jejunum, the hydrochloric acid is neutralized for absorption of the chyme's remaining nutrients into the bloodstream.

The small intestine contains billions of microbes, including "friendly" lactobacilli. The lactobacilli protect us from food poisoning, secrete anticancer substances, and manufacture vitamins. While most of the body uses glucose for energy, the small intestine uses glutamine, an amino acid, for energy, maintenance, and repair. Common health problems of the small intestine include bacterial infection and leaky gut syndrome, which contributes to food allergies and sensitivities, skin problems, osteoarthritis, migraine headaches, and chronic fatigue syndrome. Crohn's disease can involve the small and/or large intestine.

Gut-Associated Lymphatic Tissue

Current research indicates that 70 percent of the immune system is located in or around the digestive system. As mentioned, the mucosal surface of the gut is only one cell thick. Underneath this is the gut-associated lymphatic tissue, which must continually distinguish between friend and foe in the foods we eat and among our various internal bacteria.

If the digestive system is presented with a potentially harmful foreign substance, called an antigen, specialized M cells carry the antigen to the intestinal mucosa, where it is "checked out" or sampled by cells called Peyer's patches. These, in turn, alert B cells and T cells to find and process antigens in the system for removal and destruction. B and T cells carry antigens back to the intestinal lining, where they are gobbled up by cells called macrophages.

Microbes entering the digestive system are confronted with several nonspecific and antigen-specific defense mechanisms including peristalsis, bile, HCl, mucus, antibacterial peptide molecules, and the antibody immunoglobulin A (also called secretory IgA), which serves as a "sentinel" on constant alert to trigger the inflammatory process designed to rid our bodies of foreign substances. These mechanisms stop most food-borne microbes and parasites from infecting the body. Those that do get through are recognized as foreigners by toll-like receptors, which fight disease-causing types of bacteria by stimulating production of pro-inflammatory cytokines (unfortunately, this gut inflammation makes us feel sick).

The Pancreas: An Enzyme and Hormone Factory

The pancreas, located behind the stomach, manufactures bicarbonate (essentially, baking soda) and secretes it through a duct into the duodenum to neutralize hydrochloric acid. To promote the digestion and absorption of nutrients, the pancreas also produces and releases specific enzymes: lipase to break fats into fatty acids and glycerol, amylase to split carbohydrates into simple sugars, and protease to break the links between amino acids in proteins. Protease, for example, is required to separate vitamin B_{12} from its carrier molecule (intrinsic factor, described previously), so poor pancreatic function can lead directly to a B_{12} deficiency.

Most people, however, know the pancreas better for its role in regulating blood sugar levels. When blood sugar is too high, the pancreas normally manufactures and releases the hormone insulin to signal the body's cells to pull glucose from the bloodstream and store it for cellular use—but if this signaling mechanism fails, diabetes develops.

The Liver: The Body's Most Overworked Organ

The quality of virtually every bodily function depends on the liver, which is perhaps our most overworked organ. I once heard a medical school dean say he'd rather perform all of the functions of General Motors for a day than be his own liver for a day. It manufactures bile to emulsify fats for digestion; makes and breaks down many hormones including cholesterol, testosterone, and estrogens; helps regulate blood sugar levels; and processes all nutrients, drugs, and other materials that enter the bloodstream, letting them pass, breaking them down, or storing them (see the inset "Liver Life" on page 36).

Located under the lower right ribs, the liver has three lobes and is the largest abdominal organ (in an adult, it weighs about 3–5 pounds and is about the size of a football). It manufactures 13,000 substances and has 2,000 enzyme systems, plus thousands of other helpful chemicals, all of which are used by the liver to "humanize" nutrients for our cells to use. Most of the vitamins and minerals we take in, for example, need to be enzymatically processed by the liver before use, and if the liver is too congested to do this, we won't benefit from those nutrients.

Neutralizing today's environmental pollution is no small task, but the liver does an admirable job of it, even though many of the chemicals it must contend with are brand new. The human capacity to metabolize chemicals, however, varies dramatically. Our liver's ability to detoxify drugs and other substances depends on the cytochrome P-450 system of enzymes and is primarily genetically determined. We are now seeing many children and adults whose detoxification systems are overloaded; exhibiting symptoms that can resemble fatigue, pain, and mental "fogginess," they report that their condition is aggravated by everyday chemicals such as perfumes, scented shampoos, and household cleaning products.

The amazingly resilient liver can lose as much as 70 percent of its capability

Liver Life

Your liver helps you by:

- Producing quick energy when it is needed
- Manufacturing new body proteins
- Preventing shortages in body fuel by storing certain vitamins, minerals, and sugars
- Regulating transport of fat stores
- Regulating blood clotting
- Aiding in the digestive process by producing bile
- Controlling the production and excretion of cholesterol
- Neutralizing and destroying poisonous substances

- Metabolizing alcohol
- Monitoring and maintaining the proper level of many chemicals and drugs in the blood
- Cleansing the blood and discharging waste products into the bile
- Maintaining hormone balance
- Serving as the main organ of blood formation before birth
- Helping the body resist infection by producing immune factors and by removing bacteria from the bloodstream
- Regenerating its own damaged tissue
- Storing iron

—*source: American Liver Foundation, Illinois chapter, www.illinois-liver.org/*

and not show diagnosable disease. The most common liver problems are toxicity, jaundice, cirrhosis, and hepatitis. Others include pruritis (itching), Wilson's disease (a disorder in which the liver accumulates copper), and cystic fibrosis.

The Gallbladder: Bile's Holding Tank

A soaplike substance made of bile salts, cholesterol, and lecithin, bile is produced in the liver and then stored and concentrated between meals in the gallbladder, a pear-shaped organ just below the liver. When we eat a fat-containing meal or snack, bile is released into the common duct that connects the liver, gallbladder, and pancreas to the duodenum. Bile emulsifies fats, cholesterol, and fat-soluble vitamins by breaking them into tiny globules, making them more water-soluble and creating a greater surface area for fat-splitting enzymes (lipases) to act on during digestion. Along with bicarbonates from the pancreas, bile from the gallbladder also buffers the stomach acids in chyme as it enters the small intestine.

The most common problem with this organ is gallstones. Bile that becomes too concentrated may form stones, which can cause pain, nausea, and discomfort. Gallbladder disease is directly related to diet and is relatively rare in children.

The Colon: Recycling and Waste Removal

After nutrient absorption in the small intestine, the remaining chyme—which is mostly water, bacteria, and fiber—passes through the ileocecal valve (by the right hipbone) into the large intestine or colon. The large intestine is actually shorter than the small one, at only 3–5 feet long, and has three main parts: the ascending colon (up the right side of the abdomen), the transverse colon (straight across the belly under the ribs), and the descending colon (down the left side), which contains the rectum and anus. It may surprise you to learn that your appendix is an extension off the beginning of your colon, just after the ileocecal valve. Until recently, the function of this small, fingerlike sac was a mystery, but now we know that the appendix contains a great deal of lymphatic tissue, and it is thought to be part of the immune system.

The large intestine contains trillions of microbes, including "friendly" types of bacteria that help our digestion and benefit our health by lowering the colon's pH, killing disease-causing microbes, producing vitamins B and K, producing lactase for milk digestion, and enhancing peristalsis. These probiotic bacteria also ferment dietary fiber to produce short-chained fatty acids like butyric acid, which serves as the main fuel for the cells of the colon (most of the rest of the body's cells run on glucose).

The colon's job is to absorb water and final nutrients from chyme and form stool for elimination from the body. Two-and-a-half gallons of water pass through the colon each day, two-thirds of it from bodily fluids, and an efficient colon recycles 80 percent of the water back into the bloodstream. If the chyme passes through the colon too quickly, water is not absorbed, causing diarrhea, whereas material that sits too long in the colon becomes dry and hard to pass, leading to constipation.

Stool begins to form in the transverse colon. About two-thirds of stool is composed of water, undigested fiber, and other indigestible food products, and the other third of living and dead bacteria. Once the stool is well formed, it gets pushed into the descending colon and then the rectum. When sufficient fecal volume accumulates for a bowel movement, the internal sphincter relaxes, signaling your brain that it's time to relieve yourself. Recognizing this urge and bringing elimination under voluntary control is taught in toilet-training. Because the external sphincter then opens on command, you can have the urge but defer defecation until it's convenient. If the urge is ignored, however, water is continually absorbed into the body and the stool gets dry and hard. Some children are chronically constipated because they don't want to take the time or don't like to have bowel movements at school or a friend's house, so it's important to teach your child to listen when his/her body calls even if the timing is not ideal.

Many health problems arise in the colon: appendicitis, constipation, diarrhea, diverticular disease, Crohn's disease, ulcerative colitis, rectal polyps, colon cancer, irritable bowel syndrome, parasites, and hemorrhoids. A low level of butyric acid from colonic bacterial metabolism has been associated with ulcerative and active colitis, colon cancer, and inflammatory bowel disease.

WHAT GOES IN MUST COME OUT

Americans are constipated! Dennis Burkitt, M.D., father of the fiber theory, found that people eating Western diets only excreted 5 ounces of stool daily on average, whereas Africans eating traditional diets passed 16 ounces. We simply don't consume enough dietary fiber, and often, we also don't have enough magnesium and helpful bacteria to maintain adequate peristalsis.

Conversations about Poop

Well-formed stool looks like a brown banana with a point at one end, is well-hydrated, and tells us when it wants to come out; it slips out easily, and we don't need to coax it. Stool that looks like little balls wadded together has been in the colon too long. The longer waste lingers before elimination, the more concentrated its remaining bile acids become, irritating the colon's lining. Hormones that have been broken down by the body are normally excreted in feces, but if stool sits in the colon for too long, these hormones are reabsorbed into the bloodstream, increasing the risk of developing hormone-dependent cancers.

We can learn a lot about ourselves from stool. Frequency of bowel movements, for example, is an important health indicator. Two to three daily is considered an optimal number, and many children poop after each meal. How often does your child have a bowel movement?

Another good indicator of digestive health is bowel transit time: that is, the time period from the point that a food is swallowed until it emerges at "the other end." When your system is working well, bowel transit time ranges from twelve to twenty-four hours. Because we don't eat enough high-fiber foods or drink enough water, Americans have an average transit time that is way too long—forty-eight to ninety-six hours—and therefore we end up reabsorbing wastes and undoing what our body has so elegantly done.

Use this simple home test to determine your child's bowel transit time (or your own):

- Buy activated charcoal tablets (these turn stool black) at a drugstore or health food store, and use about 1,000 milligrams (mg) for a teenager and about 500 mg for a child aged five to twelve years. If you prefer, you can use beets as the testing agent, as eating one or two whole beets will turn stool a deep red. People also evaluate transit time with sesame seeds or tomato seeds.

- Note the exact time that your child takes or eats the testing agent. The testing agent is best taken with a meal.

- When the last darkened, red, or seed-marked stool is seen, calculate how many hours have passed since the testing agent was taken. That is the bowel transit time.

- A bowel transit time of twelve to twenty-four hours is optimal.

- A bowel transit time of less than twelve hours usually indicates that your child is not absorbing all the nutrients he/she should from his/her food and may have malabsorption problems.

- A bowel transit time of more than twenty-four hours indicates that wastes are sitting inside the colon for too long. Poor transit time greatly increases the risk of colon disease, and substances that were supposed to be eliminated get absorbed back into the bloodstream.

If your child has a poor bowel transit time, or is not having a daily bowel movement, there can be many causes. Act now! First, take a close look at diet, because he/she probably isn't eating enough fiber. Increase your child's intake of fruits, vegetables, whole grains, and legumes, which are all generally high in fiber and magnesium and help normalize peristalsis. Make sure that he/she is drinking enough water—soft drinks don't count—and exercising nearly every day!

CHAPTER 4

Enzymes:
The Body's Workhorses

To catalyze is to trigger a change without being changed. Enzymes are substances that catalyze biochemical reactions to speed up, slow down, or change in some other way. Enzymes are proteins, but some also have a non-protein part called a co-enzyme (a metal, vitamin, or other type of molecule) attached to them. Each enzyme binds to a specific type of substance and does a specific type of job. Enzymes conserve energy in our bodies; without them, much more heat and calories would be needed to perform the same functions. There are two main types of enzymes: metabolic and digestive. And each enzyme can only produce a relatively small change, so we need many of them.

ENZYMES IN OUR BODIES

We have 2,700 known enzymes in our bodies. They are needed for *every* chemical reaction that occurs in the human body, and none of our systems or cells can work without them. We use them for such diverse purposes as making energy, thinking, controlling blood sugar, preventing blood clots, fighting disease, and building and dissembling cells, structures, and compounds. We cannot utilize nutrients or remove wastes without enzymes. Enzymes are made in the body from the proteins we ingest and by recycling the enzymes we've used. To work properly, they need to be synthesized correctly and to be in a correct pH and temperature. And if we don't have enough of the enzymes we need, we don't feel as well as we could.

Our digestive system uses enzymes, along with HCl and bile, to break down the food we eat. Although most digestive enzymes are made in the pancreas, they are produced throughout the digestive system, beginning with those in saliva. Different enzymes break down different nutrients:

- Lipases split fats.
- Amylases split carbohydrates.

- Proteases split proteins.

- Pectinases split pectins (pectins are found in fruits such as apples and pears).

- Phytases split phytic acids (phytic acids are found primarily in grains and beans; for use by the body, they must be separated by phytases from the minerals to which they are bound. Soaking beans and grains allows the phytases to break down phytic acid, which enhances our ability to use the minerals.)

ENZYMES IN FOODS AND SUPPLEMENTS

Foods can also be a good source of enzymes—fresh foods, that is. Feed your children fresh, raw fruits and vegetables in abundance to take advantage of their enzyme content and their health-protective effects. Having your own garden can be of great benefit. Children are naturally curious and will eat nearly anything home-grown, often right off the plant! And produce has its highest enzyme activity when fresh-picked. Farmer's markets are another source of fresh, locally grown food.

By the time we are middle-aged, many of us suffer from health issues related to enzyme deficiency. Cooked, packaged, or processed foods, unfortunately, are enzyme depleted. Cooking at temperatures as low as 118°F destroys enzymes. As these foods are basically what most of our children eat, many children can benefit from enzyme supplementation. There are three major types of supplemental enzyme products: pancreatic, Aspergillus-grown, and plant-based.

Pancreatic enzymes, derived from animal pancreatic tissue, work well in assisting with digestion and also to help stabilize blood glucose levels in people with diabetes and hypoglycemia. The problem with pancreatic enzymes is that they only work at a pH of 8 or above. That limited pH range is too high (alkaline; see Chapter 7) for these enzymes to function in the stomach, where a large part of digestion takes place. And although pancreatic enzymes are commonly used in treating children with cystic fibrosis, a small percentage of these children eventually become "allergic" to them.

More recently, supplemental enzymes have been grown on a fungal base of *Aspergillus niger* and *A. oryzae* (fungus species found to be completely free of poisonous substances called mycotoxins). Such enzymes have been used in food production for centuries and clinically in Japan for more than fifty years. They have the advantage of functioning at all human pH levels (between 1 and 8), so they can begin working in the stomach and continue throughout the digestive system. They have also been found to cause fewer allergic issues in children than animal-derived enzymes do.

Plant-based enzymes such as bromelain and papain are useful for digesting protein and for reducing inflammation and pain. Supplemental enzymes that improve protein digestion also decrease the quantity of antigens leaking from the digestive system into the bloodstream, reducing issues with food sensitivities and allergies (discussed further in Chapters 11 and 12).

Enzymes are measured by their activity level rather than by their mass in milligrams or micrograms (mg or mcg). On the labels of enzyme supplements, you should see units such as DU, HUT, FCCLU, CU, IAU, and others that express the level of enzyme activity; if the label only shows measurements in mg or mcg, you cannot be certain whether or not the product contains any active enzymes. Many enzyme supplement labels do not have expiration dates, as enzymes are very stable and will last for at least three years.

ENZYMES, CHILDREN, AND DISEASE

Many of our children are enzyme deficient, and these deficiencies can play a pivotal role in the development of childhood disease. According to Dic Qie Fuller, M.D., a leader in the enzyme supplement business, the ability to manufacture enzymes develops prenatally, between the ninth and twelfth weeks in the womb (a time when many women don't even know that they are pregnant). In *How to Be Healthier with Enzymes,* Dr. Fuller states, "If anything goes wrong in that time, then that's where [children] face some of their real problems. Well, we know that cystic fibrosis and some of the other diseases that children come in with are an enzyme deficiency— that's a given. But many times people don't realize that enzyme deficiency can come out as obesity later, or these children that have their diabetes type II when they're only seven to ten years old. Those are enzyme problems."

Breast-milk is the only food that newborn babies can fully digest. Infants' digestive systems cannot handle complex carbohydrates until the age of seven months or sugars other than lactose until the age of three years. Dr. Fuller has given enzymes to babies and children of all ages preventively, and to children with digestive problems or with a failure to thrive. She has had great results, and has never seen any negative side effects from their use. When a baby or child fails to thrive and grow, enzymes are the first thing I think of to balance their systems. Because enzymes are gentle, I am using them more and more for children who have digestive issues.

Enzymes have been used clinically for treating conditions including Crohn's disease, ulcerative colitis, pulmonary fibrosis, sinusitis, multiple sclerosis, and bladder infections, as well as for breaking up and preventing blood clots (this effect is also protective against heart disease). In adults, enzyme supplements have been found more effective than drugs against several types of arthritis. They can, in fact, be effective against swelling and pain throughout the body, and can reduce the healing time of bruises by about 50 percent. In a study of soccer players, injuries were found to heal more quickly, sometimes up to twice as fast, with administration of enzymes *versus* a placebo.

Enzymes have also been used for decades as part of cancer treatment, especially in Europe. At a recent medical conference, oncologist Mahesh Kanojia reported that using aspergillus-derived enzyme supplements lessens the side effects of chemotherapy (including hair loss) and enhances the results of the treatments. Nicholas Gonzales, M.D., uses pancreatic enzyme supplements as an anti-tumor therapy, primarily with pancreatic cancer, and a study to duplicate his work has been funded by the National Institutes of Health.

In children, enzyme supplements have been used successfully to treat food allergies, eosinophilic gastroenteritis, asthma, and other illnesses, and research on enzymes for children is promising. A study of pancreatic enzyme supplementation in children diagnosed with celiac disease showed that the enzymes, along with a gluten-free diet, enhanced recovery during the first month (after that, there were no additional benefits).

About 70 percent of the world's population is sensitive to lactose, but an aspergillus-based lactase (lactose-digesting enzyme) given at a dairy-containing meal works effectively to allow children to eat dairy products. In a study of forty-eight healthy Guatemalan preschoolers, 56 percent of the children were found to be lactose sensitive. When given *A. oryzae*–derived enzymes, not only were the lactose-sensitive children better able to digest lactose, but lactose absorption also improved in the other children as well.

CHAPTER 5

Probiotics and Prebiotics: Keys to Healthful Resilience

In general, we are in great symbiotic harmony with bacteria. . . .
Our soils are filled with them. . . . They thrive in our waters and exist
in air. On a personal level, . . . they comprise 10 percent of our dry
body weight. . . . Their story is one of wonder and creation of life.
The oxygen we breathe is a result of their evolution.
They comprise the first "world wide web" and were the first
motorized vehicles! They are the initial substance of all life,
and without them plants and animals could not survive.

—ELIZABETH LIPSKI, "WONDROUS BACTERIA" (UNPUBLISHED)

Did you know that you have ten times as many bacteria in your digestive tract as you have cells in your body? The billions in your mouth, many billions in your small intestine, and hundreds of trillions in your large intestine (half of the colon's volume) have a total weight of about 3 pounds. Each day, you produce several ounces of these microbes and eliminate several ounces in stool.

These gut organisms function much like an organ and act as a major part of the immune system. They manufacture substances that influence disease risks, drug effects, fat metabolism, immune competence, nutritional status, and rate of aging. The symbiotic and antagonistic relationships of our intestinal bacteria create an ecological balance that plays a huge role in our digestive and overall health status.

OUR INTERNAL INHABITANTS

Human intestinal flora includes 400–500 types of bacteria, each type having hundreds of different strains—an almost overwhelming variety, but twenty types make up three-quarters of the total (the most common are bacteroides, bifidobacteria, eubacteria, fusobacteria, lactobacilli, peptococcaceae, rheumanococcus, and streptococcus). Not all are beneficial; some even cause acute or chronic illness. Several groups of friendly flora in our internal environment are called probiotics, organisms that "promote life" of microorganisms, in opposition to antibiotics, which kill microorganisms." The term is also commonly used in reference to supplements of these organisms.

Where Do Probiotics Come From?

Until birth, we receive predigested food from our mothers and our digestive tract is sterile. The trip down the birth canal then initiates us into the world of microbes thriving everywhere. Babies are subsequently exposed to bacteria in breast-milk and formula and when sucking on nipples, fingers, and toes. With every breath and touch, bacteria flock to an infant's skin and mucous membranes. In no time, every conceivable space in the colon is occupied by microbes.

The first two years of life are critical for our long-term immune responses. Bacterial colonization patterns set up in infancy continue to prevail throughout our entire lifetime—and the foods and drugs to which we expose our children dramatically affect this delicate balance.

Escherichia and streptococcus species colonize in the first few days of life. Within a week of birth, bifidobacteria, bacteroides, and clostridia species are established in bottle-fed babies, whereas breast-fed infants have increased numbers of lactobacillus and bifidobacteria species. The microbes set up homogeneous neighborhoods and push out competing microbes that try to break into their territories. After weaning, the dominant beneficial flora changes from *Bifidobacteria infantis* in infants to other species of bifidobacteria in children and adults.

This process normally happens in a predictable way, and, once established, the colonies flourish. Babies who are unable to properly colonize friendly flora, however, can become irritable and colicky and have gas pains, diaper rash, or eczema. Babies who don't develop the right balance of beneficial bacteria are also more susceptible to allergy and asthma.

What Do They Do?

Digestively speaking, intestinal flora manufacture many nutrients including vitamin K and several of the B-complex vitamins: biotin, thiamin (B_1), riboflavin (B_2), niacin (B_3), pantothenic acid (B_5), pyridoxine (B_6), cobalamine (B_{12}), and folic acid. Certain acid-secreting species increase our absorption of minerals including calcium, copper, iron, magnesium, and manganese. Probiotics improve peristalsis, help normalize bowel transit time, and are also important in preventing traveler's diarrhea. If you travel outside the United States, take a probiotic supplement daily, as studies show it significantly increases your ability to withstand new microbes.

Native and supplemental probiotics help us in many additional ways. Some have antitumor and anticancer effects, and others help to keep our normal population of internal fungus from proliferating out of control. Probiotics help us metabolize foreign substances like mercury and pesticides, protect us from damaging radiation and harmful pollutants, and break down and rebuild our "used" hormones. Friendly intestinal flora also plays a vital role in our ability to fight infectious disease, providing a front line in our immune system's defenses. And although the mechanism is not yet understood, bacterial balance is also essential for healthy metabolism; many super-thin people have been able to gain weight through the use of probiotic supplements.

It is impossible in a book of this scope to describe all of our probiotic species, but the following sections highlight several of the most significant.

Lactobacillus and Bifidobacteria

Our two most important groups of intestinal flora are the lactobacilli, found mainly in the small intestine, and bifidobacteria, found primarily in the colon.

Lactobacilli and bifidobacteria secrete large amounts of acetic, formic, and lactic acid, which makes the intestinal environment inhospitable to invading microbes and helps prevent, or lessen the severity of, food poisoning. In 1993, 20–40 million cases of food poisoning were reported in the United States, although the U.S. Food and Drug Administration estimates the true total to be 80 million (many cases go unreported because the symptoms closely resemble the flu); some food-borne infections lead to chronic illness, causing heart and valve problems, immune system disorders, joint disease, and possibly even cancer.

Beyond their impact on our intestinal ecology, lactobacilli have been repeatedly shown in studies to help normalize cholesterol levels, and *Lactobacillus bulgaricus* has been shown to have antitumor, antibiotic, and antiherpes effects. See the inset "Benefits of a Few Probiotic Supplements" on page 48 for details on the "talents" of particular lactobacilli and bifidobacteria.

Streptococcus, Escherichia coli, and Fungus?

Streptococcus bacteria are typically associated with strep throat, but the species *Streptococcus thermophilus* is a helpful, transient resident found in cultured dairy products or supplements. Like *Lactobacillus bulgaricus*, *S. thermophilus* enhances the production of bifidobacteria and has been shown to have antitumor effects. Similarly, *Escherichia coli* is often associated with disease and poor sanitation, but the Nissle strain of *E. coli* has been studied for its role in protection from inflammatory bowel disease and irritable bowel syndrome.

The fungus *Candida albicans* can infect the nails and eyes, the oral cavity and throat (thrush), and the urinary tract and vagina (yeast infections). *Saccharomyces boulardii,* on the other hand, is a friendly yeast (a cousin to bread yeast) that enhances our internal levels of the protective immunoglobulin called secretory IgA and helps control *C. albicans*—in France, it's called "yeast against yeast" and *C. difficile.* Well-studied and used clinically for over fifty years, *S. boulardii* is safe for people of all ages. It helps protect and restore normal flora and is antibiotic-resistant (except for antifungal medications). Most research on *S. boulardii* has focused on its benefits for people with diarrhea, but it has been shown to be helpful against salmonella and irritable bowel syndrome as well as for clearing the skin, and it also significantly reduces the number of bowel movements in people with Crohn's disease.

PROBIOTIC SUPPLEMENTS

In healthy people, the composition of the intestinal population usually remains fairly constant, but it can become unbalanced by aging, diet, disease, drugs, poor health, or stress. Health problems resulting from unbalanced flora have now become widespread. Eating cultured dairy products and other foods (see page 53) can maintain colonies of friendly flora in people who are already healthy, but once disease-producing microbes get established, probiotic supplements are necessary to rebalance the internal community. Until recently, it was believed that taking these supplements would cause the desired organisms to colonize in the gut; newer research indicates, however, that they probably don't, which makes a good argument for taking probiotics on a regular basis to increase our body's ability to protect itself.

Shopping for Probiotics

The many probiotic supplements on the market look similar but can be extremely different in their effectiveness. It is important to use well-researched probiotics that have been found useful in clinical settings. Purchase your supplements from a company known for quality, and look for a batch number and an expiration date.

Species and Strains

Look for the normal gut flora such as lactobacilli and bifidobacteria. *Bifidobacteria infantis* is the most appropriate choice for a baby (see page 50) and is also useful for children and adults. Supplements may also contain the species *Lactobacillus casei, L. reuteri, Bifidobacteria longum, B. breve, L. lactis, L. plantarum, L. rhamnosus,* and others (see Table 5.1 on page 49).

Benefits of a Few Probiotic Supplements

Lactobacillus acidophilus

- Prevents infections including candida, *Escherichia coli*, *Helicobacter pylori*, and salmonella
- Prevents and treats antibiotic-associated and traveler's diarrhea
- Aids digestion of lactose and dairy products
- Improves nutrient absorption
- Maintains integrity of intestinal tract
- Helps prevent vaginal and urinary tract infections

Lactobacillus reuteri

- Inhibits growth of disease-causing microbes including gram-negative and gram-positive bacteria, yeast, fungi, and protozoa
- Appears to inhibit adherence of pathogens in the gut
- Shortens duration of children's rotaviral infections (these cause diarrhea)
- Has protective and therapeutic effect on vaginal infections

Bifidobacteria infantis

- Helps treat colic, cradle-cap, and eczema in infants and babies
- May protect against bacteria that promote inflammatory bowel disease
- Along with *L. acidophilus*, reduces illness and deaths from necrotizing enterocolitis in infants
- Has antitumor properties in test research

Some supplements contain soil-based probiotics such as *Bacillus laterosporus, B. subtilis,* and *L. sporonges* (also known as *B. coagulous*), but research has yet to substantiate the many anecdotal stories of great success with these soil-based organisms.

Most manufacturers produce combination supplements, but different flora will compete for nourishment and even cannibalize each other within a supplement unless the product is freeze-dried. Freeze-drying keeps the probiotics dormant until they are activated by moisture within the body, where there is plenty of available food. (The only truly cooperative bacteria are the two used in making yogurt, *Lactobacillus bulgaricus* and *L. thermophilus.*)

Table 5.1. Bacteria and Yeasts Used as Probiotic Supplements			
Bifidobacteria	**Lactobacilli**	**Streptococcus**	**Other Species**
B. adolescentis	L. acidophilus	S. jacium	Enterococcus faecium
B. angulatum	L. brevis	S. jaecali	Lactococcus cremoris
B. bifidum	L. bulgaricus	S. lactis	Saccharomyces boulardii
B. breve	L. casei	S. thermophilus	
B. atenulatum	L. debreuckii		
B. infantis	L. gasseri		
B. longum	L. kefir		
B. pseudocatenulatum	L. lactis		
	L. plantarum		
	L. reuteri		
	L. rhamnosus		
	L. salavarius		
	L. yoghuni		

The most-studied strains of acidophilus are DDS-1, NCFM, and CERELA, though many others are also effective. Acid-resistant acidophilus strains can survive the stomach and reach the intestines alive. Strains that aren't acid resistant can be enterically coated for safe passage, but they have not been well researched and I don't recommend them.

Manufactured probiotics are raised on dairy products, fruit, grain, or other fermentable foods. Strains from a nondairy source are often recommended for the lactose intolerant. Although this makes sense, many people find that taking dairy-grown strains actually improves their ability to tolerate dairy products. The best test is to try them out and see what is most effective for your child.

Viability and Potency

Most probiotics supply between 1 billion and 6 billion organisms per dose, and a few supply substantially more, up to 450 billion. The number, however, isn't the most important thing, as some studies have shown supplements that contain only millions of microbes to be effective; what matters is whether the product contains living, viable organisms that adhere to the gut lining, are not destroyed by bile, and have benefit once in your body. Of twenty-five products tested by Consumer Lab (at www.consumerlab.com), eight contained less than 1 percent of the number of viable bacteria listed on the label, and six of those had less than 0.1 percent of living organisms and probably wouldn't be helpful at all. According to Consumer Lab, however, products that listed specific numbers of organisms were more likely to be alive.

These delicate bacteria must be refrigerated in shipping, at the store, and in your home to ensure their lifespan and greatest potency. Probiotics will maintain potency at room temperature for short periods of time: for instance, if you are on vacation for a week or two. Many people forget to take probiotics that are stored in the refrigerator, so I encourage you to put several days' worth on the counter where you'll remember them.

Bacteria multiply very quickly, but they need enough food and protection to survive the trip through the stomach and into the intestinal tract, so many probiotic supplements also contain prebiotics such as fructo-oligosaccharide (FOS) and inulin, which provide nourishment for the bacteria (see "Prebiotics" on page 53).

Probiotics for Babies

In a study of growth rate and probiotic supplementation, babies given bifidobacteria showed better growth during their first six months of life. In another study, supplemental *Lactobacillus acidophilus* and *L. casei* decreased the severity and incidence of bronchitis and pneumonia in babies aged six months to two years. Adding probiotics to infant formula can reduce the need for antibiotics, and can help prevent infections in preterm infants by giving their immune systems a boost. I've seen colicky babies become calm in less than twenty-four hours when given *Bifidobacteria infantis*—what a blessing! (See also Chapter 13.)

Clearly, probiotic supplementation promotes infant health in a variety of ways, which also includes:

- Enhancing digestion and mineral absorption
- Preventing diarrhea
- Preventing/lessening/curing diaper rash, eczema, and cradle-cap
- Decreasing anemia and asthma
- Diminishing/preventing cow's milk allergy
- Eliminating thrush

Powdered probiotics can be fed directly to infants and toddlers by mixing a pinch of powder with a drop of water on your hand and putting the paste on your child's tongue, or the powder can be added to bottled breast-milk, formula, juice, milk, or water. For toddlers, ¼–½ teaspoon twice daily is recommended; however, the exact dosage isn't critical.

Your baby or child may experience bloating and gas from taking probiotic supplements. If this happens, restart the supplementation process with tiny amounts, and build up his/her dosage slowly to avoid the die-off reaction (as disease-producing bacteria and fungus are killed, they release chemicals that aggravate those symptoms).

Probiotics for Older Children

As with infants, probiotics can help reduce the severity and frequency of childhood respiratory infections such as bronchitis and pneumonia. In a recent study of children aged one to six years with acute infections and taking antibiotics, those also given probiotic supplements recovered somewhat faster, were able to eat better, and had increased weight gain. Children with eczema benefit from probiotic supplements, and studies show even greater improvements in children who show other signs of allergy such as a positive IgE scratch-test.

In older children, probiotics help prevent symptoms of irritable bowel syndrome, diarrhea, and constipation; reduce intestinal inflammation; enhance growth; and generally make the child's health heartier. See the inset "Probiotic Benefits for Children and Teenagers" on page 52.

Probiotic supplements are available in capsules, but chewable tablets and powders are useful with small children. Powdered probiotics can be taken "straight" or stirred into juice, milk, or water. I used to put about a quarter-teaspoon of probiotic powder in my boys' hands and they would lick it off and say, "Give me more 'dophilus, Mommy! Tastes yummy!" Give your child or teenager 1–2 capsules or tablets or ¼–½ teaspoons of powder twice daily. Again, the exact dosage isn't critical, and if your child experiences bloating and gas from taking probiotics, restart with a low dosage and build it up slowly to avoid the die-off reaction described previously.

EATING AND FEEDING FRIENDLY FLORA

Bacteria manufacture nutrients for their own benefit, but we can reap the rewards. Compared to their fresh counterparts, bacterially cultured or fermented foods supply more probiotics and health-building enzymes. By having cottage cheese and yogurt rather than milk (see Table 5.2 on page 53), sauerkraut rather than cabbage, tofu and tempeh rather than soybeans, and wine rather than grapes, we obtain higher dietary levels of such nutrients as vitamins A, B-complex, and K.

People around the world have long recognized the health benefits of fermented foods. Traditional sauerkraut is historically eaten by Europeans to combat ulcers and digestive problems. Asian cultures serve pickled daikon radish and *kimchee* as condiments and drink a sweet rice beverage called *amasake*. Lactose-intol-

Probiotic Benefits for Children and Teenagers

Digestive

- Balances intestinal pH
- Improves or prevents irritable bowel syndrome
- Stops diarrhea
- Relieves constipation by regulating peristalsis
- Reduces intestinal inflammation

Nutritional

- Increases absorption of minerals
- Minimizes or eliminates lactose intolerance
- Aids protein digestion
- Manufactures essential fatty acids and short-chain fatty acids
- Converts flavonoids to usable forms

Immune

- Prevents and treats complications from antibiotic therapy
- Prevents infection by producing antibiotic and antifungal substances
- Prevents and alleviating eczema
- Prevents food poisoning
- Decreases severity and duration of respiratory and other infections
- Breaks down bacterial toxins
- Protects against toxic substances
- Has antitumor and anticancer effects
- Prevents and controls thrush, vaginal yeast infection, and bladder infection

Heart

- Normalizes serum cholesterol and triglycerides

Metabolic

- Breaks down and rebuilds hormones
- Promotes optimal growth
- Promotes healthy metabolism
- Breaks down bile acids

Table 5.2. Nutritionally Enhanced Dairy Foods		
Original Food	Fermented/Cultured Food	Increased Nutrition
Milk	Cheddar cheese	Vitamin B_1, 3x
Milk	Cottage cheese	Vitamin B_{12}, 5x
Milk	Yogurt	Vitamin B_{12}, 5–30x
Milk	Yogurt	Vitamin B_3, 50x
Skim milk	Low-fat yogurt	Vitamin A, 7–14x

erant people worldwide have relied for centuries on cultured dairy products such as cottage cheese, kefir, and yogurt; in India, the fermented dairy drink *lassi* is a household staple, and in Israel, yogurtlike *leban* is served daily.

The traditional Japanese diet takes advantage of several fermented soy foods with antibiotic properties. *Miso* paste, for example, contains 161 strains of aerobic bacteria, almost all of which compete successfully with the main food-poisoning agents *Escherichia coli* and *Staphylococcus aureus,* and contains many lactic-acid-producing bacteria as well. Several microbes including yeast and *Lactobacillus acidophilus* are used to brew health-giving soy sauce, also called *shoyu* or *tamari.* (In the United States, however, most soy sauce is manufactured with inorganic acids that break down the soybeans, rather than by fermentation with living microbes, so it doesn't have the same benefits.)

Certain herbs also promote the growth of friendly flora. Polyphenols, which are the enhancing substance in the positive effects of green tea (*Camellia sinensis*) against serum cholesterol, tumors, and ulcers, have been shown to increase the number of beneficial intestinal bacteria such as lactobacilli and bifidobacteria while decreasing the number of disease-causing clostridia. A significant increase in beneficial flora was also found when an extract of the herb *Panax ginseng* was tested *in vitro* on 107 types of human-dwelling bacteria.

Prebiotics

Prebiotics are saccharide (sugar) molecules that were initially developed as potential low-calorie sweeteners; eventually, however, it became apparent that these molecules could play an important role in health maintenance. Like probiotics, they acidify the intestinal environment, enhancing the absorption of essential minerals. Prebiotics also nourish "good" bacteria while promoting a reduction in disease-causing clostridia, klebsiella, and enterobacter. Prebiotics work synergistically with probiotics and can be taken together for best results (together, they are called synbiotics).

The two well-documented prebiotics fructo-oligosaccharide (FOS) and inulin have been shown to increase intestinal levels of acidophilus and bifidobacteria, and to lower serum triglycerides and normalize insulin levels as well. They also protect against colon cancer and are antagonistic to at least eight disease-causing microbes including salmonella, listeria, campylobacter, shigella, and vibrio. All this, and the research on prebiotics has just begun!

Because of their health-building qualities, inulin and FOS are being investigated worldwide as possible functional food additives, but they are naturally found in our food already. On average, we consume about 2.5 grams per day of FOS alone. Honey is a good prebiotic food, and in a recent test-tube study, worked as well as FOS, galactooligosaccharide (GOS), and inulin in promoting bifidobacteria's production of lactic and acetic acid. It just may be helpful to add a spoonful of honey to your beverages—yum!

Foods High in Prebiotic Content

• Asparagus	• Eggplant	• Kefir	• Sugar maple
• Bananas	• Fruit	• Leeks	• Yogurt
• Burdock root	• Garlic	• Legumes	• Whole rye
• Chicory	• Green tea	• Onions	• Whole wheat
• Chinese chives	• Honey	• Peas	
• Cottage cheese	• Jerusalem artichokes	• Soybeans	

Many people experience gas and bloating when they start taking prebiotics, but these symptoms usually dissipate after a week or so; if they do occur, you can either continue your child's current dosage or lower the dosage and then increase it gradually. Human studies using prebiotics show the greatest growth of helpful bacteria in the people who need it most, with benefits most evident at doses up to 10 grams daily. After your child stops taking prebiotics, his/her internal bacteria will return to previous levels in about two to three weeks.

CHAPTER 6

Dysbiosis: An Unbalanced Body Ecology

Within these regions battles rage; populations rise and fall, affected
just as we are by local environmental conditions, industry thrives
and constant defense is exercised against interlopers and dangerous
aliens who may enter unannounced; colonists roam and settle—
some permanently, some only briefly, in general we have in miniature
many of terrestrial life's vicissitudes, problems and solutions.

—LEO CHAITOW AND NATASHA TRENEV, 1990

Early in the twentieth century, Eli Metchnikoff, M.D., popularized the theory that disease begins in the digestive tract with an imbalance of intestinal bacteria. To describe this state of imbalance, he coined the term "dysbiosis," combining "dys" for "not" and "symbiosis" for "living together in mutual harmony." Dr. Metchnikoff discovered the useful properties of probiotics and won a Nobel Prize for his work on the role of lactobacilli in immune function. He found that a bacterium in yogurt (named *Lactobacillus bulgaricus* after the long-lived, yogurt-loving peasants of Bulgaria) prevented and reversed bacterial infection. His research proved that lactobacilli could displace many disease-causing organisms and reduce the toxins they generated—toxins that he believed shortened the human lifespan.

We now know that the well-developed ecological system of a healthy gut can be disrupted by various factors, enabling pathogenic microbes to take hold. The resulting irritation to the lining of the small and/or large intestine can cause many health problems including leaky gut syndrome, stomach-aches, irritable bowel syndrome, constipation, diarrhea, eczema, headache, emotional ups and downs, and even learning or behavioral difficulties. A bacterial infection can also trigger juvenile arthritis, ulcerative colitis, and Crohn's disease. (These conditions are addressed in later chapters of this book.)

Most doctors in our culture do not yet recognize dysbiosis, so they treat its symptoms with medication but may never deal with its underlying cause, and ultimately their patients with dysbiosis do not get well. Fortunately, because children are so resilient, it is often easy to rebalance a child's disrupted internal environment through dietary changes and by using probiotics and supportive nutrients, as you will learn in this chapter.

COMMON CAUSES OF DYSBIOSIS

Our ileocecal valve normally keeps waste matter in the colon from mixing with chyme that is still being digested and absorbed in the small intestine. If this valve is stuck either open or closed, dysbiotic problems can occur, which can then be alleviated by a chiropractic adjustment of the valve. But we generally bring dysbiosis upon ourselves—or our children—through ongoing stress, exposure to toxic metals and chemicals, overuse of medications, poor food choices, and other factors.

Antibiotics: Friend and Foe

The most common cause of dysbiosis in childhood is the use of antibiotic medication, which changes the balance of intestinal microbes. Most children recover fairly easily from a single round, but even those with strong constitutions have trouble rebalancing after repeated use of antibiotic drugs. Because antibiotics are not terribly specific about their targets, they simultaneously kill both harmful and helpful bacteria throughout the digestive system, vagina, urinary tract, and skin, leaving the territory open to subsequent invasion by other bacteria, parasites, viruses, and yeasts. The invaders can then produce a wide variety of toxic substances (including amines, ammonia, hydrogen sulfide, indoles, phenols, and secondary bile acids) that poison the cells around them and produce symptoms in the person they inhabit. These substances can damage the intestinal lining and thereby pass into the bloodstream, causing system-wide effects.

In the decades since Metchnikoff's work, scientists have endeavored to conquer infectious diseases with antibiotics and immunizations, but viruses and bacteria are extremely adaptable, and our eradication efforts have instead pushed some of them to evolve. It is estimated that 20 to 50 percent of all antibiotic prescriptions are written for people who actually have viral rather than bacterial infections—despite the fact that antibiotics have *no effect* against viruses! Bacteria "learn" from exposure to the indiscriminate use of antibiotics in both humans and animals. As they shuffle their components in rapid reproduction and mutation, super-strains of bacteria develop that no longer respond to any antibiotic treatment, and their resistance information is "communicated" to other types of bacteria.

In 1992, 13,300 hospital patients in North America died of bacterial infections that withstood every drug their doctors tried. Currently, 40,000 North Americans die each year from such infections. Antibiotic-resistant gonorrhea (*Neisseria gonorrhoeae*), leprosy (*Mycobacterium leprae*), staphylococcus, and streptococcus now exist. Many bacteria that cause dysentery, cholera, and other diseases of the digestive tract have also become resistant to certain antibiotic drugs. So when a doctor recommends an antibiotic for your child's ear infection or cold, think twice about the consequences to his/her internal ecology, and to the bigger picture as well!

Anti-Inflammatories Block Both Pain and Healing

Nonsteroidal anti-inflammatory drugs (NSAIDs) like aspirin, ibuprofen, and acetaminophen relieve fever and pain by interfering with prostaglandins, which are small hormonal messengers that circulate throughout the body. Some prostaglandins cause pain and inflammation, as when you twist an ankle or get a burn in the kitchen. Others cause healing and repair. Taking NSAIDs blocks them all; the symptoms are gone, but the healing process is compromised too. Short-term, occasional use of NSAIDs shouldn't cause any lasting problems for children or adults. Prolonged use, however, causes bleeding, damage, and inflammation in the mucous membranes of the intestines, which leads to a well-known dysbiotic side effect: increased intestinal permeability, or leaky gut syndrome.

"SAD" Nutrient Deficiencies

Poor food choices also contribute to dysbiosis. A diet high in fat, sugar, and processed foods—the Standard American Diet—may not provide enough nutrients to optimally nourish the body or repair and maintain the digestive organs. The nutrients most likely to be lacking are antioxidants (vitamins C and E, beta-carotene, coenzyme Q_{10}, glutathione, selenium, sulfur-containing amino acids, and zinc), B-complex vitamins, calcium, essential fatty acids, and magnesium.

CANDIDA: THE MASQUERADER

Candidiasis, a fungal infection, is the most prevalent and obvious form of dysbiosis in children. The yeast candida is found in nearly everyone, and in small amounts is compatible with good health. Its population is normally moderated by our friendly flora, immune defenses, and intestinal pH. But if the bacteria that help control candida are eliminated, the fungus can infect the nail-beds or eyes, the vagina (a yeast infection), or the mouth and throat (thrush). Candida can also colonize the digestive tract and thereby wreak havoc throughout the body.

Candida albicans is the usual offender, but other species of fungus may cause health problems as well. The powerful toxins produced by candida colonies are absorbed into the bloodstream and affect our immune system, hormone balance, and thought processes. Candidiasis has many faces and can produce many types of symptoms. The most common symptoms in children are:

- Abdominal bloating
- Anxiety
- Athlete's foot
- Attention deficit hyperactivity disorder (ADHD)
- Colic
- Constipation and/or diarrhea
- Depression
- Diaper rash, frequent
- Ear infections, recurring
- Environmental sensitivities
- Fatigue
- Feeling worse on damp or muggy days or in moldy places
- Food sensitivities
- Headaches, frequent
- Learning and behavioral problems
- Low blood sugar
- Mood swings
- Nail infections
- Sensitivities to perfume, cigarettes, or fabric odors
- Skin problems such as eczema or hives
- Thrush
- Vaginal or bladder infections, recurring

In children, candida infections are usually triggered by the use of antibiotics (which kill the helpful bacteria that normally keep candida in check) and overconsumption of sugar (which feeds the fungus). Candida quickly pushes into the intestinal lining, destroying cells in the layer of villi and microvilli. Greater numbers of candida produce greater amounts of toxins, which further irritate and break down the lining. This damage allows partially digested food to pass through as macromolecules that are the perfect size to trigger an antibody response. Your child's immune system then goes on alert for these specific foods, so the next time he/she eats them, antibodies will be waiting to sound the alarm for an immune reaction. The net result is increased sensitivity to foods and other substances in the environment.

American physicians recognize candida in many forms, but in general they have been unwilling to recognize systemic candidiasis. For those doctors who do, it is a common diagnosis. In his preface to *The Yeast Syndrome,* Abraham Hoffer, M.D., states that one-third of the world's population is affected by candidiasis. In my clinical experience, I have found candida infections to be an underlying cause of numerous, diverse symptoms and health issues.

Functional Laboratory Testing for Children with Dysbiosis

Screening questionnaires and diagnostic tests can be used to discover the underlying causes of your child's health issues. See Appendix A for details on testing. If your child scores high on the yeast questionnaire in this chapter (see the "Yeast Questionnaire for Children" on page 60), or if you suspect that a bacterial, fungal, or parasitic infection may be affecting his/her health, consider obtaining one or more of the following:

1. Small bowel bacterial overgrowth test

2. Lactose intolerance test

3. Comprehensive digestive and stool analysis with parasite screening

4. Candida antibody test (if you've had a stool analysis, this will have been done already)

Treating Candidiasis

Many options, starting with dietary modifications, exist for people who wish to rid themselves of candida. If your child scores high on the yeast questionnaire, have him/her follow the anti-candida diet and other therapeutic recommendations described below. Most people begin to feel dramatically better within two weeks of beginning an anti-candida treatment; if your child doesn't, then the problem probably isn't candidiasis, and you should consult a healthcare professional.

The standard anti-candida diet allows beef, chicken, fish, eggs, poultry, yogurt, vegetables, oils, nuts, and seeds. No fruit or dried fruit, flours, grains, mushrooms, sugar, vinegar, or yeasted items are allowed, as these foods would promote candida's growth and colonization. The idea behind this diet is to starve the fungus and help restore the normal digestive environment. Parents who suspect their child has candida are advised to limit the child's diet to the allowed foods for at least three weeks and then reintroduce foods one at a time to test for reactions. If a child is sensitive to a specific food, he/she should avoid it completely.

Alternatively, an alkalizing diet and monitoring your child's acid-alkaline balance through daily urinary pH testing (see Chapter 7) can be very useful tools in fighting candidiasis.

Candida often causes bowel problems—diarrhea, constipation, or both alternately—so it is essential to normalize bowel transit time by adding probiotics and a fiber supplement to your child's diet. Probiotic supplements also help keep candida in check (see Chapter 5). Several other natural substances are valuable candida-killing agents as well: garlic, oleic acid (from olive oil), oregano oil, thyme oil, the herb *pau d'arco,* olive leaf extract, biotin, and grapefruit-seed extract.

Yeast Questionnaire for Children

Record the score for each question in the space provided, and total the score at the end of the questionnaire.

1. During the two years before your child was born, were you bothered by recurrent vaginitis, menstrual irregularities, premenstrual tension, fatigue, headache, depression, digestive disorders, or "feeling bad all over"? Score 30 if yes.   _____

2. Was your child bothered by thrush? Score 10 if mild, 20 if severe or persistent.   _____

3. In infancy, was your child bothered by frequent diaper rashes? Score 10 if mild, 20 if severe or persistent.   _____

4. In infancy, was your child bothered by colic and irritability lasting over three months? Score 10 if mild, 20 if moderate or severe.   _____

5. Are his/her symptoms worse on damp days or in damp or moldy places? Score 20 if yes.   _____

6. Has your child been bothered by recurrent or persistent "athlete's foot" or chronic fungus infections of his/her skin or nails? Score 30 if yes.   _____

7. Has your child been bothered by recurrent hives, eczema, or other skin problems? Score 10 if yes.   _____

8. Has your child received:

   a. Four or more courses of antibiotic drugs during the past year? Or, continuous "prophylactic" courses of antibiotic drugs? Score 80 if yes.   _____

   b. Eight or more courses of broad-spectrum antibiotics (such as amoxicillin, Keflex, Septra, Bactrim, or Ceclora) during the past three years? Score 50 if yes.   _____

9. Has your child experienced recurrent ear problems? Score 10 if yes.   _____

10. Has your child had tubes inserted in his/her ears? Score 10 if yes.   _____

11. Has your child been labeled "hyperactive"? Score 10 if mild, 20 if moderate or severe.   _____

12. Is your child bothered by learning problems, even though his/her early developmental history was normal? Score 10 if yes.   _____

13. Does your child have a short attention-span? Score 10 if yes.   _____

14. Is your child persistently irritable, unhappy, and hard to please?
    Score 10 if yes. _____

15. Has your child been bothered by persistent or recurrent digestive
    problems such as constipation, diarrhea, bloating, or excessive
    gas? Score 10 if mild, 20 if moderate, 30 if severe. _____

16. Has he/she been bothered by persistent nasal congestion, cough,
    and/or wheezing? Score 10 if yes. _____

17. Is your child unusually tired or unhappy or depressed? Score 10
    if mild, 20 if severe. _____

18. Has your child been bothered by recurrent headaches, abdominal
    pain, or muscle aches? Score 10 if mild, 20 if severe. _____

19. Does your child crave sweets? Score 10 if yes. _____

20. Does exposure to perfume, insecticides, gas, or other chemicals
    provoke moderate to severe symptoms in your child? Score 30 if yes. _____

21. Does tobacco smoke really bother your child? Score 20 if yes. _____

22. Do you feel that your child isn't well, and yet diagnostic tests/
    studies haven't revealed the cause? Score 10 if yes. _____

TOTAL SCORE _____

Interpreting the Score
Scores of 60 or higher: yeasts possibly play a role in causing child's health problems.
Scores of 100 or higher: yeasts probably play a role in causing child's health problems.
Scores of 140 or higher: y
easts almost certainly play a role in causing child's health problems.

—adapted from *The Yeast Connection and Women's Health* by William G. Crook

These are often found as liquid tinctures that can be added to juice or water. They aren't manufactured specifically for children, so you need to adjust the dosage according to your child's size. Many of these anti-candida agents are available as combination products at health food stores or through healthcare professionals.

The protein fragments and endotoxins released from killed candida trigger an antibody response commonly known as a die-off reaction, which can initially worsen your child's symptoms. It is therefore important to begin administering anti-candida therapeutics gently, in small doses that are gradually increased. If symptoms are still initially aggravated, cut back the dosage of the supplements or other agents and gradually increase it again.

CHAPTER 7

Acid–Alkaline Balance: Optimizing Cellular Function

Metabolic acidosis underlies chronic disease and makes people more likely to be resistant to treatment and to feel helpless and hopeless.

—RUSSELL JAFFE, M.D., 1993

Having just read about dysbiosis and candidiasis in Chapter 6, you're probably wondering how you can protect your child's system from getting so out of balance, and wondering what you can do to correct and prevent these health problems for your whole family. The answer? Learn the information and use the simple tools in this chapter. It's easy for the body to be healthy when it is in acid-alkaline balance.

THE IMPORTANCE OF PH BALANCE IN HEALTH

Our acid-alkaline balance is regulated by the body's mineral management. Our bodies strive to maintain our blood pH between 7.3 and 7.5, which corresponds to a urinary pH of about 7.0. Our metabolism, enzymes, immune system, and repair mechanisms work most effectively within this narrow pH range. The body is very sensitive to changes in blood pH, so that always has to stay fairly constant, or else we are rushed to the emergency room. To balance blood pH, minerals are drawn from elsewhere in the body. Sodium and potassium are pulled into the bloodstream from the reservoirs of fluid outside of our cells (extracellular fluid); when these extracellular stores have been used up, the body then resorts to pulling calcium, magnesium, and other alkalizing minerals from the bones.

A urinary pH of 7.0 indicates that we have enough buffering (alkalizing) minerals to balance our acids. Alkaline-forming minerals include sodium, potassium, calcium, and magnesium. Acid-forming minerals include chlorine, sulfur, phosphorus, and iodine. Many children are deficient in potassium, calcium, and magnesium, although they do get plenty of sodium-chloride (salt). Optimal cellular health and resistance to bacterial infections are promoted by all of these minerals, but especially by abundant supplies of sodium and calcium.

Why Are We Acidic?

Most of us unknowingly have a slightly acidic body environment. An excess of carbon dioxide and carbonic acid is created and accumulated in our blood through:

- Eating an acid-forming diet
- Stress
- Toxins
- Immune system reactions
- Metabolic regulatory mechanisms that create acid by-products

It's essential that our foods contain buffering minerals to offset this naturally acidic internal state. Fruit, vegetables, seaweed, and some other foods help alkalize our systems—but we don't usually eat enough of these. Unfortunately, the standard American diet contributes to our overall acid load, as proteins, fats, sugars, grains (generally speaking), and refined foods are acid producing. Stress, alcohol, and cigarettes further compound the problem.

When our diet is high in protein and low in fruit and vegetables, as is often the case today, we have a greater need for buffering minerals. (Eating a high-protein diet temporarily causes an "alkaline tide," but the net result is not alkalizing.) When we are under stress, we have a greater need for buffering minerals. And

Soft Drinks Demineralize Bones and Teeth

One 12-ounce can of cola contains enough phosphoric acid to dramatically change our pH. The pH of the cola is between 2.8 and 3.2, but the kidneys cannot excrete urine that is more acidic than about 5.0; in order to dilute this can of cola to an appropriate urinary pH, you'd need to produce 33 liters of urine! So, the body turns to its stores of alkalizing minerals. If there aren't enough reserves of potassium and magnesium in the extracellular fluid, then calcium will be taken from bone. But the amount of minerals needed for this particular task is equivalent to the buffering capability of four Tums! Thus, a lifetime of consuming soft drinks contributes to bone loss and joint degeneration. Studies also show that soft drink consumption in children is directly linked to tooth decay.

So what's a parent to do? Instead of buying soda, give your children sparkling water with juice. It's healthful and alkalizing.

when we drink soft drinks, we *really* need more buffering minerals; see the inset "Soft Drinks Demineralize Bones and Teeth" on page 63 for an eye-opening example.

Acid Woes

Imagine how much harder it would be for us to function if the air were filled with sulfuric acid; the more caustic the environment, the more detrimental it would be to our health. Similarly, our cells react to an acidic internal environment by becoming sluggish and unable to function properly. A change of 0.1 in either direction outside of the optimal blood pH range of 7.3–7.5 can produce up to a tenfold reduction in enzyme activity. This happens for *each* tenth of a point, so the more out of line pH is, the less cellular activity occurs. Wastes build up, toxins aren't excreted, cellular messages aren't sent, and nutrients aren't properly utilized—it's kind of like a labor strike!

Acidity contributes to disease: constipation, diarrhea, kidney and liver problems, and the fatigue that accompanies most health problems. What's more, most of us are continually "borrowing" minerals from bone to stabilize our cellular and blood pH. If we don't replenish these minerals, the long-term effects are osteoporosis, osteoarthritis, and overall poor health. (See Figure 7.1 below.)

An acidic internal environment is also a microbe's playground, in which bacteria, fungi, and parasites flourish and replicate with abandon; but when this over-acidity is neutralized, these organisms cannot thrive. Many healthcare practitioners recommend killing parasitic, fungal, and bacterial infections with medications and herbs. Nutritionists often find, however, that simply rebalancing internal pH can achieve the same antimicrobial effect without using any drugs.

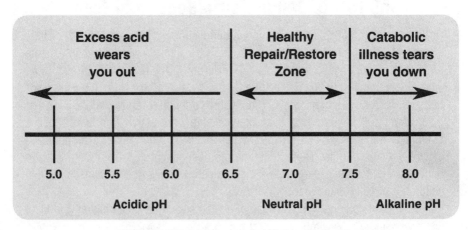

Figure 7.1. The Importance of pH Balance in Health

TENDING TO pH

Getting your child's pH properly balanced is an important accompaniment to other healthful dietary changes. It's easy and inexpensive, and you can do it at home—even as a fun "experiment" for the whole family's participation and benefit.

Reading the Morning pH Paper

Purchase a packet of pH test paper with a testing range of 5.5–8.0 (available at most health food stores; see also Resources). You or your child can then perform the test by simply dipping a 2 to 3-inch strip of pH paper into your child's first morning urine stream and "reading" it by matching the color of the test strip with the color chart on the back of the packet. Optimally, urinary pH will be between 6.5 and 7.5, which is fairly neutral. The pH of water, 7.0, is best. Any number below 7.0 indicates that your child's urine is on the acid side. The lower the number, the more acidic, and the pH scale is logarithmic: That is, 6.0 is ten times more acidic than 7.0, and 5.0 is 100 times more acidic than 7.0.

Rebalancing Your Child's pH

If your child's readings fall consistently below 6.5, begin to make dietary changes to bring his/her urinary pH back into the optimal range (6.5–7.5). Be sure to include lots of fresh fruits and vegetables in your child's meals and snacks. Use Table 7.1 on pages 66–67 to identify alkalizing foods; the further to the left on the chart, the more alkalizing the foods are (see Chapter 9 for more dietary details). Have your child take a mineral supplement daily and use a fully buffered vitamin C-mineral ascorbate to promote alkalinity.

In addition to nutrition, incorporate stress-reducing habits in your child's routine to normalize his/her pH: meditation, spending time outdoors, gardening, playing catch together, and taking gentle walks around the block or in the woods. At bath time, dissolve ½ cup each of baking soda and Epsom salts in your child's bathwater to alkalize, gently detoxify, and relax the body as they cleanse the skin.

What should you do if your child's urinary pH is *above* 7.5? An occasional reading of 7.5–8.0 is acceptable. Readings that are typically between 7.5 and 8.0, however, likely represent a "false alkalinity" that may indicate an active inflammation or other health issue; if this occurs, see your child's healthcare practitioner.

Foods Affect the Body's pH

Many people assume that if the pH of a specific food, say lemons, is acidic, the food will be acid-producing in the body—but this assumption is inaccurate. In

Table 7.1. Food & Chemical Effects on Acid/Alkaline Body Chemical Balance

Food Category	Most Alkaline	More Alkaline	Low Alkaline	Lowest Alkaline
Spice/Herb	Baking Soda*	Spices/Cinnamon Valerian Licorice Black Cohash*	Herbs* (most): Arnica, Bergamot, Echinacea, Chrysanthemum, Ephedra, Fevefew, Goldenseal, Lemongrass	White Willow Bark Slippery Elm Artemesia Annua
Preservative	Sea Salt			*Sulfite*
Beverage	Mineral Water	Kambucha*	Green or Mu Tea*	Ginger Tea
Sweetener		Molasses	Rice Syrup	Sucanat*
Vinegar		Soy Sauce	Apple Cider Vinegar	Umeboshi Vinegar*
Therapeutic	Umeboshi Plum		Sake	Algae, Blue-Green*
Processed Dairy				Ghee (Clarified Butter)*
Cow/Human				Human Breast Milk
Soy				
Goat/Sheep				
Egg			Quail Egg	Duck Egg
Meat				
Game				
Fish/Shell Fish				
Fowl				
Grain				Oat "Grain Coffee"
Cereal				Quinoa*
Grass				Wild Rice Japonica Rice
Nut		Poppy Seed	Primrose Oil	Avocado Oil
Seed/Sprout	Pumpkin Seed	Cashew	Sesame Seed	Seeds (most)
Oil	*Hydrogenated* Oil	Chestnut Pepper	Cod Liver Oil Almond Sprout*	Coconut Oil Olive Oil Linseed/Flax Oil
	Lentil	Kohlrabi	Potato/Bell Pepper	Brussels Sprout*
Bean	Brocoflower	Parsnip/Taro	Mushroom/Fungi	Beet
Vegetable	Seaweed*	Garlic	Cauliflower	Chive/Cilantro
	Nori/Kombu/Wakame/Hijiki	Asparagus	Cabbage	Celery/Scallion
Legume	Onion/Miso	Kale/Parsley	Rutabaga	Okra/Cucumber
Pulse	Daikon/Taro Root*	Endive/Arugula	Salsify/Ginseng*	Turnip Greens
Root	Sea Vegetables (other)*	Mustard Greens	Eggplant	Squash
	Burdock/Lotus Root*	Ginger Root	Pumpkin	Lettuce
	Sweet Potato/Yam	Broccoli	Collard Greens	Jicama
Citrus Fruit	Lime	Grapefruit	Lemon	Orange
	Nectarine	Cantaloupe	Pear	Apricot
	Persimmon	Honeydew	Avocado	Banana
	Raspberry	Citrus	Apple	Blueberry
Fruit	Watermelon	Olive	Blackberry	Pineapple Juice
	Tangerine	Dewberry*	Cherry	Raisin, Currant
	Pineapple	Loganberry	Peach	Grape
		Mango	Papaya	Strawberry

* Therapeutic, gourmet, or exotic items   *Italicized* items are NOT recommended.

Food Category	Lowest Acid	Low Acid	More Acid	Most Acid
Spice/Herb	Curry	Vanilla Stevia	Nutmeg	Pudding/Jam/Jelly
Preservative	MSG	*Benzoate*	*Aspartame*	*Table Salt (NaCl)*
Beverage	*Kona Coffee*	Alcohol Black Tea	Coffee	Beer, *"Soda"'* Yeast/Hops/Malt
Sweetener	Honey/Maple Syrup		*Saccharin*	Sugar/Cocoa
Vinegar	Rice Vinegar	Balsamic Vinegar		White/Acetic Vinegar
Therapeutic		*Antihistamines*	*Psychotropics*	*Antibiotics*
Processed Dairy	Cream/Butter	Cow Milk	Casein, Milk Protein, *Processed Cheese* Cottage Cheese	
Cow/Human	Yogurt	Aged Cheese	New Cheese	Ice Cream
Soy		Soy Cheese	Soy Milk	
Goat/Sheep	Goat/Sheep Cheese	Goat Milk		
Egg	Chicken Egg			
Meat	Gelatin/Organs	Lamb/Mutton	Pork/Veal	Beef
Game	Venison*	Boar/Elk/Game Meat	Bear	
Fish/Shell Fish	Fish	Shell Fish/Mollusks	Mussel/Squid*	Lobster
Fowl	Wild Duck	Goose/Turkey	Chicken	Pheasant*
	Triticale*	Buckwheat	Maize	Barley
Grain	Millet	Wheat	Barley Groat	*Processed Flour*
Cereal	Kasha	Spelt/Teff/Kamut*	Corn	
Grass	Amaranth*	Farina/Semolina	Rye	
	Brown Rice	White Rice	Oat Bran	
Nut	Pumpkin Seed Oil	Almond Oil	Pistachio Seed	*Cottonseed Oil/Meal**
Seed/Sprout	Grape Seed Oil	Sesame Oil	Chestnut Oil	Hazelnut
Oil	Sunflower Oil	Safflower Oil	*Lard*	Walnut
	Pine Nut	Tapioca	Pecan	Brazil Nut
	Canola Oil	Seitan or Tofu*	Palm Kernel Oil	*Fried Food*
	Spinach	Split Pea	Green Pea	Soybean
Bean	Fava Bean	Pinto Bean	Peanut	Carob
Vegetable	Kidney Bean	White Bean	Snow Pea	
	Black-eyed Pea	Navy/Red Bean		
Legume	String/Wax Bean	Aduki Bean	Legumes (other)	
Pulse	Zucchini	Lima or Mung Bean	Carrot	
Root	Chutney	Chard	Chick Pea/Garbanzo	
	Rhubarb			
Citrus Fruit	Coconut			
	Guava	Plum	Cranberry	
	Pickled Fruit*	Prune	Pomegranate	
	Dry Fruit	Tomato		
Fruit	Fig			
	Persimmon Juice			
	Cherimoya*			
	Date			

Prepared by Dr. Russell Jaffe, Fellow, Health Studies Collegium. Reprints available from ELISA/ACT Biotechnologies. 14 Pidgeon Hill, #300, Sterling, VA 20 165. Sources include USDA food data base (Rev 9 & 10), Food & Nutrition Encyclopedia; Nutrition Applied Personally by M.Walczak; Acid & Alkaline by H.Aihara. Food growth, transport, storage, processing, preparation, combination, & assimilation influence effect Intensity. Thanks to Hank Liers for his original work. (Rev 6/0 1] the 1920s and 1930s, scientists with the U.S. Department of Agriculture (USDA) began burning foods and measuring the pH of the ash residue. Later, realizing that this technique didn't yield sufficient information about what occurred inside the body, the USDA performed tests to see what would happen if someone ate only a specific food for fourteen days. (How would you like to eat only carrots for two weeks?)

Subsequently, Russell Jaffe, M.D., a former researcher for the National Institutes of Health, found a way to calculate the body's net response to a food by using a formula based on that food's mineral, sugar, fat, and amino acid composition. Dr. Jaffe's formula correlates with the results of the USDA's few mono-diet studies. It is the most accurate system I have seen for predicting the effect on pH of eating a particular food.

If your child is healthy and has a urinary pH of 6.5–7.5, have him/her eat 60 percent of his/her foods from the alkalizing side of Table 7.1 and 40 percent from the acid-producing side of the chart. If your child needs to rebuild health, has a chronic ailment, or has a urinary pH consistently lower than 6.5, have him/her eat 80 percent alkalizing foods and 20 percent acid-producing foods. Eating fruits and vegetables in abundance helps maintain a healthful acid-alkaline balance. And insist that your child avoid brown-colored soft drinks! Lemon or lime juice in water makes a refreshing and alkalizing drink, as does ginger tea with rice syrup and lemon. Fresh vegetable juices flood the body with alkalizing minerals.

Here are additional tips for healthful feeding and eating:

- Switch to quinoa, oats, and wild rice as your main grains.

- Use sucanat, molasses, and rice syrup as your main sweeteners.

- Eating daikon radish and steamed greens daily is strongly recommended.

- Lentils, miso soup, and yams are extremely alkalizing.

Apple-Cider Vinegar Is Actually Alkalizing!

Use apple-cider vinegar in salad dressings, mix it into sweet juices (like apple juice), and drizzle it over vegetables, chicken, or fish. It helps promote healthy digestion, increase blood oxygen levels, prevent intestinal putrefaction of food, regulate calcium metabolism, reduce frequent urination, and regulate menstrual cycles. Along with many essential enzymes and minerals, it also contains malic acid, which helps neutralize toxins. Always buy organic apple-cider vinegar; it's most beneficial raw, unfiltered, and unpasteurized.

PART TWO

Healing Your Child with Food

CHAPTER 8

We Are
What We Eat!

We are what we repeatedly do.
Excellence, then, is not an act, but a habit.

—ARISTOTLE

Most diets focus on fats, carbohydrates, protein, fiber, sugar, and sodium. Although these are important, it's time to begin thinking of food differently. Food is information for our bodies and brains. Each time we eat, we produce neurotransmitters that regulate mood and behavior. Our foods also contain chemical messengers that tell our cells to replicate, excrete wastes, accept nutrients, and more. When we eat healthful foods, these messages are healthful and appropriate. But when we eat foods laden with chemicals, pesticides, and synthetic ingredients (such as food colorings and restructured fats), we probably aren't giving our cells the right messages. Research in this area is young, but fascinating.

Why create biochemical roadblocks to health? Eat natural, real food nearly all of the time. It's what our children's bodies need to set them up for a life of good health. Once you make the decision to rely on natural foods, your family's bodies and minds will adjust so that natural foods taste more delicious than manufactured derivatives. Once their sugar and salt taste-buds calm down, fresh fruit will taste sweet again and they won't need that salt-shaker as much. Ninety percent of your food should be excellent for your body, and 10 percent excellent for your soul.

The general information about food and diet that you will find in this chapter and the next can be modified as necessary or desirable to fit your family's needs. For instance, someone with Crohn's disease will probably want to avoid grains and dairy products completely. Children who get recurrent ear infections, allergies, and colds often benefit from a dairy-free diet. If you have older children, you may have to change your family's food plan gradually. In our house, our "three out of four" rule means that if three people like something, it can be served, and the fourth person has to make do or substitute something else. But whatever your restrictions are, you should be able to identify and provide a variety of foods that you and your family love to eat.

DIET = A WAY OF LIVING

The word "diet" comes from Greek and means "a manner of living" or "way of life"; the Latin root means "a day's journey." Several years ago, at a seminar I organized to demonstrate how different diets work for different people, one presenter spoke on low-carbohydrate programs, another on macrobiotics, another on vegan (total vegetarian) eating, another on the blood-type diet, and another on Ayurvedic eating. What is common to all of these diets? They rely upon natural, home-cooked, genuine-food meals; they are devoid of artificial colors and flavors, trans fatty acids, and refined sugar; and they are loaded with phytonutrients (health-protective substances found in plant foods) as well as fiber and good-quality fats.

Those are a handful of the many healthful ways to eat. You need to find a digestion-enhancing, health-supporting diet that works for you and your family. The key is to make real changes—changes you can live with successfully on a long-term basis—in the way you approach food and your lifestyle in general.

Your Child's Food Diary

Write down everything your child eats and drinks in a Food Diary and keep track of how he/she feels. If he/she has diarrhea or pain after eating, or seems happy and full of energy, write it down. See whether you can correlate specific foods to the way your child feels and behaves. A sample Food Diary appears on the next page.

Keep the Food Diary for at least three days, then examine it and answer the following questions to gain insight on your child's eating habits—good and bad.

- Does your child eat breakfast every day? "Breaking the fast" provides much-needed fuel.

- Is your child's digestion better or worse at specific times of the day? Timing can be a clue to causes of indigestion (what, when, where, how fast, how much, and the like).

- How often does your child eat? Most children feel best with three meals daily plus at least one or two snacks. For small children, you can consider it a success if they've eaten at least two "real" meals plus snacks. (See rule #3 on page 75.)

- Do certain foods and/or beverages provoke symptoms? Eliminate suspicious foods for a week and note any differences in how your child feels. The usual suspects include sugar, dairy products, wheat, and artificial colorings.

Sample Food Diary		
DAY 1		
Time of day	What did my child eat/drink?	How did he/she feel and act?
DAY 2		
Time of day	What did my child eat/drink?	How did he/she feel and act?
DAY 3		
Time of day	What did my child eat/drink?	How did he/she feel and act?

- Are your child's mealtimes relaxed or rushed? It's important to schedule meals with enough time so your child doesn't feel rushed. (See rule #5 on page 75.)

- Does your child eat at least five servings of fruits and vegetables each day? A typical serving size is a piece of fruit, a half-cup of most vegetables, or a cup of lettuce; for small children, however, servings are much smaller. (See rule #8 on page 77.)

- What percentage of your child's foods and drinks are high-sugar, high-fat, low-fiber, or highly processed? Replace these with fresh, wholesome foods.

- Does your child consume enough high-fiber foods? Fiber is consumed in whole grains, fruits, vegetables, and legumes. (See rule #10 on page 79.)

- Does your child drink enough water? Teenagers should have at least 6–8 cups of water, herbal tea, or 100-percent fruit juice daily. Smaller children should have at least three 8-ounce cups daily. (See rule #11 on page 81.)

RULES TO EAT, COOK, AND LIVE BY

We eat several times each day, but few of us have studied nutrition. Most of our nutritional information has probably come from our mothers, a health class in high school, or the media—and if we believe media reports, we'll be more confused than ever. By learning more about food, you can make a healthful food plan that will allow you and your family to enjoy eating and to feel better. Read on for some basics on eating well and incorporating more natural foods into your family's diet.

1. The life in foods gives us life.

Fresh foods have the greatest enzyme activity. Enzymes are to the body what spark-plugs are to the engine of a car. If we eat foods with little enzyme activity, they don't "spark" our body to work correctly. Eating foods that have natural vibrancy gives vibrant energy to our own bodies. So if it won't rot or spoil, don't eat it!

2. Plan ahead and carry food with you.

Planning ahead and carrying your own food are great tools for healthful eating. Planning ahead of time helps you create balanced meals and saves shopping time. Carrying snacks for yourself and your kids helps keep your moods and blood sugar levels even. It also saves you money and time, and you can ensure that the snacks are healthful. (See also rule #3.)

An extension of this rule is to make bag lunches for your children. That way you have some control (or at least the illusion of control!) about what your children eat at school. Just put in some leftovers or a sandwich with a salad and/or a piece of fruit, add a beverage, and you've got lunch. Lidded containers and zip-lock bags simplify the process. To save time, I often begin making tomorrow's bag lunch while putting away leftovers from dinner.

3. Eat small, frequent meals.

Snacking is a great strategy for boosting and sustaining energy. Snacking keeps blood sugar levels even and facilitates digestion. People in Europe, South America, and Japan take time in the middle of the afternoon to have tea. Only American adults are "too busy" to stop for a snack. Our children have the sense to rush home from school and raid the refrigerator. Make snacking, especially in the mid-afternoon, a regular part of your family's lives. You'll all find that your energy levels will stay more constant throughout the day and your moods will be more consistently pleasurable!

Here are a few quick snack ideas:

- Half a sandwich saved from lunch plus a piece of fruit
- Bagel and cream cheese with tomatoes
- Rice cake with peanut butter and apples
- Baby carrots and salsa or ranch dressing.
- Cup of soup and several pretzels
- Handful of nuts and raisins
- Banana or apple with peanut or almond butter.

4. Eat when you are hungry and stop when you are satisfied.

From the time babies are born, they let us know when they're hungry; they drink as much formula or breast-milk as they want, and then they stop sucking when they're satisfied. As they begin eating solid foods and thereon through childhood, children know when they are hungry or full, but then we start encouraging them to just eat a little bit more or to taste something because "it's yummy," or we treat them with cookies or ice-cream to reward them for eating their meals. We've got to learn to just leave them alone. It's our job to put a variety of healthful foods on the table, and it's our children's job to decide how much to eat.

Emotional overeating is one of the reasons for obesity in this country. We regularly turn to food when we want love and support. Don't push your children to eat if they aren't hungry. Do try to train them to be hungry at meals by reminding them that food is on the way and making sure to be pretty regular about mealtimes. If dinner is going to be late, put out a plate of carrots and cucumbers, or some fresh peas in pods, for your kids to snack on while they wait.

5. Relax while eating.

Many times we don't even stop what we're doing long enough to sit down when we eat. Remember that eating is a time for rejuvenation of body and spirit and a time to connect with your children. (See also "The Family Meal" in Chapter 10.) Turn the television off and have a family dinner almost every night. One way I've found to encourage peace of mind during meals is to say grace. It puts me in touch with the bounty of our earth, directs my attention to the people I am with and to my gratitude for their presence in my life, helps me thank the people who produced the food, and reminds me that we all depend upon each other and community.

6. Eat local foods in season.

Local produce is the freshest and has the highest levels of nutrients. Ask your supermarket's produce manager to purchase locally grown products whenever possible. Incorporate farm-stands and farmer's markets into your food-shopping routine. This has the added benefits of supporting the local economy and helping the environment by cutting food-transportation costs and consumption of fossil fuels. Act locally, think globally!

Eating foods in season also reduces the amount of pesticides and herbicides we consume.

7. Choose organically grown foods whenever possible.

Organic foods generally have higher nutrient levels because farmers who use organic methods add more nutrients to the soil, knowing that healthy plants can better fend off pests and that the nutrients end up in the crops. A study from Doctor's Data, for example, showed that mineral levels in organically grown apples, pears, potatoes, wheat, and wheat-berries were twice as high as in their commercially grown counterparts. Italian researchers found that levels of polyphenols, which are active antioxidant nutrients, were about a third higher in organic peaches and about three times higher in organic pears. Another recent study found that wild berries had twice the antioxidant level as commercially grown berries. As consumer awareness of such benefits increases, organically grown foods are becoming more plentiful and are now stocked in many supermarkets.

Organic food production also protects soils and water, treats animals more humanely, and helps prevent antibiotic resistance. Conventionally (non-organically) raised animals are routinely given growth-promoting antibiotics and hormones, and animal production accounts for an estimated 70 percent, or 25 million pounds, of the antibiotics used annually in the United States. When we eat non-organic dairy, poultry, eggs, and meats, we ingest small amounts of these drugs. Antibiotics in animal feed also create the perfect environment for bacteria to develop resistance; as stronger and newer antibiotics are developed, some bacteria survive by adaptation, and these strains can then pass to humans in our food and through contact with farm animals. Conventional animal production thereby lessens the effectiveness of drugs that we so rely on.

Although nearly all countries in Europe have banned antibiotic growth-promoters, they are still widely used in the United States. Many beef, pork, and poultry producers (including Tyson Foods, Cargill, Perdue Farms, Foster Farms, and Smith Food) claim to use them only for treating sick animals, but the line between antibiotic growth-promotion and antibiotic treatment is unclear and largely determined by individual farmers. The elderly, infants, small children, and people with chronic illnesses are most at risk from resistant bacteria. For more information about this, read *The Killers Within: The Deadly Rise of Drug-Resistant Bacteria* by Michael Shnayerson & Mark J. Plotkin (Back Bay Books, 2003). For information on organic and antibiotic-free products in your area, visit the website www.keepantibioticsworking.org/ pages/consumers.cfm.

8. Eat as many fruits and vegetables as possible.

The available research on the positive benefits of eating fruits and vegetables is overwhelming. They are chockfull of vitamins, minerals, fiber, and phytochemicals (plant-produced substances) that protect us from heart disease, cancer, degenerative diseases, and other common health problems. High-fiber diets also protect our colons (see rule #10).

It's good for children and adults to eat at least five servings of fruits and vegetables a day, but more is even better: try to get your family up to nine, ten, or eleven servings. Children love to shell fresh peas, pick vegetables and berries right out of the garden, and snack on vegetables with healthy dips. Cut up vegetables for small hands to hold easily. If you present veggies and fruits as fun, they will be!

Benefits of Sea Vegetables

Although we have been exposed to them through macrobiotics and Japanese cuisine, seaweeds are highly nutritious foods that are often neglected in the American diet. Marine algae and sea vegetables contain small amounts of well-balanced protein and easily absorbed vitamins and minerals, and also offer significant amounts of the essential fats EPA and DHA. Many people find that eating sea vegetables gives them a tremendous energy boost, probably because the seaweed fills some minute but critical nutrient need.

9. Eat lean protein and high-EPA/DHA seafood.

Meat and poultry are delicious and can be nutritious, but are generally high in fat, contain unwanted dietary cholesterol, and contribute to the development of chronic degenerative disease. (It is recognized that vegetarians are statistically healthier than meat-eaters.) Focus on lean protein sources such as legumes, fish, eggs, and skinless poultry. Fish are nearly ideal, as they contain easily digestible protein, many trace nutrients, and not much cholesterol or saturated fat.

Coldwater fish are also an excellent source of the omega-3 fatty acids that are essential to our good health and promote neurological development in babies and children—hence the old saying, "Fish is brain food." The fatty acids eicosapentaenoic acid (EPA) and docosahexaenoic acid (DHA), found in all of our cells, are especially critical for the eyes, brain, nervous system, heart, and glands. Although many of us can manufacture DHA in our bodies from other fats, others lack the enzymes and nutrients necessary for this conversion and must obtain DHA through diet. The fish richest in EPA and DHA are salmon, halibut, tuna, mackerel, trout, sardines, eel, and herring. Low-fat fish or fish from tropical waters are still healthful to eat but do not contain significant levels of EPA and DHA.

Studies show that people who eat coldwater fish twice a week have a reduced risk of heart disease, cancer, and stroke. Other studies have found fish oils to be protective against, or therapeutic for, allergy, Alzheimer's disease, angina, asthma, attention deficit disorder, cancer, depression, eczema, high blood pressure, high serum cholesterol, hyperactivity, inflammatory disorders, kidney disease, lupus, migraine, multiple sclerosis, psoriasis, rheumatoid arthritis, and schizophrenia. Although supplementation with fish-oil capsules is beneficial, the best way to get

The Environmental Impact of Eating Meat

Environmentally speaking, animals raised for meat are a disaster. Most water pollution is runoff from animal farming. The antibiotics given to farmed animals go into our rivers, streams, fields, crops, and bodies. The hormones they are fed affect us after we eat their meat. It takes 16 pounds of grain to produce 1 pound of beef. If our nation consumed just 10 percent less meat, the resulting additional stores of grain could feed 60 million people each year. Countries that switch from a grain-based to a meat-based economy become poorer, have more hunger and starvation, and strip their land of its natural resources.

these oils is to eat the fish itself, but not more than two to three times a week due to the mercury content of many fish.

Eggs got a bad rap when they were linked to high cholesterol levels, but many researchers now believe that eating eggs has little or no effect on normal serum cholesterol. Recent studies show no significant change in the cholesterol of healthy people after six weeks of consuming two hard-boiled eggs daily, and other studies show that eating eggs can actually raise levels of "good" cholesterol (high-density lipoprotein, or HDL; "bad" cholesterol is low-density lipoprotein, or LDL). Current thinking is that if your cholesterol level is normal, eating egg yolks that have not been oxidized (that is, eating hard-boiled, soft-boiled, or poached eggs) is probably more healthful than harmful. Eggs also contain high amounts of phospholipids that are integral to our cell membranes and are a precursor to the important neurotransmitter acetylcholine.

Other recommended protein sources include beans, nuts, and seeds. Use a handful of nuts and seeds for a snack, or sprinkle them as a garnish on salads or vegetables. They add a lot of flavor and nutrients, but too much of this good thing can put on unwanted pounds. A cup of nuts contains 800–1,200 calories, mostly from fat. (Chestnuts, which are delicious steamed or roasted, are an exception to this rule.)

10. Eat more high-fiber foods.

Researcher Dennis Burkitt, M.D., noticed in the 1970s that rural Africans eating a traditional diet had almost no colon cancer, constipation, diabetes, diverticular disease, heart disease, or irritable bowel syndrome, whereas Africans consuming a Western diet had a heightened incidence of these problems. In a hospital in India, he found that the incidence of appendicitis was only 2 percent of that in a similar American hospital and that there was virtually no hiatal hernia, which affects nearly 30 percent of Americans over fifty years old. After examining many factors, Dr. Burkitt concluded that the large amount of fiber in traditional diets was crucial for health maintenance.

We have since learned much more about fiber and its contributions to health:

• Diets high in soluble fiber help with Crohn's disease, hiatal hernia, irritable bowel syndrome, and peptic ulcer.

• High-fiber diets reduce the risk of heart disease, high blood pressure, and certain types of cancer including colon cancer.

• Fiber has been shown to normalize serum cholesterol levels.

• High-fiber diets reduce the incidence of colon polyps and bowel disease.

• Dietary fiber helps prevent obesity by slowing digestion and the release of insulin and stored glucose into the bloodstream.

• Improving bowel function can help prevent diverticulosis, appendicitis, hemorrhoids, and varicose veins.

We also know that low-fiber diets lead to the digestive disorders suffered by one out of four Americans. We eat an average of 14–15 grams (g) of fiber per day, but adults should actually eat 25–30 g of fiber daily (the same amount that Americans ate in 1850). Children older than two years should consume at least an amount in grams equal to their age plus five, daily: so a four-year-old ought to get at least 9 g of fiber per day, and a twelve-year-old at least 17 g. To estimate the grams of fiber in foods, see Table 8.1 below.

The richest food sources of fiber are also the four food groups that make up the bulk of a healthful eating plan: whole grains (such as brown rice, wheat, millet, buckwheat, rye, barley, spelt, and oats), legumes (all beans except string

Table 8.1. Amount of Fiber in Selected Foods			
Fruits (raw)	Fiber	Legumes/Starchy Vegetables (cooked)	Fiber
Apple with skin	1 medium = 4 g	Baked beans, canned	$1/2$ cup = 6.5 g
Peach	1 medium = 2 g	Kidney beans, fresh	$1/2$ cup = 8 g
Pear	1 medium = 4 g	Lima beans, fresh	$1/2$ cup = 6.5 g
Tangerine	1 medium = 2 g	Potato, fresh	1 = 3 g
Vegetables (fresh)	Fiber	Grains	Fiber
Asparagus, cooked	4 spears = 1 g	Bread, whole wheat	1 slice = 2 g
Broccoli, cooked	$1/2$ cup = 2.5 g	Brown rice, cooked	1 cup = 2.5 g
Brussels sprouts, cooked	$1/2$ cup = 2 g	Cereal, bran flake	$3/4$ cup = 5 g
Cabbage, cooked	$1/2$ cup = 1.5 g	Oatmeal, cooked	$3/4$ cup = 3 g
Carrot, cooked	$1/2$ cup = 2.5 g	White rice, cooked	1 cup = 1 g
Cauliflower, cooked	$1/2$ cup = 1.5 g		
Romaine lettuce, raw	1 cup = 1 g		
Spinach, cooked	$1/2$ cup = 2 g		
Summer squash, cooked	1 cup = 3 g		
Tomato, raw	1 = 1 g		
Winter squash, cooked	1 cup = 6 g		

beans), vegetables, and fruits. Soluble and insoluble fibers, which work differently inside the body, are mixed in foods, so if you eat a wide variety of high-fiber foods you will get both types of fiber.

A high-fiber cereal for breakfast is an excellent way to increase your child's fiber intake. Unfortunately, the bulk of breakfast cereals and other baked goods contain too much sugar, hydrogenated and/or cottonseed oil, and other unhealthful ingredients. With careful screening, however, you can find nutritious cereals and other grain products (see Chapter 9).

11. Drink lots of clean water.

Our bodies are 70 percent water. If we don't adequately hydrate our cells, they cannot function properly. Moreover, the water we drink and consume in food is an essential carrier, bringing in nutrients and taking away wastes. In *Your Body's Many Cries for Water,* F. Batmanghelidj, M.D., describes the numerous, even fantastic roles that water plays in the body. Good hydration can help prevent many health problems from gout to asthma; for example, Dr. Batmanghelidj believes water is the best cure for ulcers. Drinking plenty of clean, pure water every day is one of the most promising routes to digestive wellness.

Unfortunately, any chemical we use will show up in our water supply, as groundwater is easily contaminated by runoff. The U.S. Environmental Protection Agency estimates that 1.5 *trillion* gallons of pollutants leak into the ground each year, with the highest incidence of contamination by lead, radon, and nitrates (from fertilizers). Over 700 chemicals have been found in tap water, but testing is commonly done for fewer than 200 of these, and the significance of chemicals in such low concentrations as parts per trillion is often unknown.

Many cities fail to provide good-quality water, and there is much controversy today about chlorination. The level of chlorine needed to kill water-borne bacteria is rising because of increasing bacterial resistance, but chlorine is strongly associated with elevated cancer risks. Inexpensive charcoal filters can remove chlorine and many pollutants from tap water. A pitcher with a simple carbon filter such as Britta or Pur can help purify your drinking water at little cost.

In Europe, bottled water is preferred for its high mineral content. Bottled water isn't always better than tap water, however, especially if it's just tap water that's been filtered. Water from plastic containers may also contain small amounts of plastics that are known to have hormone-disrupting effects. If you regularly buy bottled water, ask the manufacturer for information on water source, type of plastics used, mineral content per 8 ounces of water, and levels of toxic substances. If you rely on local tap water, find out where it originally comes from, how it's processed, and what's been added to it, and ask your water department for an analysis. If you have a well, get a water sample tested for bacterial content and pollutants. *Caution:* Distillation removes all minerals from water, so the regular consumption of distilled water leads to a leaching of minerals from the body. Although distilled water is recommended by many health experts and may be a beneficial part of a detoxification program, I cannot recommend its regular use.

12. Respect your own biochemical uniqueness.

The foods that are best for any person are those that agree with his/her body and unique biochemistry. Many people with digestive problems benefit from avoiding all grains and dairy. About half of the people in my clinical nutrition practice benefit most from a high-complex-carbohydrate, high-fiber, natural-foods diet, and the other half from a low-carbohydrate, relatively high-protein diet high in fruits and vegetables.

If your child has a problem eating wheat, dairy, or any other food or food type, it's best for him/her to avoid it. Most people will support a friend's or family member's unique dietary needs. This is important if your child is going to a "play-date" or a birthday party. With advance notice, your child may be able to eat nearly everything that will be served. If not, give your child a snack beforehand or send food along with him/her. Perhaps you can bring a suitable dish. One of the mothers I work with prepares a muffin-sized, wheatless replica of a birthday cake when her son is invited to a birthday party, so he has something special to eat when the other kids do. Remember that restaurants are there to cater to you, so tell the server if you need a menu item prepared a special way. Restaurants are becoming more used to accommodating people with special dietary needs.

You will probably need to experiment with your own diet and your family's diet to find out what works best for all of you specifically and over the long term. Whether it's the Zone, the blood-type diet, macrobiotics, a vegan diet, Ayurvedic eating, natural hygiene/food-combining, or some other well-balanced program, a proper diet ought to make us feel energetic and keep our immune system strong. Our bodies run best on real foods; a natural-foods diet is the ultimate direction in eating for all of us, no matter exactly how we shape it.

CHAPTER 9

Making the Change

They always say time changes things,
but you actually have to change them yourself.

—ANDY WARHOL

The temptation to use packaged and processed foods is high because they are abundant and heavily marketed. From preschool, children are bombarded with marketing on television, in movie advertising, at fast food restaurants, and in grocery stores. Fruit roll-ups come in Spider-Man, Winnie the Pooh, Cat in the Hat, Sports Illustrated Kids, Lion King, Care Bears, Loony Tunes, Clifford the Big Red Dog, and so on. Today's marketplace is buzzing with low-carbohydrate "foods"; a few years ago, ads were all about low-fat "foods" like Snackwells that are loaded with sugar. The pendulum swings back and forth. Our children are cherished gifts and we want to feed them properly, but it's very confusing! In this chapter, you'll learn how to stick to real foods.

FOOD LABELS: SMOKE AND MIRRORS

Eating is our most intimate contact with our environment. Each day we eat several pounds of food, and our bodies needs to decide if that food is friend or foe. Nutrients signal our cells to grow, develop, and repair themselves, and tell old cells when they need to die. But our modern food supply also contains ingredients and contaminants that contribute to poor health: trans fats, coal tar, dyes, artificial flavors and colors, preservatives, pesticides, herbicides, and other stray toxins like mercury and aluminum. Food labels can be "smoke and mirrors," so you must read them very carefully in order to better understand what's really in your family's food. If you don't, you are sure to eat ingredients that you probably don't want. Stick with products that contain ingredients similar to what they would be if you made the food from scratch—for example, you probably wouldn't put shortening or preservatives in your own home-made soup!

Nutrition Facts Panel

Check out the Nutrition Facts panel on packaged foods. It's one of the only places on the label that is guaranteed by law to be true. The rules for the rest of the package are pretty loose, and labels can be quite deceptive: "natural" is meaningless, "no sugar" nearly always denotes Splenda or another artificial sweetener, and "whole grain" or "honey" may signify only tiny bits of those ingredients.

The top of the Nutrition Facts panel lists the amounts of major nutrient groups such as fat, carbohydrates, sugar, protein, fiber, and a few vitamins and minerals. Look first at sodium content; daily sodium intake should not exceed 1,500 milligrams for your child or yourself. The National Academy of Sciences recommends 325–975 milligrams (mg) of sodium daily for children aged one to three years old. Look next at fiber content; daily fiber intake ought to be 25–40 grams (g) for adults and 15–20 g for children. As for sugar content, understand that 4 g of sugar is 1 teaspoon. Some sugars may occur naturally as in milk, fruit, or fruit juice, but most sugars are added. Look also at the amount of trans fats; if this number is more than *zero,* don't buy the product! (See page 85 for more about trans fats.) Aso, put it back on the shelf if it contains hormone-disrupting cottonseed oil.

Ingredients List Subtleties

Below the Nutrients Facts panel is a list of all ingredients ordered by weight from most to least. This list must also be accurate by law. Look for hydrogenated, partially hydrogenated, or cottonseed oil; these ingredients are detrimental to your family's health, so if such oils are present, don't buy the product! Look for sugar, which also goes by names including corn syrup, dextrose, fructose, and many others. Manufacturers often use several types of sugars in a product in order to make sugar appear less abundant on the label. Look also for preservatives and additives. A basic rule: If it doesn't look like a list of ingredients for something you'd make from scratch, leave it on the shelf.

Notice the use of parentheses in that cereal label. Sugar, the third ingredient, is also the first ingredient in the sub-list for "oat clusters"; within the oat clusters are "toasted oats," and sugar is the second-highest ingredient in that sub-list, followed by corn syrup, plus honey and molasses; and if you keep reading, you'll find more sugar, corn syrup, high-fructose corn syrup, polydextrose, and honey.

Other ingredients issues include:

- Corn and soy—Nearly all corn and soy products are now genetically modified (see Chapter 2). There is no data yet on whether these genetically modified foods are harmful or benign in the long term. Avoid all products that contain

corn, corn syrup, modified corn syrup, corn starch, soy, soybean oil, other soy derivatives, and tofu *unless they are labeled organic.*

- Juice—Only a product that is 100-percent juice can be called "juice." Any less juice than 100 percent must be specified on the label, and the product will be called "drink," "nectar," "punch," "blend," or something other than juice. Many "juice drinks" contain only 10 percent actual juice; the rest is corn syrup or other sugars and flavorings, colorings, and preservatives. If you look carefully at the container, you'll see information that tells you the actual percentage of juice that it contains. It will say: "Contains X% juice." If it's not 100 percent, put it back on the shelf.

- Low-carb products and artificial sweeteners—These days when you look in the store, you can find many labels that say "low carb" and "no sugar added." You will probably think that means they are naturally sweetened or contain no sweeteners at all. Only yesterday my husband came home with a "no sugar added" product. The ingredient list included aspartame. My husband was shocked, as many people are. Artificial sweeteners such as aspartame (Nutrasweet), sucralose (Splenda), and saccharine (Sweet'N Low) have not been tested on children and are not intended for children's use on a regular basis. Artificial sweeteners are added to microwave popcorn, jams, salad dressings, frozen desserts, ice cream, and many other foods that you would never suspect. This is another reason to be watchful and read all labels carefully!

- Percentage of fat—Some foods such as dairy products and cold-cuts present themselves as lean by announcing "97-percent fat free" or "4-percent milk" on the front label, so the consumer thinks that 3 or 4 percent of the product's total calories are from fat—but the label is actually presenting the volume of the product, not the calorie content; for instance, 2-percent milk is indeed mostly water, but 28 percent of its calories come from fat. In whole milk, which contains 4 percent milk fat, the total amount of calories from fat is 56 percent. So don't be fooled. If something sounds too good to be true, look at the nutrition facts; it will tell you specifically the percentage of calories that come from fat.

Toss the "Bad" Fats and the Low-Nutrient Foods

Some "bad" fats, known scientifically as trans fats, are listed on ingredients labels as hydrogenated or partially hydrogenated vegetable oil or vegetable shortening. Hydrogenated oils are cheap, have a long shelf-life, and give a buttery texture to foods, but are extremely unhealthful. Trans fats increase risk of inflammatory diseases like arthritis, cancer, diabetes, eczema, and irritable bowel syndrome, and recent research indicates that these fats play at least as large a role as saturated fats in heart disease. Trans fats also block nerve transmission and normal biochemical reactions, inhibit the function of enzymes involved in synthesizing cholesterol and needed fatty acids, and interfere with liver detoxification pathways.

Our body tissues incorporate the types of fats that we eat—and the average American consumes 6 to 8 percent of his/her total daily calories in trans fats! The U.S. Food and Drug Administration (FDA) has declared that these fats are unhealthful, and new labeling laws require that all trans fats be listed on food labels by January 1, 2006. Fortunately, most food manufacturers are responding by removing these fats from their products.

Removing trans fats from your family's diet is the most important dietary change you can make.

Begin to put your new knowledge of nutrition and food labels to work and "make the change." Start by raiding your cabinets, refrigerator, and freezer and getting rid of any packaged foods that contain trans fats. You'll find these fats in margarine, cookies, crackers, cereals, frozen items, breads, snack foods, salad dressings, mayonnaise, and so on. Because they are used so widely, your cupboards may end up looking like Old Mother Hubbard's once you've thrown them all out.

Next, turn your attention to any foods that contain cottonseed oil. You'll find this inexpensive oil in crackers, cookies, chips, frozen items, and other processed foods. Cottonseed extracts, however, have been known to cause hormone disruption. A chemical in cottonseed called gossypol has been researched extensively as a male contraceptive because it destroys sperm. Cows fed cottonseed meal have decreased fertility and more miscarriages. Given those facts, do you really want your children to be eating any cottonseed?

While you're purging your pantry, toss out the following items: high-sugar foods, highly processed foods including white-flour products and enriched foods, foods that contain a lot of colorings and other additives, and foods with a shelf-life that extends beyond a year. If you feel guilty about throwing these foods away, donate them to a food pantry. If you feel angry, write to the manufacturers and tell them to improve the quality of their products.

A HEALTHFUL GROCERY LIST

Now you're ready to go shopping! Reading labels and being choosy about your groceries will take longer the first few times you shop, but soon you'll be zipping through the store with your new food-recognition skills. If you're careful to bring home foods that provide excellent nourishment, then the treats your family eats at parties and restaurants will be occasional indulgences that you don't have to feel bad about. The idea isn't to be perfect, but rather to make progress and build good health habits that will last a lifetime.

In your local market and health food store are great treasures waiting to be uncovered that will add flavor, variety, and fun to your food. The following shopping list includes some brand names that I happen to know, but hundreds of other brands are equally good. If you've never been to a health food store, the salespeople will be happy to show you around and steer you toward products that meet your specific needs. It's a bit more expensive to eat healthfully, but you and your children are worth it! And we can spend money on excellent food, or we can spend it on medication and medical bills... Because natural and organic foods are often less available and sometimes more expensive, many people form informal food co-ops so they can buy natural foods in large quantities from wholesale distributors. Buying foods in bulk saves time and money, and most stores are willing to give a discount on cases.

Fruits and Vegetables

In terms of mere quantity, fruits and vegetables ought to constitute about half of our daily food intake. Fresh (and local, if possible) is always best. In a culture that imports and ships fresh foods so widely, it's easy to obtain fresh produce. It's the life in foods that gives us life! Processing by freezing or canning destroys many of the enzymes and bacteria that make food "alive." Dried fruits are a good source of nutrients, but it's important to remember that one prune equals one un-dried plum. You might eat three or four fresh plums, but it's easy to eat twenty prunes at a time; that's a concentrated batch of antioxidants, which is terrific, but also of sugar, which can cause people with digestive issues a great deal of gas and bloating.

Legumes

Beans and lentils are a hidden food treasure. Laden with protective antioxidants, protein, and fiber, they are also quite inexpensive. Beans are one food that is often reasonable to purchase in cans because the processing isn't that different from what you'd have to do at home with dried beans. Dried beans require twelve hours of soaking followed by several hours of cooking. If I'm making chili, I'll use dry beans, but for tossing into a salad, making hummus, or eating with rice, it's easier to use a can or two.

When purchasing soy products, choose only those that were organically grown. Eighty percent of the non-organically grown soy in the United States is primarily genetically modified.

- Beans (black, fava, garbanzo, great northern, kidney, lima, navy, pinto, red, white)
- Lentils (green, orange, yellow)

Seasonal Foods

This list of seasonal foods will vary a bit from region to region, but it will give you a general idea of what you can expect to find in your markets.

Apples	Late summer through fall		Pears	Fall
			Peas	Late fall
Asparagus	Spring		Peppers	Summer
Beans	Summer through early fall		Plums	Summer
			Potato	Summer to fall
Blackberries	Late Summer through fall		Pumpkin	Fall
			Raspberries	Summer
Blueberries	Mid-summer		Rhubarb	Spring
Broccoli	Fall		Spinach	Spring to early summer
Cabbage	Fall			
Carrots	Summer through fall		Strawberries	Winter to early summer
Cauliflower	Fall			
Cherries	Summer		Squash, summer	Summer
Corn	Summer		Squash, winter	Fall
Kale	Fall to early winter		Swiss chard	Spring through summer
Lettuce	Spring through early fall			
			Tomatoes	Summer till frost

- Soybeans (*edamame, miso,* soy flour, soy grits, *tempeh,* tofu)
- Split peas (green, yellow)

Whole Grains and Grain Products

Try to use only organically grown grain products; even more important is to use whole grains. Basmati rice, for example, is a whole grain that your whole family will enjoy (it's white naturally, not as a result of stripping). Experiment with whole-oat groats, steel-cut oats, quinoa, millet, and amaranth, which can all be used like rice.

In the following list, an asterisk (*) indicates a gluten-containing grain (many people are sensitive or allergic to gluten). Many people with digestive issues (celiac disease, Crohn's disease, irritable bowel syndrome, ulcerative colitis, and the like) find grains difficult to tolerate.

- Corn (corn bran, corn flour, corn meal, polenta, popcorn)

- Oats* (oat bran, oatmeal, whole oats, and such)

- Rice (basmati, brown, wild, black, red)

- Wheat* (bulgur, couscous, cracked wheat, wheat-berries, wheat bran, whole-wheat flour)

- Other grains (amaranth, barley*, buckwheat, kamut*, millet, quinoa, rye*, spelt*)

Whole-grain products can be found in natural food stores as well as some grocery stores and some bakeries. Look for the terms "whole-wheat" or "stone-ground wheat" on the label; if it says "wheat flour" or "enriched flour," it's just white flour (see Table 9.1 on page 91). Dense, heavy breads usually contain the most nutrients and fiber. Many stores carry gluten-free breads and pastas made with quinoa, rice, millet, and soy flours, which are terrific for people with gluten sensitivity.

- Bread

- Crackers (Akmak, Barbara's pretzels and breadsticks, Finn Crisp, Hain, Health Valley, rice cakes, Ry-Krisp, Wasa rye, whole-wheat matzoh)

- English muffins and other muffins

- Pancakes and waffles

- Pasta (cellophane noodles, corn, Jerusalem artichoke, quinoa, rice, semolina, soba, udon, whole-wheat)

- Pita bread

- Tortillas (corn or whole-wheat)

Read cereal labels carefully, checking for the amounts of sugar and fiber. Healthful cereals are those made from the whole grain, so look for brown rice instead of white and for whole corn instead of de-germed. Some cereals have organically grown ingredients like oatmeal and bulgur, and there are many delicious blends like seven-grain cereal and granola. Is anyone in your family sensitive to gluten? You can find non-gluten breakfast cereals in natural food stores or progressive grocery stores.

- Cereal (All-Bran, Barbara's, Erewhon, Health Valley, Kashi, Nature's Path, New Morning, Perky's, Shredded Wheat with bran, Uncle Sam's)

- Oatmeal (McCann's)

Dairy Products

As a rule, stick with low-fat dairy products unless you are buying organic dairy products. Because of the antibiotic and hormonal growth-promoters used in conventionally raised dairy cows, organic dairy products are preferable. Cheese is best used as a condiment rather than as a main food or snack.

- Butter and ghee (clarified butter often used in Indian foods)
- Cheese (cow's milk feta, farmer's cheese, goat's milk cheese, hoop cheese, Mexican cheese, parmesan, ricotta, sheep's milk feta, and yogurt cheese are all lower-fat than most other cheeses)
- Cottage cheese
- Kefir
- Milk (buttermilk, goat's milk, skim milk)
- Sour cream
- Yogurt

Eggs

It's best to buy organic eggs at your local grocery store, farmer's market, or farm-stand. If you believe that the quality of a seed determines the health and vibrancy of the plant it produces, then consider this: What is the quality of eggs produced by commercially raised chickens living in unnatural settings and pumped with hormones and antibiotics?

- Eggs (chicken, duck, free-range, organic)

Meat and Poultry

If you choose to eat meat, be sure to select lean cuts, and if you choose to eat poultry, remove any skin (the skin contains most of the fat and half of the calories, so by removing it you can eat twice as much poultry and stay within the same calorie count). Pork is marketed as "the other white meat," but the only truly low-fat cut of pork is the tenderloin. To avoid consuming antibiotic and hormonal growth-promoters, look for organically raised meat and poultry.

- Beef (lean cuts, lean hamburger)
- Buffalo
- Chicken
- Leg of lamb

Table 9.1. Whole Grains versus Enriched Refined Grains						
	Wheat Flour per 1 cup			Rice per 1 cup		
Nutrient	Whole	Enriched Refined	% Loss or Gain	Whole	Enriched Refined	% Loss or Gain
Protein	16.0 g	11.6 g	–27%	14.8 g	13.1 g	–11.4%
Fiber	2.8 g	0.3 g	–89%	1.6 g	0.4 g	–75%
Vitamin B$_1$	0.66 mg	0.48 mg	–27%	0.68 mg	0.86 mg	+21%
Vitamin B$_2$	0.14 mg	0.28 mg	+100%	0.08 mg	0.06 mg	–25%
Vitamin B$_6$	0.41 mg	0.066 mg	–84%	1.0 mg	0.3 mg	–70%
Biotin	6.0 mcg	1.1 mcg	–82%	18.0 mcg	5.86 mcg	–67%
Niacin	5.2 mg	3.9 mg	–25%	9.2 mg	6.8 mg	–26%
Vitamin B$_5$	1.32 mg	0.51 mg	–62%	2.1 mg	1.26 mg	–40%
Folic acid	65.0 mcg	24.0 mcg	–63%	32.0 mcg	20.0 mcg	–37%
Vitamin E	3.12 IU	1.87 IU	–40%	3.0 IU	0.7 IU	–77%
Calcium	49.0 mg	18.0 mg	–63%	64.0 mg	47.0 mg	–27%
Copper	0.6 mg	0.21 mg	–65%	0.4 mg	0.2 mg	–50%
Iron	4.0 mg	3.2 mg	–20%	3.2 mg	5.7 mg	+56%
Magnesium	136.0 mg	28.0 mg	–79%	172.0 mg	13.0 mg	–92%
Manganese	—	—	—	3.2 mg	2.1 mg	–34%
Phosphorus	446.0 mg	96.0 mg	–78%	432.0 mg	183.0 mg	–58%
Vitamin K	444.0 IU	105.0 IU	–76%	420.0 IU	179.0 IU	–57%
Selenium	77.4 mcg	21.7 mcg	–72%	77.2 mcg	65.1 mcg	–13%
Sodium	4.0 mg	2.0 mg	–50%	16.0 mg	10.0 mg	–37%
Zinc	2.88 mg	0.77 mg	–73%	3.6 mg	2.5 mg	–28%
Fat	2.4 g	1.1 g	–54%	3.6 g	1.5 g	–58%

(g = grams, mg = milligrams, mcg = micrograms, IU = international units)

Note: Where nutrients have increased, it's because they were added to the wheat or rice.

—Data from *Agricultural Handbook,* 1–23, U.S. Dept. of Agriculture.

- Pork tenderloin
- Turkey (light meat)
- Venison

Fish and Seafood

All fish and shellfish are good low-fat protein choices. When possible, choose the fish highest in omega-3 fatty acids (see Chapter 8). It's also important to know where your seafood comes from. Farm-raised fish contain lower levels of omega-3 fatty acids because those beneficial fats tend to go rancid and are not typically included in their feed. However, they do have lower levels of mercury in them. Do not eat seafood from polluted or questionable waters—which includes most freshwater lakes, streams, and rivers. Even ocean fish are contaminated with mercury. Fish and shellfish found close to shore, in rivers, or in lakes are virtually all tainted with mercury and other environmental toxins (see Chapter 2). Water-filtering mollusks like oysters, clams, mussels, and scallops can concentrate mercury and pesticides up to 70,000 times their concentration in seawater. The EPA and FDA recommend eating only one serving of albacore tuna per week, and recommend against eating high-mercury fish: bluefish, king mackerel, shark, swordfish, and tilefish.

- Low-mercury seafood (anchovies, catfish, light tuna, pollock, salmon, sardines, shrimp)
- Other seafood (Atlantic sturgeon, bluefin tuna, eel, herring, farm-raised trout, non-king mackerel, sablefish)
- Bluefish (only sparingly)
- Seaweed and other sea vegetables

Beverages

Water is the most healthful beverage. Make certain your drinking water is uncontaminated, as discussed in Chapter 8. Fresh juices and herbal teas offer delicious and healthful options; buy organic juices and teas whenever possible. Check all beverage labels carefully for juice percentages and added sugars.

- Pure water/carbonated water
- 100-percent fruit juice
- 100-percent vegetable juice
- Grain coffee-substitute(s)
- Tea (green, herbal, rooibus)

Oils

Use only extra-virgin, cold-pressed, or expeller-pressed oils, and organic whenever possible. Use olive oil frequently, except for stir-frying or baking. Most other oils in grocery stores have been treated with solvents, heated to temperatures that destroy all natural antioxidants, deodorized, bleached, refined, de-gummed, de-foamed, and chemically preserved.

Organic and/or cold-pressed oils can be found at progressive grocery stores, health food stores, and some gourmet food shops. Extra-virgin olive oil is widely available and retains many of the original benefits of the olives themselves: beta-sitosterols, which balance serum cholesterol, and beta-carotene, a flavonoid that benefits the liver, gallbladder, pancreas, brain, and blood. Keep all oils except olive oil in the refrigerator so they don't go rancid. You'll find it's best to use less of the stronger-flavored oils.

Remember to avoid all trans fats: hydrogenated or partially hydrogenated oil, margarine, or vegetable shortening. (*Author's note:* Some new margarines contain no trans fats, but most of their ingredients lists don't really fit my definition of "food"; I did, however, find some margarine in the health food store that had real food ingredients.)

- Olive oil
- Other oils (almond, coconut, corn, macadamia, peanut, rice bran, safflower, sesame, soybean, sunflower, walnut)

Nuts and Seeds

Buy raw or roasted nuts and seeds that have not been seasoned, dry-roasted, or coated with sugar and/or salt. You can find these in health food stores and in the baking section of most grocery stores. Be sure to buy only the old-fashioned kind of peanut-butter: ground-up peanuts and salt. Other nut-butters and sesame *tahini* are good alternatives. Store nuts and seeds in the refrigerator or freezer to keep them fresh.

A note about peanuts: Peanuts are called nuts but are actually legumes. As they grow underground, they can acquire a toxic, carcinogenic mold called afla-toxin, which is also tasteless, so it's impossible to tell if it's in your peanuts or peanut-butter. Healthy people should be able to handle aflatoxin exposure, but a sick person may have a difficult time with it.

- Coconut (unsweetened)
- Nuts and nut-butters (almond, Brazil nut, cashew, chestnut, hazelnut, macadamia, peanut, pecan, pine, pistachio, walnut)
- Seeds (pumpkin, sesame, sunflower)

Condiments

Many delicious condiments add great flavor to foods without adding lots of calories or fat. Read condiment labels carefully, however, as sauces and dressings are often salty, fatty, sugary, or filled with chemicals. Homemade salad dressings are, of course, best.

- Anchovy paste, seaweed flakes
- Capers, olives, pickles, sun-dried tomatoes
- Catsup, horseradish, mustard, relish, salsa, sauerkraut
- Gomasio (toasted sesame seeds ground up with sea salt)
- Herbs
- Pepper (black, green, red, white) and other spices
- Vinegar (balsamic, rice, apple-cider, other fruit)
- Worcestershire sauce, soy or tamari or shoyu sauce

YOU'RE ON YOUR WAY

Hopefully, you've now discovered several new foods to try with your family. Now that your pantry is filled with nutrient-dense foods, you'll be inspired to use and eat them! You'll soon develop a new list of healthful recipes featuring your new favorites.

CHAPTER 10

How to Feed Your Kids So They'll Be Happy and You'll Be Happy

It is your job as a parent to avoid, whenever possible, making
the inevitable battles of the toddler period battles over food . . .
If you emphasize or enforce eating too much, you will arouse
her need to exert her individuality and the battle will be on . . .
Successfully negotiating this demands a division of responsibility:
You are responsible for what your child is presented to eat,
she is responsible for what and how much she eats.

—ELLEN SATTER, *CHILD OF MINE: FEEDING WITH LOVE AND GOOD SENSE*

Our children eat what we expose them to. If we bring only healthful food into our homes, that's what they'll eat; but if we dine on fast foods and ready-made meals, that's what they'll eat. Setting the stage for our children's future health and habits begins early, and the foods and lifestyles that we choose to grow our children on have great impact on their lifelong health. Breast-fed babies, for example, have fewer incidences of hospitalization throughout childhood and adolescence. Vegetarian families have a lower risk of developing diabetes, obesity, and heart disease, but vegetarian children are more likely than meat-eating children to become anemic. Children who regularly drink sodas erode their tooth enamel and are more likely to be obese. Children who live with parents who smoke are more likely to get asthma and have more colds. When children watch television during meals, they eat fewer fruits and vegetables.

Teaching children good eating habits from early childhood helps them develop into healthier and more balanced adults. In families where meals are planned, children have higher intakes of fruits and vegetables and lower intakes of low-nutrient foods. And the vanishing custom of eating sit-down meals together has far-reaching benefits. Family dinners have even been shown to reduce aggressive behavior in children and to help prevent juvenile delinquency in girls and in children from single-family homes.

FEEDING BABIES

You will know when your baby is ready to try solid foods because he/she will begin to show an interest, perhaps trying to grab something from your plate when sitting in your lap. This can happen at any time from four to eight months of age, around when your baby gets his/her first teeth. In general, it's good to begin with hypoallergenic foods like whole-grain rice cereal, well-cooked puréed vegetables, and puréed fruits. Unsweetened applesauce and mashed bananas are two other simple "starter" foods. Stick with organic foods, as your baby's metabolism takes in everything (nutrients, chemicals, contaminants) at a higher rate than adults do.

Puréed foods can be purchased or home-made. Mills for transforming home-cooked food into baby-food are very useful for your child's first few months of food-eating, and can help you save time and money. I found that often I could simply purée some of what the rest of the family was having. The nutritional content of a baby's food isn't primary at first, as babies will still get most of their nutrients from breast-milk or formula until later; the experience of eating and swallowing is the important thing.

After two to three months of puréed foods, your baby will have the hang of swallowing, using his/her tongue, and eating in general. At this point you can begin to pile some "real" food on the tray. Babies love to feed themselves, so let your baby pretty much feed himself/herself by the age of eight months or so (expect this to be a messy process that will get neater over time). It's amazing what a relatively toothless baby can gum successfully! Give well-cooked vegetables such as carrots, broccoli, peas, mashed potatoes, and cauliflower, and easily gummed foods like banana, blueberries, raspberries, and applesauce; try rice, raw tofu squares, and a few canned beans or cooked lentils. Just let babies "go to town" with their hands. They will find this entertaining, and you will have time to eat yourself!

It is recommended that you avoid giving dairy, wheat, eggs, honey, and citrus until your child is at least one year old. These foods are difficult to digest; given too early, they can cause lifelong food sensitivities or allergies and other health issues. Allow your baby's digestive system ample time to grow into them. Of course, many babies are given milk-based infant formula; if they do well with it, that's great, but babies often develop reactions to dairy products, with symptoms varying from hives and rashes to recurrent ear infections, crankiness, constipation and/or diarrhea, gas, and asthma.

Additional Notes on Feeding Babies

- Give your newborn the probiotic bacteria *Bifidobacteria infantis* (see Chapter 5) to prevent gas, colic, cradle-cap, and other problems.

- If you give juice, dilute it with at least three or four parts water. Organic apple juice is a great one to start with.

- Do not give your baby any food that contains honey until he/she is at least one year old. Honey in newborns can cause infant botulism (as they get older, this becomes a non-issue).

FEEDING PRESCHOOLERS

The preschool years can be a trying time for parents, as toddlers are beginning to assert their independent ideas about the way they live—and food is a fertile battle-ground. After all, children begin "deciding" at birth when they're hungry and satisfied, when to eat and when to stop. As mentioned earlier, your job as the parent of a preschooler is to offer a variety of wonderful foods, and your child's job is to decide what to eat. When my boys were small, I considered it a success if they ate two real meals a day, plus some snacks. Try not to make a big deal about what your children do and do not eat, or you'll just end up fighting about food as they try to exert their own will. Instead, relax. Know that if you provide them with healthful foods, they'll choose wisely.

Children, like babies, need to eat often, usually every two to three hours. They have fast metabolisms and small tummies, and they use up many more calories per pound of body weight than adults do. When children's blood sugar levels drop, they get tired, cranky, or downright impossible. So think about an eating schedule that includes breakfast, a mid-morning snack, lunch, a mid-afternoon snack, a late-afternoon snack or early dinner, and then dinner or a bedtime snack. Carrying healthful foods with you when you leave the house really helps. It cuts down on not only the cost of stopping to buy whatever's convenient and handy, but also the frequency that your child has a "melt-down" from low blood sugar.

Small children are under our control—they eat what we feed them. So, they only love French fries because we give them French fries. They only love sodas because we give them sodas, and candy because we give them candy. If you are wise, you will give your kids healthful foods only. You can control this pretty well for the first few years. This is easy to do with a first child, but more difficult with subsequent siblings. My older son, Kyle, came up to me with a handful of M&M's

and asked if he could have them. I said no, so he just put them back in the bowl. Since he'd never tasted them, it wasn't any issue at all. But by the time his younger brother was two, his big brother could show him the ropes!

As children begin going to preschool and to other people's homes, they are exposed to foods that may be different than what you keep at home. If your child has specific dietary needs (for example, is a vegetarian, or doesn't do well with sweets, or has a food allergy), let the school's staff know about it. Your child can also be trained to ask if a food is okay for him/her to eat. Once a neighbor's three-year-old stopped by, and I asked him if he'd like some orange slices. He asked me if they had dairy or wheat in them. When I said no, he was happy to eat them.

Keep in mind that, generally, children like simple foods. Some children's plates have three sections because many kids don't like their foods to touch or mix with each other. Respect this; instead of tuna casserole, give tuna, noodles, cheese, and peas. It takes a while for kids to develop more sophisticated tastes. If they like what they see or smell, they are likely to be willing to try it; but if they dislike the sight or odor, they may refuse to eat it.

It's important with children to be easygoing about food. Cake and ice cream at a birthday party are not cause for panic, unless your child is allergic to the ingredients. Remember, though, that bribing a child with desserts creates a monster. In our house, we never had dessert unless we had company. If we baked cookies, we ate them and then they were gone until we baked cookies again, which could be a long time! There wasn't ice cream in the freezer on a regular basis, and there wasn't candy or soda in the house. But we did have plenty of fresh fruits, peas in shells, juice popsicles, healthful chips, and food fresh from the garden. When we went grocery shopping, we'd stop at the produce section first, I'd buy a carton of blueberries, raspberries, or strawberries, and the kids kept themselves busy with those while I shopped.

Make a Snack Cabinet

Take a lower cabinet and make it your children's snack cabinet. Stock it with cereals, crackers, raisins, and other ready-to eat foods along with plastic bowls, cups, plates, and utensils. You can also put a bowl in the cabinet that has plastic bags filled with snack-sized portions that your child can easily take. This gives preschoolers the ability to eat when they're hungry and helps them become independent—and it gives you flexibility, because once they get the idea, they'll get many of their own snacks.

FEEDING BIGGER KIDS

Continue feeding older children with the same ideas described in the previous section for younger ones. Keep a big bowl of fruit out on the counter so it will be the first thing your children see when they look for something easy to eat. Big kids also like chips and nuts; consider nuts in shells that they can open with nutcrackers. Stock fresh juices and herbal iced tea sweetened with apple juice. Freeze juice into popsicles. Make sure your child goes to school with breakfast in his/her tummy. Continue to make bag lunches for your school-aged children, even in their teen years. If you do, they'll most likely eat them, but if you don't, who knows?

As your children become teenagers, you'll be amazed at how much food they can consume. Their metabolic rates are soaring and they can probably eat two to three times what you eat. A houseful of teenage boys can hit a kitchen like a natural disaster—and if you're well stocked with mainly healthful food, that's what they'll be happy to make and eat. Keep some easy-to-prepare frozen products on hand: small pizzas, burritos, pot-pies, and fish sticks. Supply the ingredients for nachos: refried beans, natural chips, salsa, olives, and cheese. If you don't have good snack-foods in your kitchen, teenagers will go to the local mini-mart and buy junk. If they do spend their allowance on candy bars occasionally, don't make a big deal about it.

Teach Your Children to Cook

From the time children are five years old or so, they can begin helping in the kitchen. Slowly teach your children to cook: how to cut vegetables with a knife, how to wash lettuce for a salad. As your children get bigger, teach them how to make a fruit smoothie in the blender. By the time children are eight or nine, they can make the whole salad, or the steamed vegetables. And by the time children are twelve or so, they can easily be taught to cook a simple dinner like pasta with sauce and steamed broccoli—or, a batch of cookies or brownies!

At first, teaching your children to cook will seem like it's just not worth the effort. It's so much easier to do it yourself. But over time and with patience, they'll improve. When my sons were in high school, they each cooked dinner one night a week and I helped if they needed it. Soon they were both at ease in the kitchen, and now they're really great cooks.

Clean up Your Child's Diet

Let's take a look at what your child is eating! Keep a Food Diary for your child for several days (see page 73). Then, get out some crayons or markers and do the following:

- Circle these in red: sugar, caffeine, alcohol, junk foods, fried foods, high-fat foods, highly processed foods, diet foods, pastries, donuts, chips, microwaved popcorn, soft drinks.

- Circle these in blue: dairy products (milk, cheese, yogurt, ice cream, frozen yogurt, ice milk).
- Circle these in green: fruits and vegetables.
- Circle these in yellow: protein foods (fish, poultry, beef, pork, lamb, veal, legumes, soy products).
- Circle these in purple: nuts and seeds, oils, butter, margarine.
- Circle these in black: grains (wheat, bread, corn, non-microwaved popcorn, rice, millet, buckwheat, bulgur, quinoa, amaranth, barley, oats, rye).

Now look at what you've circled. Is there one food group that dominates your child's Food Diary? Does your child crave specific foods? Sometimes we need the foods we crave, but at other times they make us sick, and when we take those foods away, the experience can be like withdrawal from a drug addiction.

Choose one area at a time to make a change. You may decide to eliminate refined sugars and corn syrup or to decrease dairy products and/or wheat; you may choose to increase fruits and vegetables, or increase other high-fiber foods, or cut down on junk foods, or stop going to fast-food restaurants; you may choose to make your child's lunch rather than depend on the school-lunch program. Each week, pick another healthful dietary change. If your child is old enough to be educated about what you are doing, enlist him/her in the process (by first grade, a child can usually begin to understand it).

THE FAMILY MEAL

Meals are a time for getting the family together to eat and to talk. When children are included in conversation about the day and discussions of community and world events, they develop skills that they'll carry into social situations later in life. Meals are also times when children learn about manners. When my boys were smaller, we'd have specific meals that were "manners nights" so they would know how to eat appropriately when in a social situation away from home. Make time to have a family meal nearly every night! Admittedly, this gets harder as children get older. Some things to remember at family meals:

- Meals are for togetherness. Pick some other time to criticize or punish your children. Make the dinner table a safe and welcoming place to be.
- Give everyone a task. Teach small children to help set the table or help you cook. Older children can also help clean up the kitchen.
- Say grace. In our house, we hold hands, close our eyes, and have a silent moment or two.

- Serve desserts only for special occasions. Never bribe your children with dessert in order to get them to eat something else.
- Don't insist that your children finish everything on their plates.
- Ask everyone to tell about something that happened during his/her day. Make it fun to be together. On some nights, you may find yourselves sitting at the table laughing and talking for hours.
- Turn the television off. Don't take phone calls. Make the meal itself the event.

Digestive Health Issues in Children

Introduction
to Part Three

This part covers the most common digestive problems in children, and the next covers some additional health conditions that people don't always associate with digestive issues. Each chapter provides a comprehensive list of self-care ideas, in order (loosely) of what works best. Some of these Healing Options alleviate particular symptoms, whereas others address the problem's underlying cause. The remedies presented are mostly nutritional and herbal, with other modalities occasionally included. Nutrients and herbs can be found separately and in combination products. You may want to work with a healthcare professional to tailor a program that best suits your child's needs. You'll notice that some recommendations are repeated for many different problems. Although each health condition has unique characteristics, many share symptoms or origins that respond to similar treatments.

Health care is both a science and an art. You may first enlist the science in a full evaluation including laboratory testing and medical diagnosis. Information is included in these chapters about customary lab tests as well as others that may be unfamiliar to your child's physician (Appendix A will help you and the doctor connect with the appropriate labs). The art of health care then comes into play in determining which paths to follow, which therapeutic ideas have the most merit, and which dosages are appropriate.

Healing often happens in layers. Sometimes you try the right thing at the wrong time and it isn't effective, but then later you may try it again with great results because the initial obstacle has since been removed. If the first Healing Option you try doesn't work or only works partially, try another. Be persistent and patient. Symptoms are the body's way of telling us to pay attention because something is out of balance. By listening, we often have the inner wisdom to know exactly what our children need.

CHAPTER 11

Food and Environmental Sensitivities

Each day we are bombarded with sensory input including advertising, email, newspapers, phone calls, and conversations, and somehow we filter most of it, usually letting just the most useful bits into our awareness to be acted upon and remembered. In much the same way, we are exposed daily to an enormous variety of foods and chemicals, and somehow our bodies must determine what is friend and what is foe. The basis of our immune system's purpose and function is to distinguish between self and non-self by continually sampling our environment, blocking potentially dangerous substances, and welcoming others. And as you learned in Chapter 3, two-thirds of the immune system is actually located in the digestive system.

For most of what we are exposed to, our immune system makes protective antibodies that signal "safety" and allow us to accept foreign foods and substances into our bodies without mounting an attack against them. Tolerance of foods and other environmental exposures is based on many factors including genetics, age, gender, and gut ecology as well as the type and dose of the particular foreign substance (antigen). When a child's body has a reaction to his/her food or environment, it's a sign of diminished tolerance. As parents, we must help build our children's tolerance to their world so they can live normal and active lives.

In allergies and intolerances, the immune system produces antibodies in response to its recognition that the body is being attacked in some way. Such allergic and sensitivity responses can be provoked by foods, molds, pollens, chemicals, metals, and nearly any other substance. Throughout the wide variety of autoimmune conditions, however, the immune system seems to turn on its own body for no obvious reason. The analogy I like is that every time birthday candles are lit, someone quickly quenches them with a fire extinguisher. In cases of allergies, sensitivities, and other immune system over-reactions, we must teach the body to reset itself (to learn that a birthday candle doesn't require a fire extin-

guisher). Avoiding the offending foods and substances and using nutrients, probiotics, and herbs can rebuild gut health; along with making time for relaxation, this
can help reset the immune system's reactions.

FIVE LINES OF IMMUNE PROTECTION

When we are healthy, our immune system handles the challenges it's continually
faced with, and we may never even know about them. Our first line of defense is
on our skin and mucous membranes, in the form of nonspecific substances called
opsonins and mucins that mobilize against everything "foreign," mainly bacteria.
Our second line of defense is the dendritic system: granulocytes, macrophages,
astrocytes, and other specialized cells that gobble up foreign materials. Residing
primarily in our skin and mucous membranes, these dendritic cells are also found
in the blood when they are immature; when the cells become active, they migrate
into the lymphatic tissues. Our third line of defense, immunoglobulin A (IgA), acts
as a sentry on skin, in saliva, lungs, eyes, nose, ears, vagina, and throughout the
digestive tract. IgA antibodies prevent bacteria, food residue, fungus, parasites,
and viruses from attaching to our mucous membranes and neutralize these potential invaders before they can cause problems.

Line Four: Food and Environmental Sensitivity Reactions

When the first three lines of immune defense are overloaded, the body begins producing additional antibodies, immunoglobulins M and G (IgM and IgG). IgM antibodies circulate temporarily for about three months until longer-lasting IgG
antibodies mobilize to take over the fight. We keep producing IgG antibodies as
long as we eat the offending foods or are exposed to chemicals, bacterial toxins, or
other antigens that challenge the immune system. These IgM and IgG responses
are called delayed or "hidden" sensitivity reactions because their symptoms can
take from several hours to several days to appear, making it very difficult to track
down the trigger food or substance.

Although we may inhale only a mere teaspoon of pollen in an entire year, we
eat pounds of food every day. As it turns out, the most common antibody responses are IgG reactions to mold and foods. In Western countries, 10 to 20 percent of children have delayed food sensitivities. Almost any food can cause a
sensitivity reaction, but beef, citrus, dairy products, egg, pork, and wheat provoke
80 percent of them. Food sensitivities can underlie a huge variety of symptoms
(see the inset "Sensitivity Symptoms" on page 107). In addition to discovering
which foods your child is reacting to, it is important to identify other underlying
factors such as parasites; bacterial, viral, or candida infection; pancreatic insuffi-
ciency; enzyme deficiency; medications; or poor lifestyle habits.

Sensitivity Symptoms

Professional evaluation is necessary to determine whether the following symptoms, which can be caused by many health conditions, are in fact due to food and/or environmental sensitivities:

- Head—chronic headaches, difficulty sleeping, dizziness, migraines

- Mouth and throat—coughing, frequent need to clear throat, gagging, hoarseness, pain, sores on gums/lips/tongue, sore throat, swelling

- Eyes, ears, nose—blurred vision, dark under-eye circles, ear infections, excessive mucus, hay fever, hearing loss, postnasal drip, ringing in ears, runny/stuffy nose, sinus problems, sneezing attacks, swollen/red/sticky eyelids, watery and itchy eyes

- Heart and lungs—asthma, bronchitis, chest pain and congestion, difficulty breathing, irregular heartbeat (palpitations, arrhythmia), rapid heartbeat, shortness of breath

- Gastrointestinal tract—bloating, constipation, cramping, diarrhea, heartburn, indigestion, irritable bowel syndrome, nausea and vomiting, passing gas, stomach pain

- Skin—acne, dryness, eczema, excessive sweating, hair loss, hives, irritation around eyes, psoriasis, rashes

- Muscles and joints—aches/pains, arthritis, general weakness, stiffness, swelling

- Energy and activity—apathy, depression, difficulty getting work done, fatigue, hyperactivity, memory lapses, mental dullness, restlessness

- Emotions and mind—aggressive behavior, anger, anxiety, binge eating or drinking, confusion, depression, difficulty learning, fear, food cravings, irritability, mood swings, nervousness, poor comprehension, poor concentration, tension

- Other—dizziness, fluid retention, frequent urination, genital itch, insomnia, overweight, underweight

In addition to the symptoms listed above, children with food and/or environmental sensitivities may have:

- Attention deficit disorder

- Behavior problems

- Learning problems

- Recurring ear infections

Children with these problems will often benefit from a dietary evaluation and environmental sensitivity testing.

Line Five: True Allergic Reactions

When the four previously described lines of immune system defense have been over-whelmed, the body begins to make immunoglobulin E (IgE). IgE antibodies attach to our mast cells in mucous membranes and connective tissues, stimulating the release of inflammatory substances called cytokines and histamines. This is called a true allergic reaction. It produces symptoms within minutes to two hours after the food is eaten or the environmental allergen is encountered: closing of the throat, fatigue, hives, itching, itchy eyes or ears, respiratory distress, runny nose, skin rashes, tearing, and sometimes severe reactions of asthma or anaphylactic shock.

True food allergy is rare, affecting only 0.3 to 7.5 percent of American children and 1 to 2 percent of American adults. The foods that most often trigger true allergic reactions are cow's milk, eggs, nuts, shellfish, soy, wheat, and fish. Within the last five years, allergy to peanuts has doubled in children under the age of five years. Peanut allergy can be so severe that a child may have a reaction simply if someone else has recently eaten peanuts or peanut butter in the room—that's why peanuts are no longer served on airplanes. As of January 2006, food manufacturers must note if a product contains any of the eight major food allergens.

Environmental Illness

Chronic exposure to food additives, household chemicals, building materials, contaminated recirculating air, and impure water can so depress and weaken a person's immune system that eventually, exposure to even a small amount of a toxin makes him/her acutely or chronically ill. This condition, called environmental illness or multiple chemical sensitivities, is becoming increasingly common; two recent studies put its incidence at 12.9 and 15.9 percent in adults.

If blood tests show that your child has environmental allergies, or if you know that specific substances make your child ill, it is essential that he/she avoid those antigens. Malic acid can be helpful in neutralizing some of the reactions. It is also important to work with a healthcare provider who is educated in this area, so look for a doctor familiar with environmental medicine or clinical ecology. Multiple chemical sensitivities can be overcome, but it takes guidance and persistence.

Functional Laboratory Testing for Children with Sensitivities and Allergies

Most doctors can easily screen your child for food allergies by using either a blood test called the modified RAST or a scratch test. Testing for food sensitivities and IgG antibodies is not as widely done. A few labs additionally perform IgA and IgM antibody tests, which give a more comprehensive picture. See Appendix A for details on testing.

Some Recommended Tests

1. Food sensitivity/allergy test(s)

2. Comprehensive digestive and stool analysis with parasite screening

3. Candida antibody test through blood or stool, CDSA, lactose breath test, and/or intestinal permeability test

4. Intestinal permeability test

5. Lactose intolerance test

Self-Testing with an Elimination/Provocation Diet

If you wish to investigate your child's possible food sensitivities on your own, you can try an elimination/provocation diet. The idea behind it is simple: For a week or two, have your child eat only foods that he/she is unlikely to be sensitive to (listed below), and then gradually reintroduce other foods that he/she normally eats. The removal of offending foods calms symptoms, and the careful addition of a single food each few days makes it easier to identify any that provoke a symptomatic reaction.

Here is a typical list of foods that can be eaten during the initial elimination phase:

- All vegetables

- All fruits (except citrus)

- Rice and rice products (for example, rice milk, rice cereal, and rice bread/crackers/cakes)

- Fish or chicken

- Olive oil

- Water and herbal tea to drink

- Salt, pepper, and herbs to make the food tastier

All dairy products and all grains other than rice are to be avoided during the elimination phase. If you don't notice a big improvement in your child's health or symptoms during this phase, your child either doesn't have food sensitivities or has other issues that are masking the benefit of the restricted diet. If you do notice changes in your child's behavior and physical well-being after ten days to two weeks of the elimination phase, begin the provocation phase with one new food at a time. Give your child that food at least two or three times daily for a few days to see whether it provokes symptoms; if it does not, you can allow him/her to continue eating that food. Meanwhile, add another food and follow the same procedure.

Although the elimination/provocation diet sounds simple, it can be challenging. Most people find it fairly easy to follow a restricted food plan for a week or two, but the slow reintroduction of foods into your child's diet may be more difficult. Recipes and restaurant foods include many ingredients, and sometimes it's hard to determine which one causes the distress, especially when reactions are delayed for a day or two. If you experience these complications in the provocation phase, remove all suspected foods from your child's diet for four days and then introduce those foods again one at a time. You'll know you've found the culprit if a reaction results each time you add a particular food.

It is common to be sensitive to more than one food or food "family." If your child is sensitive to a food, he/she will often be sensitive to all foods in that same family; for example, some people who are sensitive to milk are also sensitive to cheese, yogurt, and other dairy products. If your child is sensitive to cherries, also avoid apples, peaches, pears, nectarines, plums, and apricots.

Healing Options for Children with Sensitivities and Allergies

With a holistic treatment program, a child can become increasingly less reactive to foods and environmental antigens over time. Begin by having your child avoid all substances to which he/she is sensitive or allergic. The reactions will gradually stop and his/her body (especially the liver) will have the opportunity to detoxify. Using the probiotics, anti-inflammatory nutrients, and herbs listed below will speed the process. Eating organically grown, nutrient-rich, natural foods promotes self-repair. An exercise program and stress management also play a part in recovery. See Appendix B for more details on the following nutrients, herbs, and supplements. For best results, follow at least the first four of the recommendations below.

Avoidance—of all substances that cause your child to have a sensitivity or allergic reaction, for a period of four to six months. To substitute for these, check out the health food store's plethora of special foods for people with food allergies. If chemical sensitivity is an issue, use natural household-cleaning products (it's good to use these anyway). Some people react to mattresses, gas-stoves, paints, carpeting, and upholstery, which can make avoidance difficult. Consult a healthcare professional who can help with the details.

Glutamine—to heal the intestinal tract. Dosage for children: ½–4 teaspoons daily, mixed in juice or water.

Probiotics—to protect the digestive tract's mucosal lining and limit damage caused by pathogenic bacteria. Dosage for children: capsules, two to six daily; or powder, ¼–½ teaspoon twice daily.

Enzymes—to help normalize allergies. Digestive enzymes taken with meals help foods to be broken down more completely, and proteolytic (protein-splitting) enzymes taken between meals help cleanse the bloodstream of food molecules and other debris. Dosage for children: digestive enzymes, one or two capsules with each meal and snack; proteolytic enzymes, one capsule at bedtime and another upon arising.

Quercetin—to reduce pain and inflammatory responses and control allergies. Dosage for children: 250–1,000 milligrams (mg) three or four times daily.

Milk Thistle, Dandelion Root, Burdock, and Similar Herbs—to support the liver. These can be used singly or in combination. Dosage for children: tea, 1–3 cups daily; tincture and capsules, as directed on label; for children younger than four years old, half of suggested regular dosage.

Vitamin C—to help flush toxins from the body. Dosage for children: 250–3,000 mg buffered ascorbate or Ester-C daily.

Mineral Salts—containing bicarbonates of calcium, magnesium, and/or potassium (for example, Alka-Seltzer Gold), to alkalize and to help minimize reactions. Dosage for children: as directed on label; for children younger than four years old, half of suggested regular dosage.

Malic Acid—to stop or slow reactions if your child has eaten something questionable. Dosage for children: as directed on label. Malic acid is also found naturally in fruits and apple-cider vinegar.

Multivitamin-mineral Supplement—for general nutritional support. Be sure to purchase a good-quality, allergen-free supplement. Dosage for children: for children up to eight years old, a daily child's chewable; for children eight to twelve years old, a daily half-dose of an adult supplement; for children over the age of twelve years, a full daily adult supplement.

Four-Day Food-Rotation Diet—to help a child with sensitivities or allergies to a large number of foods and/or food families. Such a child often becomes reactive to more and more foods, but a rotation diet prevents the development of an ever-widening set of sensitivities. In this protocol, the child avoids eating any foods to which he/she had strong antibody reactions, and eats the remaining foods in a rotating pattern that "tricks" the body into being more tolerant.

As described earlier, eating a food to which we are sensitive results in the production of antibodies against it for the next twenty-four hours. Therefore, if we eat that food again the next day, we'll have symptoms from our immune system's reaction to it; however, if we don't eat that food for several days, the antibodies that were ready for a fight will have disappeared as though it were a false alarm.

Then, when we restart the rotation and resume eating that food, antibody production also starts again, but symptoms don't develop because the appropriate antibodies are never present at the time that the offending food is eaten.

To set up the rotation, list all the foods that your child tolerates; then, divide
that list into four groups, with each group getting a quarter of the tolerable fruits,
vegetables, grains, proteins, oils, nuts, seeds, and beverages. Keep all foods from
the same food family, however, in the same group (for example, apples, blackber-
ries, raspberries, peaches, apricots, and pears are all in the same food family, and
dairy products are all one family). The foods in the first group will be eaten on
Day 1 of the four-day rotation diet; those in the second group on Day 2; those in
the third group on Day 3; and those in the fourth on Day 4. The rotation restarts on
the fifth day with the first food group (Day 1 again). You may find it helpful to
have specific shelves in your cabinets and refrigerator for each of the four groups,
or to identify the foods in the four groups with colored stickers.

Laboratories supply sample lists of food groups with test results, and you can
easily find these lists in the many good books on the four-day food-rotation diet.
My favorites are by Sally Rockwell, Ph.D.: *Dr. Sally's Allergy Recipes* (Seattle,
WA: Diet Design Publishing, 1996) and *The Rotation Game* (Seattle, WA: Diet
Design Publishing, 1989). Dr. Rockwell also offers a wonderful computer pro-
gram that creates rotation diets for your child's specific needs.

CHAPTER 12

Leaky Gut Syndrome

Imagine that your body's cells are screaming, "Hey, send me a kernel of corn." The bloodstream replies, "I have a can of corn, but I don't have a can-opener" (think of digestive enzymes as the can-opener). So the can circulates around and around, while the cells starve for corn. Finally, your immune system reacts to the can of corn by identifying corn as a foreign invader and producing antibodies against it. The next time you eat corn, these antibodies are at the ready to trigger an immune system response to what was formerly a perfectly acceptable food. That, essentially, is what happens in leaky gut syndrome. And as time passes, people with a leaky gut tend to become more and more sensitive to a wider variety of foods and environmental contaminants.

WHAT CAUSES A GUT TO LEAK?

Leaky gut syndrome is a nickname for the more formal term "increased intestinal permeability." There is no single cause, but some of the most common contributing factors are chronic stress, environmental contaminants, gastrointestinal disease, immune system overload, poor food choices, infection with bacteria or parasites or yeasts, and prolonged or repeated use of antibiotics and pain medications. As knowledge of the synergy between digestion and immune function increases, the list of health problems associated with leaky gut also grows. Although the syndrome itself is not a disease, it underlies an enormous variety of illnesses and symptoms.

The Dual Functions of the Small Intestine

A healthy gastrointestinal lining allows properly digested fats, proteins, and starches in the gut to pass through to the bloodstream for circulation and assimilation into the body. At the same time, it serves as a barrier to prevent bacterial products, foreign substances, and large undigested molecules from entering the bloodstream. Substances can move across that barrier, however, in several ways. Free fatty acids and ions of chloride, magnesium, potassium, and sodium pass through by the simple process of diffusion, which equalizes the concentrations of various particles inside and outside of cells. Most other fatty acids, amino acids, glucose, minerals, and vitamins move through the lining by a process called active transport, in which low-molecular-weight carrier molecules take nutrients across cell membranes like molecular taxis.

A third form of particle movement through the intestinal lining is between cell junctions called desmosomes. Normally, these are tight junctions that do not permit the passage of large molecules, but when an area in the mucosal membrane is irritated and inflamed, the desmosomes there become loose. Large molecules of food and other substances can pass through the loosened junctions and are seen by our immune system as foreign, stimulating an "alarm" reaction that activates antibodies and cytokines. Cytokines create inflammation in the gastrointestinal (GI) tract and elsewhere in the body. In addition, when the GI tract has been damaged, free radicals (molecules missing an electron, which cause harm by grabbing electrons from cell membranes) are often produced in quantities too large to process, causing more inflammation and irritation that further exacerbate a leaky gut. See Figure 12.1 below for an illustration of a leaky gut versus a normal gut.

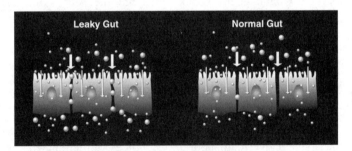

Figure 12.1. Leaky Gut versus Normal Gut

Depending upon our individual susceptibilities, we may develop a wide variety of health problems in response to increased intestinal permeability. The conditions and symptoms listed in the inset "Common Symptoms and Conditions Associated with Leaky Gut" on page 115 can arise from a variety of causes, but leaky gut syndrome may underlie many diseases. When the gut is healed, many of these issues improve dramatically.

Increased intestinal permeability puts an extra burden on the liver, which is in charge of handling all toxic or foreign substances. Water-soluble toxins are easily excreted, but the breakdown of fat-soluble toxins is a two-stage process, and a

Common Symptoms and Conditions Associated with Leaky Gut

Common clinical conditions associated with leaky gut in children include:

- Allergy
- Arthritis
- Asthma
- Autism
- Bronchitis
- Burn (severe burn damage can cause leaky gut)
- Cancer treatment (can cause leaky gut)
- Celiac disease
- Chronic fatigue syndrome
- Crohn's disease
- Cystic fibrosis
- Eczema
- Ear infection (recurring)
- Environmental illness
- Food sensitivity and/or allergy
- Giardia and/or other parasite
- Hives
- HIV infection
- Hyperactivity
- Intestinal infection
- Irritable bowel syndrome
- Learning and behavior problems
- Malabsorption/ malnutrition
- Multiple chemical sensitivity
- Psoriasis
- Reiter's syndrome
- Schizophrenia
- Trauma
- Ulcerative colitis

The following list is applicable to both children and adults:

- Abdominal pain
- Aggressive behavior
- Anxiety
- Asthma
- Autoimmune disease
- Bed-wetting
- Bloating
- Chronic joint pain
- Chronic muscle pain
- Confusion
- Constipation
- Diarrhea
- Fatigue and malaise
- Fever of unknown origin
- Fuzzy thinking
- Gas
- Indigestion
- Mood swings
- Nervousness
- Poor exercise tolerance
- Poor immune function
- Poor memory
- Recurrent bladder infection
- Recurrent vaginal infection
- Shortness of breath
- Skin rash
- "Toxic feelings"

liver bombarded by inflammatory irritants from incomplete digestion has less energy to do this; when overwhelmed, it resorts to storing toxins in fat cells. The liver may be able to deal with these stored toxins later, but most commonly, it is too busy with what is newly coming in and never catches up. These toxins are then a continuing source of inflammation to the body. Liver-detoxifying cleanses are advisable for adults with leaky gut syndrome, but I hesitate to recommend them for children.

Functional Laboratory Testing for Children with Leaky Gut Syndrome

If your child has any of the common symptoms or disorders associated with leaky gut, ask his/her physician to order an intestinal permeability test. The best diagnostic test for leaky gut is the mannitol-lactulose test. See Appendix A for details on testing.

Healing Options for Children with Leaky Gut Syndrome

Leaky gut syndrome is a cry for repair, and, if left untended, can become the root of many illnesses and symptoms. If you believe that your child suffers from leaky gut, it's best to work with a healthcare professional to determine the underlying factors. Fortunately, there are many ways to restore gut integrity. One simple step is to chew food more completely. Supplements and herbs can be taken to quench the "fires" of free radical production and inflammation, and others to help the body repair itself. At the very least, you should try the first four suggestions below. See Appendix B for more details on the following nutrients, herbs, and supplements.

Avoidance—of foods that your child is sensitive to. Consistently remove these foods from his/her diet.

Probiotics and Prebiotics—to replenish beneficial intestinal flora. Dosage for children: ¼–½ teaspoon two or three times daily, or one or two capsules twice daily.

Digestive Enzymes—to encourage more complete digestion of food. Plant-based enzymes are preferable. Dosage for children: one capsule with each meal.

Proteolytic Enzymes—to reduce inflammation and sensitivity reactions. Plant-based enzymes are preferable. Dosage for children: one capsule two to four times daily on an empty stomach.

Consider Food Sensitivity/Allergy—see Chapter 11.

Consider Dysbiosis or Infection with Bacteria, Candida, or Parasites—see Chapters 6 and 15.

Antioxidant Supplement—to assist the body in processing excess free radicals. Dosage for children: a children's antioxidant formula, use as directed.

Glutamine—to repair the mucosal lining directly. Dosage for children: 1–30 grams daily, according to the child's needs. Caution: Too much glutamine will constipate your child.

Zinc—possibly an essential nutrient for gut repair. Dosage for children: 5–10 milligrams.

Other nutrients and supplements that soothe and help heal the gut lining include gamma-oryzanol, Seacure, vitamins A and C, pantothenic acid (vitamin B_5), deglycyrrhized (DGL) licorice, folic acid, whey concentrate, colostrum, transfer factor, schizandra, and *Aloe vera*.

CHAPTER 13

Care and Feeding of Infants and Toddlers

A t birth, a previously dormant digestive system becomes responsible for your baby's sustenance and development. Fortunately, many of the common digestive problems that babies experience are easily solved and often self-limiting. The ideas presented in this chapter are what you can use first when your infant or toddler gets ill. (In rare cases, newborns have serious digestive problems that require medical intervention and even surgery; with the exception of an intestinal condition called Hirschsprung's disease, this chapter does not cover these problems.)

Simple, gentle remedies often give quick and lasting results. For example, many digestive issues in infants can be resolved with supplemental *Bifidobacteria infantis.* I recommend giving this probiotic to all newborns, as it helps prevent many health problems during infancy. Although it's frightening for parents when babies get sick, children are pliable and resilient, and they do get well pretty quickly. Whether this is your first or last baby, you'll find tips here that can help prevent sleepless nights—for all of you!

COLIC

Most babies fuss at times, but a baby with colic is upset for more than three hours each day. Colic is pretty common, affecting 10 to 20 percent of all infants. It usually begins at two to three weeks of age, often peaks between four to twelve weeks, and often occurs at about the same time each day, usually in the late afternoon or during the evening. Colicky babies typically clench their fists and draw up their legs, and have distended bellies, flailing arms, and arched backs—in other words, they look like they are in pain. An episode can last for a few minutes or for hours, and sometimes the baby will simply cry until exhausted.

Although you think you'll go mad from the exhaustion of days and nights spent trying to soothe your unhappy baby, colic usually ends by three to four months of age, so stay calm and be assured that it will pass. Colic isn't caused by a medical condition and isn't harmful. You haven't done anything wrong, and you aren't a horrible parent. When babies are uncomfortable, they cry; it's just their way of letting you know.

Healing Options for Babies with Colic

Passing gas or having a bowel movement will usually relieve a colicky baby, but this doesn't happen on cue. Experiment with several remedies and techniques to give your baby—and yourself—some relief. See Appendix B for more details on the following nutrients, herbs, and supplements.

Bifidobacteria infantis—to populate a baby's formerly sterile digestive system with microbes that can deal with the sudden influx of milk, formula, germs, and other substances. The result can seem like a small miracle. I have normalized several colicky babies with this approach in twenty-four hours or less, but be patient, as it could take several days. Dosage for children: ⅛ teaspoon powder three times daily, mixed with a few drops water and put on your baby's tongue or added to your baby's bottle. If you are breast-feeding, take ¼ teaspoon two or three times daily yourself to pass through your milk.

Fennel, Catnip, Chamomile, Lemon Balm, or Dill Tea—to calm the baby and soothe his/her digestive system. Use commercially available herbal tea (noncaffeinated), or make it yourself. Dosage for children: 1 teaspoon four times daily, given in a dropper, teaspoon, or bottle. If you are breast-feeding, drink at least 2 cups daily yourself to calm your system and pass through your milk. Also, try calming a colicky baby with a bath in catnip, fennel, hops, lavender, linden flower, or chamomile tea (cooled to the appropriate safe temperature).

Check the Bottle Nipple—in case your baby is swallowing too much air or over-feeding. The holes in the bottle nipple should be relatively small, and your baby should take at least twenty minutes to finish a small bottle.

Remember to Burp Your Baby—after each feeding, to release gas from the stomach and aid digestion. Holding your baby upright allows him/her to burp more easily.

Consider Food Sensitivity/Allergy—see Chapter 11. Some babies are sensitive to certain proteins in formula; alternatives to milk-based formula are lactose-free, soy-based, or elemental formula. If you are breast-feeding, empty one breast completely before offering the second, as the hind-milk contains more fat and is often soothing to your baby's digestive system.

For breastfed babies, gassy moms sometimes make gassy babies, so look at your own digestion as well. The most commonly problematic foods are caffeine-containing foods, chocolate, nuts, dairy products, peppers, spicy foods, cucumbers, melons, citrus foods, and cabbage-family foods such as broccoli, Brussels sprouts, and cauliflower, although any food can cause a reaction. Keeping a Food Diary may help you draw connections between your foods (or your medications) and your baby's discomfort. Try changing your diet to improve your baby's digestion.

Hold Your Baby More—in your arms, lap, a sling, or other carrier. The more you hold your baby throughout the day, the less likely that he/she will be colicky. I used to cook dinner and shop for groceries with my babies in a sling or pack.

Belly Massage—to release gas and relieve distention.

Relax—when you nurse or feed your baby. Be calm and view feeding time as a "time out" for yourself. Some babies are colicky because their mom is stressed. Some babies also react to family tension with colic, so think about your own family's dynamics.

CRADLE-CAP AND ECZEMA

Cradle-cap is a crusty, scaly rash that appears between the ages of two and twelve weeks and is usually found on the scalp. When found on other places such as eyebrows, eyelids, behind the ears, the sides of the nose, and the groin area, this type of rash is called eczema or seborrheic dermatitis. It is caused by overactive sebaceous glands that secrete oil that dries and flakes, plugging up the glands; they keep making oil, and the build-up can be quite thick. The rash may be red, inflamed, and greasy, but although it may look bad, it doesn't itch or hurt. It is usually gone before the age of one year. Many experts believe cradle-cap is triggered by hormones that the baby receives during pregnancy and birth.

Additional Ideas for Colic

- Some babies like having a warm hot-water bottle or heating pad placed on their tummies.

- Some babies love to sleep and swing in a baby hammock. The gentle rocking motion is soothing, perhaps recreating the movement inside the womb.

- Most babies love to be sung to and rocked, or walked and walked and walked.

- Sometimes the noise from a vacuum, the vibration from a washing machine or dishwasher, or the motion of riding in a car can be comforting.

- Pacifiers may also be calming for some babies.

Healing Options for Babies with Cradle-Cap and Eczema

See Appendix B for more details on the following nutrients, herbs, and supplements. (See also "Healing Options for Babies with Colic" on page 119.)

Bifidobacteria infantis—to establish normal gut flora for balancing effects on your baby's digestive system, scalp, and skin. (*Author's note:* My son Kyle's cradle-cap and eczema-type diaper rash appeared at ten days of age, and by three months he looked like a burn victim from groin to belly. After I tried other things without success, both conditions were resolved easily by *B. infantis.*) Dosage for children: ¼ teaspoon powder mixed with a few drops water and put on your baby's tongue, twice daily. If you are breast-feeding, take ½ teaspoon twice daily yourself to pass through your milk.

Oil and Shampoo—to soothe and cleanse. Massage the scalp with calendula lotion, butter, vitamin E oil, olive oil, sesame oil, or almond oil (commercially available oils containing vitamin E, chamomile, and/or calendula may also be of benefit). Let the oil sit a few minutes, loosen the scales with a soft brush or washcloth—*do not pick* at the scales, or they may bleed or become infected—and then wash with a mild baby shampoo, rubbing very gently.

Dietary Changes—can be especially helpful for a baby in a family with a history of hay fever, asthma, and allergies. Sometimes changing a baby's formula—or changing the breast-feeding mom's diet—will reduce cradle-cap and eczema.

Consider Candida Infection—see Chapter 6. Candida is a possible trigger of cradle-cap and/or eczema, and thrives on sugar, so a breast-feeding mom may improve the condition by avoiding sugar and sweets.

DIAPER RASH

Moisture, urine, and feces are irritating to a baby's skin, and diapers can chafe where they meet the waist and legs, so most babies have diaper rash at some time. It is usually self-limiting, not painful, and not a big deal (see the inset "The Main Types of Diaper Rash" on page 123). Once a diaper rash has lasted more than three days, however, there is a good chance that you are now dealing with a fungal or yeast infection.

Healing Options for Children with Diaper Rash

Diaper rash can occur at any time but is most common around nine months of age. This is also when a baby's diet is becoming more varied. Coincidence? I don't think so. Food sensitivities and allergies can play a large role in rashes of all sorts. See Appendix B for more details on the following nutrients, herbs, and supplements.

Change Diapers Often—to prevent the irritation caused by leaving wet or soiled diapers on for long periods. This precaution is the single most important one! Change your baby's diapers often, and always change a poopy diaper right away.

Air Out—to give the skin a chance to really dry. Leaving diapers off for twenty to thirty minutes can help substantially, especially in sunlight, so let the baby air outdoors if the weather is warm or by a sunny window if the weather is cool.

Keep Clean—to prevent irritation and infection. Carefully wash your baby's diaper area with warm water—this seems obvious, but sometimes you're in a hurry. Keep a squeeze-bottle of water with a couple teaspoons white apple-cider vinegar (it's antiseptic) at the changing station.

Bifidobacteria infantis—to normalize your baby's digestive flora and make him/her inhospitable to yeast infection. This can clear up diaper rash within a couple of days. Dosage for children: ¼ teaspoon powder mixed with a few drops water and put on your baby's tongue, two or three times daily. If you are breast-feeding, take ½ teaspoon two or three times a day yourself to pass through your milk.

Topical Calendula—to keep your baby dry, soothe irritated skin, and prevent infection. Use calendula ointment or cream instead of chemical cream.

Avoid Baby Powder, Talcum Powder, and Cornstarch—because baby powder can aggravate diaper rashes, talcum powder is naturally contaminated with small amounts of asbestos, and cornstarch can worsen a yeast infection (many babies are allergic to corn).

Hydrate—to dilute the urine so it is less irritating to the skin. Make sure your baby gets plenty of water by bottle and/or sippy-cup.

Consider Food Sensitivity/Allergy—see Chapter 11. An irritated anus is usually a sign of food sensitivity. As mentioned earlier, it is likely that your baby is reacting to one or more new foods. The probiotic *B. infantis* (see above) will really aid digestion. If you are breast-feeding, you may need to restrict your diet; if your baby is beginning to eat solid foods, you'll need to track down the offenders. The foods most commonly causing irritation are dairy products, wheat, yeasted breads, beer and wine, sugar, caffeine, and a high intake of fruit and fruit juice. Once your baby's digestive system matures, he/she will be able to tolerate most of these.

SPITTING UP/GASTROESOPHAGEAL REFLUX

The medical term for spitting up is gastroesophageal reflux. We adults don't do this much, but it's normal and typical for babies and children. The cause of this reflux in babies is usually an immature digestive system. When babies are overfed,

The Main Types of Diaper Rash

- Friction Rash—the most common type, found on the baby's waist or where the diaper meets the leg. Frequently changing diapers and "airing out" the baby resolve this quickly.

- Irritation Rash—in response to irritants such as soaps, powders, cleansers, detergent residue, wipes, and topical medicines. This type is usually found in the baby's skin-folds.

- Allergic Rash—due to food sensitivity or allergy. You may see an inflamed ring around the baby's anus. You'll need to figure out which food is causing the problem; if the baby is breast-feeding, it may be something mom is eating.

- Yeast Rash—very common, and occurs especially after use of antibiotics. This rash can be smooth, shiny, and very red and inflamed, possibly with a cottage-cheesy discharge.

- Intertrigo—in the baby's skin-folds, worsened by heat, moisture, friction, and lack of air circulation, and common in hot, moist climates. The skin looks like it has lost layers; it is very smooth, inflamed, and looks burned. Intertrigo is often complicated by an accompanying fungal, bacterial, or viral infection.

- Certain rare diseases can also cause chronic rashes. If diaper rash persists and is severe, seek medical advice.

they spit up because the sphincter muscle between their stomach and esophagus is a bit immature; eating is a new activity and this formerly unused muscle needs practice. Spitting up peaks around three to four months of age and disappears between six and twelve months of age. As long as your baby is gaining weight appropriately, spitting up is usually not any reason for concern.

Healing Options for Children Who Are Spitting Up

It's helpful to burp your baby more frequently and give smaller feedings. Remember not to put pressure on his/her tummy after feeding. (See also "Healing Options for Children with Projectile Vomiting" on page 124.)

PROJECTILE VOMITING

Unlike regular throwing up, projectile vomiting is very sudden and unusually forceful. I remember my son Kyle projectile vomiting at a restaurant and hitting a friend of mine across the table! It can be a sign that your baby's body is trying to get rid of a poison, or it can indicate a concussion after a head injury. If projectile vomiting is accompanied by diarrhea, it's probably a sign of influenza or other infection. It can also occur up to twice a day in an infant who is overfed and/or bounced around.

This problem is usually short lived, thank goodness. Frequent projectile vomiting, however, may point toward something more serious. This could be gastroesophageal reflux disease (GERD), which is similar to heartburn in adults, or pyloric stenosis, which occurs when the sphincter muscle between the small intestine and stomach is closed so tightly that digested food cannot pass through, so the food backs up and shoots out through the mouth—sometimes for a good distance. Pyloric stenosis occurs in one in 500 children, mainly boys, and usually shows up around three to four weeks of age. It appears that erythromycin, an antibiotic commonly used for ear infections, can cause pyloric stenosis in babies between three and thirteen days old, or in breast-fed infants whose mothers are taking the medication.

If your child's projectile vomiting is persistent or frequent, seek medical advice. Additional reasons to call your child's doctor are if your baby is continuously hungry, dehydrated, losing weight, or has a huge tummy bulge before the vomiting occurs. In the most extreme cases of projectile vomiting caused by pyloric stenosis or GERD, corrective surgery may be needed.

Healing Options for Children with Projectile Vomiting

See Appendix B for more details on the following nutrients, herbs, and supplements.

Consider Food Sensitivity/Allergy—see Chapter 11. It may be that your infant is intolerant of his/her formula, as many babies are sensitive to both dairy and soy, so try an elemental formula and watch for possible improvement. If you are breast-feeding, change your own diet to avoid dairy products, wheat, sugar, eggs, or other foods that you believe may be causing a problem.

Aethusa—to stop projectile vomiting by calming your child. This homeopathic remedy might be most useful for a baby who is fussy and restless. Dosage for children: a few pellets as needed under the tongue if possible, or in the mouth if not.

Digestive Enzymes—Give your baby digestive enzymes at each feeding. Dosage: ¼ teaspoon. Take as powder and mix with a bit of water or juice. You can also place it mixed with a bit of water right on your baby's tongue.

Osteopathic or Chiropractic Adjustment—to open the pyloric sphincter. These manipulations are very gentle and may be an effective cure.

Licorice Tea—to soothe and calm the digestive system. Drinking licorice tea (or teething on a licorice root) can be especially helpful in cases of GERD/gastric reflux. Dosage for children: ½–1 cup in your baby's bottle one or two times a day.

Surgery—if all else fails. Although it is a worrisome experience for the patient's parents, correction of pyloric stenosis is not a difficult surgery and solves the problem permanently.

TEETHING

Teething is a normal, natural process that begins as early as three months of age and continues intermittently until the child is about three years old. You'll know your baby is teething when he/she starts chewing on anything available, and there will probably be quite a bit of drooling. Typically, the first two teeth appear on the bottom gums between four and seven months; between one and two months later, the first upper teeth appear, soon followed by the next set on the bottom and top, and so forth. By the age of three years, most children have twenty teeth.

For many babies, teething isn't a big deal and most of the teeth come in painlessly; but for some, it can be a time of fussing, clinging, and irritability that nothing seems to soothe. You know how uncomfortable a sore inside your mouth can be? Gums can be equally tender when teeth are erupting. Your teething baby may have a mild fever, trouble sleeping, difficulty eating, or a drippy nose, or may be cranky for no reason, or may be putting fingers into his/her mouth more often. Diarrhea, high fever, and rashes, however, are not normal teething companions; if these occur along with the other symptoms of teething, contact your child's doctor.

Healing Options for Babies Who Are Teething

If the teething tablets described below don't do the trick (and they most often will), you can always use baby-formulated acetaminophen or ibuprofen for the pain and inflammation. See Appendix B for more details on the following nutrients, herbs, and supplements.

Gum Massage—with a clean finger, to relieve gum pressure. Fingers seem to have just the right texture for this to feel really good to your baby.

Teething Biscuits and Teething Toys—to relieve gum pressure. Make sure that the biscuits or whatever you give your baby to "chew" on—such as a teething ring, a toy, or the end of a hairbrush—are too big for him/her to choke on or swallow. Some teething rings are designed for chilling in the freezer or refrigerator, and the coldness helps your baby's swelling and pain; a dampened, chilled washcloth will also do.

Homeopathic Teething Tablets—to counter the various symptoms of teething. This sweet-flavored product from Hyland contains several different homeopathic remedies, each for different symptoms. Dosage for children: three or four tablets under your baby's tongue as needed. These were a lifesaver when my son Arthur was teething and fussy for days at a time. If I gave him these tablets, he'd settle down almost immediately, so I used them any time he was irritable until he was about four years old—when he ate the whole bottle! I wasn't worried, because they are completely safe, even a whole bottle; I just didn't buy any more because he was past teething.

Gummy Rub—to relieve pain by numbing the gums temporarily and reducing inflammation. This product from Gaia Herbs combines kava, meadowsweet, willow bark, clove bud, California poppy, yellow jasmine, and clove and peppermint oils. Dosage for children: apply as needed to your baby's gums with a cotton-swab or your finger.

Clove—to numb the gums. Dosage for children: ⅛ cup tea in your baby's bottle or sippy cup; one drop oil diluted in 1 tablespoon olive or safflower oil and rubbed on the gums; or ¼ teaspoon powder mixed into a paste with a few drops water and rubbed on the gums, then wiped off after one or two minutes. Use as needed.

Chamomile Tea Ice-Cubes—to calm your baby and relieve gum discomfort. Ice applied directly is a little too cold for babies, so place the cubes in a wet washcloth for your baby to suck as needed.

Wipe the Drool—to prevent rash. When your baby is sleeping, you may also want to put a diaper under his/her head to catch the drool so you won't need to change the sheets.

THRUSH/MONILIASIS

Thrush, an infection of the yeast *Candida albicans* in the mouth or throat, usually occurs in the first six months of life but can occur in older children whose immune systems are compromised. Symptoms of thrush are white, cheesy-looking patches on the tongue and gums, inside the cheeks and lips, and sometimes on the outside of the cheeks and lips. Most babies with thrush usually have a yeasty diaper rash as well (see the inset "The Main Types of Diaper Rash" on page 123). Candida can also cause a rash of red lesions or sores with pus on the thighs, vagina, or tummy. If you are breast-feeding, your baby's yeast infection can spread to your nipples; they will be red and tender and may crack or itch.

The most likely causes of thrush in an infant are antibiotics, steroid medications (such as prednisone), and a poor immune response. Dirty baby-bottle nipples and pacifiers also contribute to thrush, so clean your baby's bottle nipples and bottles in the dishwasher or with hydrogen peroxide followed by a water rinse. If you are breast-feeding, remove sugar, beer, wine, and dried fruits from your diet, increase your use of fresh garlic to several cloves daily if possible, and make sure your nipples dry out thoroughly between feedings.

Healing Options for Babies with Thrush/Moniliasis

Don't pick at your baby's thrush patches, because they don't come off easily and they leave a red mark if removed, and they can really hurt. Your baby may fuss or stop eating because of the pain; if so, do what is needed to keep him/her from becoming dehydrated, such as administering a fleet enema (a salt-water solution, available at any pharmacy, easily given to babies as a rehydrating enema). See Appendix B for more details on the following nutrients, herbs, and supplements.

Bifidobacteria infantis—to compete with candida and normalize the GI tract. Dosage for children: for ingestion, ¼ teaspoon powder mixed with a few drops water and put on your baby's tongue, three times daily; for topical use, one capsule or ½ teaspoon powder mixed in 4 ounces water and swabbed inside your baby's mouth with your finger, several times daily. If you are breast-feeding, take ½ teaspoon two or three times daily yourself to pass through your milk.

Grapefruit-Seed Extract—to help heal the infection. Highly effective against yeast infections and quite safe, it comes in a liquid form that can be diluted but is *extremely* bitter. Dosage for children: one or two drops in 1 cup water swabbed in the mouth two or three times daily. If you are breast-feeding, take it yourself at doses of up to 1,500 milligrams (mg) daily, or about ten drops per 1 cup water two or three times daily. You can also use this dilute solution in your baby's mouth (if he/she doesn't refuse it).

Nystatin—to help heal the infection. The most commonly used anti-thrush medication, nystatin is safe for babies and breast-feeding moms (unfortunately, because of nystatin's decades of use, some strains of *C. albicans* are now resistant to it). Pediatrician-prescribed, it comes in a liquid suspension that can be dabbed on the sores or put into your baby's mouth with an eyedropper or medicine syringe. Dosage for children: as directed by the doctor. If you are breast-feeding, take nystatin yourself to pass through your milk.

Gentian Violet—to help heal the infection. It works really well, but it's messy and socially awkward because it stains your baby a dark purple color, starting with the inside of his/her mouth and usually spreading from there. You can also use it for a yeast-related diaper rash; it will, however, stain cloth diapers purple. Dosage for children: dab a 1% solution on your baby's skin once; repeat if needed. If you are breast-feeding, put it on your nipples as well.

EAR INFECTION

Nearly two-thirds of our children have had an ear infection by the age of two years. Most ear infections accompany colds; you may also see additional symptoms such as tugging on an ear, fever, runny nose, excessive crying, and/or waking up many times each night. A baby with an ear infection often just seems wiped out. When infection is suspected, a pediatrician will look inside your child's ear with an otoscope to assess the ear's condition and make a diagnosis. Ear infections are scary for parents and children alike, and account for about half of all visits to pediatricians

Ear infection is also by far the most common reason for prescription of antibiotics to children in the United States. Rising costs and concern about antibiotic resistance have now focused attention on this issue. As we continue to use antibiotics indiscriminately, we find that more expensive, broader-spectrum antibiotics must be used to achieve the same results. And for a child whose infection is viral, antibiotics are useless.

Could there be another way? Yes: taking a "wait and see" approach and using ear-drops and natural solutions before resorting to antibiotic treatment. In some European countries, for example, it is standard practice to treat the symptoms of ear infection without antibiotics, reserving these drugs for later use if necessary.

Ear Pain, Fever, and When to Use Antibiotics

If your child is in pain, treat the pain appropriately. Natural healers have soothed ear pain with mullein and garlic oil for centuries. A recent study found Otikon solution, an Israeli-made formula containing garlic, mullein, calendula, and St. John's wort in an olive-oil base (similar products are widely available at health food stores), to be as useful as standard commercial ear-drops against ear pain. Tylenol is also effective. Antibiotics will *not* help with the pain of an ear infection in the first twenty-four hours, and will only alleviate it in a limited way after that.

Fever is nature's way of "burning out" an infection. The viruses and bacteria that cause infections live best at around 98.6°F, so raising the body's temperature above this point is an effective way to destroy most of them. A fever is usually a sign that your child's immune system is doing its work. If your child's fever or other symptoms are causing you concern, however, you should feel free to call your child's doctor for advice.

Robert Menselsohn, M.D., a pediatrician and author well known for common-sense wisdom, suggests the following guidelines for when to bring down a fever:

- If your infant is less than two months old and his/her temperature is higher than 100°F

- If there is fever for more than three days, or if fever is accompanied by vomiting, respiratory distress, or persistent cough

- If your child is listless or irritable, or looks seriously ill

- If your child is making strange twitching movements

If your child does require antibiotics for an ear infection, give him/her a probiotic supplement such as *Saccharomyces boulardii;* taken during the course of antibiotic treatment, this beneficial yeast can help prevent the diarrhea and the changes in gut ecology that would otherwise be caused by the medication.

Medical Perspective on Ear Infection and Antibiotics

The medical term for ear infection is otitis media (OM). The most common type is called otitis media with effusion (OME), in which the ear is pink but not inflamed, and there is germ-filled fluid in the inner ear. A more severe type is called acute otitis media (AOM), which comes on suddenly, with extreme redness inside the ear, fluid in the ear, and an inflamed eardrum.

In March 2004, the American Academy of Pediatrics and the American Academy of Family Physicians issued new guidelines on the use of antibiotics for ear infection. In summary, antibiotics are generally not recommended for OME; it is recommended that antibiotics only be given to a child whose ear infection meets the strict criteria for AOM. The details of these guidelines are as follows:

- If the diagnosis of AOM is certain and the child is between six months and two years of age, a ten-day course of antibiotics is recommended.

- If the diagnosis of AOM is uncertain, the recommendation is to treat the pain and then wait and see. If the child develops severe symptoms or a fever over 102.2°F, antibiotics are recommended.

- Antibiotics are recommended for children older than two years who have a fever above 102.2°F or who have severe symptoms and a diagnosis of AOM.

- For a child with chronic health issues that could be aggravated by an ear infection less severe than AOM, antibiotics might be recommended.

An Ounce of Prevention

Commonly recognized contributors to ear infections include attendance at a day-care center, exposure to wood-burning stoves, exposure to second-hand smoke, having food allergies, and being a formula-fed baby. Interestingly, breast-fed babies have a reduced incidence of ear infections; this could be due to the high levels of essential fatty acids and protective antibodies in breast-milk.

Here are some simple tips for preventing ear infection:

• Keep your child away from cigarette smoke.

• If your baby still drinks from a bottle, make sure his/her head is elevated when drinking.

• Massage your baby's ears and neck to keep the Eustachian tubes open.

• If your child has allergies, make his/her bedroom an allergen-free and dust-free haven for sleeping—remove down pillows and blankets, keep pets out, and clean thoroughly.

Recurring Ear Infections

If your child has recurring ear infection, your pediatrician will probably recommend antibiotics at first and finally a tympanostomy, which is the insertion of tubes into the ears to keep them open and draining. There are, however, other options. First, make sure your child is adequately nourished with a wide variety of healthful foods and a multivitamin-mineral supplement, as deficiencies in vitamins A, C, and E, zinc, and essential fatty acids have been shown to increase the risk of ear infection.

Second, have your child checked for allergies, as allergic children are more likely than others to have recurring ear infection. In addition to typical allergies such as dust, pollen, mold, and animal dander, it is essential to look for delayed reactions to specific foods with IgG and possibly IgM and IgA antibody testing. Many clinicians and researchers have documented dramatic and swift improvement in children when foods to which they are sensitive were eliminated from their diets. I have seen this many times in my own practice. Dairy products are the most common offender; according to one study, the other most common food culprits include chocolate, cola, corn, citrus, egg, soy, peanuts and other nuts, shellfish, sugar, and yeast. Environmental allergies can play a role in recurring ear infection as well.

Healing Options for Children with Ear Infection

See Appendix B for more details on the following nutrients, herbs, and supplements. The last five suggestions in the list below apply particularly to recurring ear infection.

Mullein/Garlic Oil Ear-Drops—to relieve pain associated with ear infection. These drops, which may contain additional herbs such as calendula and St. John's wort, are widely available at health food stores and some pharmacies. Dosage for children: at the first sign of ear infection, use two or three drops in the affected ear(s) three times daily or as directed on bottle.

Homeopathic Remedies—to relieve other symptoms associated with ear infection. Silica is most often used for children who have discharge from the ear and are anxious and sensitive. Belladonna is used for children who have red, hot, and inflamed conditions, typically with fever and sudden onset of symptoms; heat usually makes them feel better. Chamomile is used for children who also have pain and red cheeks; they are angry and whiny, but feel better when carried; heat makes them feel worse. Dozens of specific remedies are available, but homeopathic companies often combine the several most likely to be useful into one product that is intended to best suit whatever your child's needs may be. Dosage for children: typical doses for acute health issues are 6x, 6c, 30x, and 30c, given every thirty to sixty minutes under your child's tongue until he/she begins to improve, and then stopped. If your child stops improving, give some more.

Hydrate—to prevent dehydration (obviously). Make sure that your child gets plenty of fluids: water, herbal tea, diluted juices, broths, and the like. If you are breast-feeding, nurse often.

Vitamin C—to fight inflammation and viral infection. Choose an ascorbate product that also provides extra minerals (for example, zinc, magnesium, calcium, potassium, and/or sodium). Dosage for children: 200–1,000 mg four or five times daily, according to child's size and age.

Quercetin—instead of a decongestant, to help dry nasal passages and ear canals. Dosage for children: 100–1,000 mg three or four times daily.

Echinacea and Goldenseal—to support the immune system. These herbs can be taken preventively and also during an ear or respiratory infection. Dosage for children: varies; use according to package instructions.

Healing Options for Children with Recurring Ear Infections

Multivitamin with Zinc—to fight recurring ear infection. Dosage for children: one daily.

Essential Fatty Acids—to fight recurring ear infection. Nuts, seeds, and fish high in omega-3 fatty acids (like salmon, trout, and sardines) can provide good-quality fats in your child's diet. Supplements can be given to babies, and breast-feeding mothers can take fish oil supplements to increase the fatty acid composition of their breast-milk. Cod liver oil supplies vitamins A and D as well as essential fatty acids. Dosage for children: 1 teaspoon daily.

Consider Sensitivities/Allergies—see Chapter 11 and Appendix A. Have your child extensively tested for allergies and delayed hypersensitivities to foods, inhalants, and chemicals, and then change his/her diet and environment accordingly. You may also want to remove all dairy from your child's diet for at least a month and look for behavioral and health changes; dairy-intolerant children often have chronic stuffy noses, which clear when dairy is avoided.

Larch arabinogalactan—to fight recurring ear infection. This sugar and fiber molecule derived from the wood of the larch tree has been shown to have immune-protective effects in a wide variety of illnesses and to encourage growth of *Lactobacillus* and *Bifidobacteria* in the gut. Peter D'Adamo, N.D., reports that its use decreases incidence and severity of ear infection. Dosage: 1,000–3,000 mg daily as needed.

Chiropractic, Acupuncture, or Craniosacral Therapy—to fight recurring ear infection. Chiropractic manipulation of the spine and cranium gently gives the Eustachian tubes more room and puts the child into better alignment. Pediatric acupuncturists often use a tapping method rather than inserting needles to balance the five elements and twelve meridians, promoting a healthier energy flow and a more flexible immune response. Craniosacral therapy gently opens the Eustachian tubes.

HIRSCHSPRUNG'S DISEASE

A baby born with Hirschsprung's disease, which is also called congenital mega-colon, lacks full nerve cell development in the bowel wall. Because these nerve cells are essential for peristalsis, children with Hirschsprung's disease fail to have normal bowel movements. The sections of the bowel that don't have proper nerve distribution basically collapse and block passage of the stool, so the stool backs up, and this can eventually cause a life-threatening enterocolitis infection.

One in 5,000 children has Hirschsprung's disease. It is often apparent soon after birth; 80 percent of cases are diagnosed within the first six weeks of life, and the rest usually by the age of five years. It occurs four times more often in boys than in girls, and more often in children with Down's syndrome. There is a genetic component, in that a child who has a sibling with Hirschsprung's disease has a 3 to

12 percent chance of having it too; the likelihood also increases if a parent, especially the mother, has the disease.

Fortunately, Hirschsprung's disease usually occurs only in a part of the large intestine, such as the last foot or two of the colon and rectum, with the rest being normal tissue; only rarely is it found in the entire colon. There is, however, a wide variation in the disease's presentation and severity. Doctors begin to suspect the problem if babies don't pass their first sticky, tarry bowel movement, called meconium, within twenty-four to forty-eight hours after birth. Bowel obstruction can also be indicated by a bloated belly and vomiting after an infant's very first feedings.

Some children display symptoms more gradually, with constipation, diarrhea, anemia, and failure to grow properly. Some are only mildly affected, with chronic constipation, bloated bellies, visible peristalsis, and ribbonlike, foul-smelling stools. These children are commonly poorly nourished and anemic, but don't otherwise seem ill, and they can be fairly old before the illness is discovered. In the most severe cases, serious bowel infection and inflammation develop, with explosive watery diarrhea, exhaustion, and fever; if your child has these symptoms, see his/her doctor immediately.

Medical Testing for Children with Hirschsprung's Disease

First, a barium-enema X-ray is used to look for the telltale collapsed segment(s) of the bowel. If that is seen, a small sample of intestinal tissue taken from an inch above the anus is examined; if the nerve ganglia are not developed, a diagnosis of Hirschsprung's disease is made. A painless anorectal manometry or motility test, in which a small, plastic tube is inserted into the child's rectum to measure rectal contractions, is often used to confirm the diagnosis.

Healing Options for Children with Hirschsprung's Disease

Once diagnosed, Hirschsprung's disease is always treated surgically. The affected part of the bowel is removed and the healthy segments are joined together. Seventy to 85 percent of these surgical cases are a complete success and put an end to the issue. Fifteen to 20 percent of cases, however, continue with chronic constipation, fecal incontinence, and fecal soiling, and 5 to 10 percent entail ongoing, severe constipation and encopresis. Children with Down's syndrome tend to have poorer resolution of these problems than other children do.

There is virtually no research on alternatives to surgery. However, if this were my child, I'd begin with probiotic digestive enzyme and proteolytic enzyme supplements to see if it might normalize the tissues. One 1999 study indicated that using probiotic supplements in children with Hirschsprung's disease (and other bowel-obstructive illnesses) increased the amount of helpful bifidobacteria, lowered the amount of potentially pathogenic bacteria, and reduced levels of endotoxins, which are toxic substances produced inside the body, often by disease-causing bacteria. That study used the probiotics *Streptococcus faecalis, Clostridium butyricum,* and *Bacillus mesentericus;* as these are not readily available to the public, try *Bifido-bacteria infantis.* (See also "Healing Options for Children with Constipation" on page 163.)

CHAPTER 14

Issues of the Mouth, Esophagus, and Stomach

W e'll start at the mouth and move south. The health of teeth, tongue, and gums is integral to the rest of the digestive process. Enzymes in saliva begin digesting carbohydrates, chewing facilitates swallowing and signals the brain to tell the stomach that food is on the way, and thorough chewing is an important aid to digestion. As the mouth is our first point of contact with ingested allergens, oral irritation and inflammation can be signs of food or chemical sensitivities or allergies. Careful investigation of the mouth yields additional helpful information about a person's nutritional status. Cracks along the center of the tongue, for example, indicate a need for B-complex vitamins; scalloped tongue can indicate a need for folic acid; and bleeding gums indicate a need for vitamin C and bioflavonoids.

CANKER SORES/MOUTH ULCERS

Canker sores, also called aphthous stomatitis or aphthous ulcers, are common in children. Usually found inside the mouth, these small red dots eventually produce a white-yellowish head, and they really hurt. Often, the sores result from imbalanced intestinal flora, food sensitivities/allergies, stress, hormonal changes, and nutritional deficiencies. In one study of people with a low zinc level or low zinc-to-copper ratio, zinc supplementation helped heal canker sores 81 percent of the time. Deficiencies in vitamins B_1, B_2, B_6, and B_{12} and folic acid have been associated with recurrent canker sores, and three months of supplementation was shown to significantly improve mouth ulcers in people with B-complex deficiencies. Canker sores are also sometimes triggered by eating high-sugar, high-acid foods like pineapples, citrus, and tomatoes.

Because people with celiac disease often have chronic mouth sores, a considerable amount of research has focused on the connection between these sores and intolerance of gluten, a protein fraction found in several grains. About 25 percent of people with chronic canker sores have elevated antibodies to gluten, indicating a specific sensitivity; and when gluten is avoided, their mouth ulcers go away.

Healing Options for Children with Canker Sores/Mouth Ulcers

Your child may not want to eat when his/her mouth hurts, so offer soups and soft steamed vegetables, or give nutritious beverages through a straw. If the sores don't resolve after several weeks, take your child to a doctor and ask the physician to test for anemia, as some children with recurrent canker sores become anemic. This anemia usually responds to iron supplementation. Floradix is a gentle, effective, herbal iron supplement; cooking in cast-iron pots is also an easy way to add iron to your child's diet. See Appendix B for more details on the following nutrients, herbs, and supplements.

Consider Chemical Sensitivity/Allergy—see Chapters 2 and 11. To determine whether toothpaste, mouthwash, or flavored dental floss is the source of the problem, switch brands or have your child brush with water only.

Consider Food Sensitivity/Allergy—see Chapter 11. Canker sores are often related to food sensitivities, so investigate carefully with the elimination/provocation diet and/or blood testing. Gluten-avoidance, in particular, is certainly worth a try.

Lactobacillus acidophilus—to prevent and treat canker sores. Dosage for children: one or two capsules, or ¼ – ½ teaspoon powder, two or three times daily.

B-Complex Vitamins—to address possible underlying nutrient deficiencies. Dosage for children: one daily supplement containing 10–50 milligrams (mg) of most of the B-complex vitamins.

Chlorophyll—to soothe and heal canker sores. Dosage for children: one or two tablets two or three times daily; the liquid form can be gargled or applied directly to the sores two or three times daily.

Zinc—to help the body heal wounds and to support tissue growth in children. Dosage for children: 5–10 mg daily.

Black Teabag Poultice—to draw out infection and soothe the tissue. Put a wet teabag right on the sore (the tea's tannins do the job).

Ice—to soothe the pain and dry canker sores quickly. Apply directly, either once a day for forty-five minutes or several times a day for five minutes each, and allow the resulting scab to heal.

Myrrh—to soothe canker sore pain. Often combined with goldenseal (below). Dosage for children: one to four capsules daily; alternatively, use myrrh chewing gum or apply a topical glycerin tincture of myrrh as needed.

Goldenseal Tea—to soothe canker sore pain. Dosage for children: ½ cup twice daily; alternatively, dab directly on sores as needed.

Castor Oil—on a cotton swab, to heal canker sores. An old topical remedy from Edgar Cayce.

THRUSH/MONILIASIS

See Chapters 6 and 13.

EOSINOPHILIC ESOPHAGITIS AND/OR EOSINOPHILIC GASTROENTERITIS

Eosinophilic esophagitis (EE) is a chronic inflammatory condition of the esophagus. Officially identified in 1993, this disease is emerging in many developed countries including the United States, England, Japan, Spain, Australia, Switzerland, and Italy. It first came to medical attention in children, but now that physicians are looking, they are finding EE in adults as well. One article suggests that EE is becoming the most prevalent inflammatory digestive condition, more common than Crohn's disease or ulcerative colitis. Despite this explosion, very little information on the disease is available, and much of the research on EE so far has gone into simply figuring out what the problem is and how to recognize it. Because the symptoms are similar to those of gastroesophageal reflux and gastroesophageal reflux disease, many children with EE are incorrectly diagnosed and treated for those other conditions instead.

Symptoms of EE in children include vomiting, stomach or chest pain, regurgitation, painful swallowing, and nausea. Children may not want to eat because it hurts, and scarring from untreated EE can make it difficult to swallow, so some of these children are under-height and underweight because they fail to eat enough. The disease is diagnosed by an endoscopy, which is a visual check using a scope down the esophagus, followed by a biopsy to extract a tissue sample for further examination. Many children with EE have white specks or plaques in the esophagus, which tend to occur when the condition is severe.

Eosinophilic esophagitis is being called "asthma of the esophagus" because allergic reactions to foods and also environment allergens such as mold, dust, and pollen appear to play a big role; and interestingly, one study found asthma in one-third of children with EE. Children with EE are advised to avoid eating all foods to which they are allergic. Physicians also encourage the use of the Elemental Diet, a manufactured, nonallergenic food product that supplies essential nutrients; children with EE who eat only this product for several months show great improvement in symptoms and at repeat endoscopy and biopsy.

One study showed an atypically alkaline esophageal environment in nine children with EE. More research on this subject is needed, but if your child's pH is low, you may wish to try increasing his/her level of stomach acid (see page 140) to see whether this relieves the symptoms.

My current small client with EE is a little boy whose problems began immediately after an immunization—a story commonly heard from parents of autistic children. I hypothesize that children with EE have detoxification problems like children with autism do, but that they manifest a different set of symptoms. The theory that heavy metals such as mercury play a role in this problem will either be validated or tossed out as it is put to the test.

Eosinophilic gastroenteritis (EG) is similar to EE, but takes place in the stomach and/or small intestine rather than in the esophagus. The condition is likewise called eosinophilic gastritis when it occurs only in the stomach and eosinophilic enteritis when it is confined to the small intestine. First identified in 1937 by a researcher named Kaijser, EG is far less prevalent than EE, with only about 300 cases diagnosed since Kaijser's time.

As in EE, typical symptoms of EG include abdominal pain, diarrhea, and pain with swallowing; cramping and abdominal pain may be accompanied by nausea and vomiting; and a child with EG will often refuse to eat because it hurts. Half of the children with EG have a history of eczema, asthma, or food allergies. Many of them also have more typical allergies to dust, pollen, and mold. Are you noticing a theme here? Again, as in EE, it is essential to test children with EG for food allergies and sensitivities, especially to gluten and dairy products.

Enzymes to the Rescue for Eosinophilic Conditions?

Forty-one years ago, when Dr. DicQie Fuller's baby daughter Colleen was failing to thrive, Dr. Fuller was told Colleen was going to die of eosinophilic gastritis. She began giving her baby supplemental digestive and proteolytic enzymes—and Colleen has been living healthfully ever since. Meanwhile, Dr. Fuller's passion for saving her daughter's life led her to found an enzyme supplement company in the hopes of providing others with the same benefits.

Functional Laboratory Testing for Children with Eosinophilic Esophagitis and/or Eosinophilic Gastroenteritis

If EE or EG is suspected, your child's gut health should be explored with comprehensive testing, because there is little understanding of the disease's cause(s). Regular IgE scratch-tests or modified RASTs do not reveal the allergies in most cases, so follow-up testing for delayed hypersensitivities is advised. See Appendix A for details on testing.

1. Comprehensive digestive and stool analysis with parasite screening

2. Food sensitivity/allergy test(s)

3. Provoked urine test for heavy metals

4. Intestinal permeability test

5. pH test, quantitative fluid analysis, or Heidelberg test

Healing Options for Children with Eosinophilic Esophagitis and/or Eosinophilic Gastroenteritis

Drugs currently used for EE include steroid medications, cromolyn sodium, and leukotriene inhibitors. Initial research shows that even with medication, restriction of allergy-inducing foods is still necessary to achieve full benefit. The natural healing options presented herein are my own ideas, as no research has been conducted on natural therapies for EE. See Appendix B for more details on the following nutrients, herbs, and supplements.

Elimination/Provocation Diet—see Chapter 11. The most obvious foods to eliminate are dairy, eggs, soy, corn, wheat, beef, nuts, fish, and shellfish, in conjunction with IgG and IgE testing.

Digestive Enzymes—to prevent foods from becoming allergens by promoting their complete digestion. Dosage for children: one capsule each time your child eats; if your baby is bottle-feeding, add one capsule to each bottle.

Proteolytic Enzymes—to minimize inflammation and calm the immune system by cleaning up proteins (possible antigens) in the bloodstream. Dosage for children: one to three capsules two or three times daily on an empty stomach. The best times are often upon rising and before bed.

Quercetin—to diminish, relieve, and prevent allergy symptoms and protect esophageal tissue. Dosage for children: 200–1,000 mg three to six times daily, according to child's size and symptom severity. May be combined with grapeseed extract (pycnogenol).

Probiotics—to balance gut ecology and immune system function. Dosage for children: ¼–½ teaspoon two or three times daily, or one or two capsules twice daily.

Consider Heavy-Metal Toxicity—see Chapter 2 and Appendix A.

Deglycyrrhized Licorice—to soothe inflammation and stimulate repair. Dosage for children: one or two tablets or capsules before meals. You could also consider using the demulcent herbs marshmallow, meadowsweet, and slippery elm.

Folic Acid—to protect mucous membranes from inflammation elsewhere in the gastrointestinal tract. Dosage for children: 0.8 micrograms–10 mg daily.

Vinegar or Betaine HCl—to relieve symptoms by increasing stomach acid. Dilute one part apple-cider vinegar in ten parts water and sweeten with honey or apple juice; alternatively, use betaine HCl. If the treatment produces a heartburn sensation, this indicates that the child does *not* need more HCl (if the burning is uncomfortable, neutralize the acid by giving some milk, baking soda in water, or Alka Seltzer). If EE symptoms are improved, however, the child does need more HCl. Dosage for children: vinegar mixture, 1–2 teaspoons for babies, $1/4$ cup for toddlers, and $1/2$–1 cup for older children with protein containing meals; betaine HCl, one-half to two tablets with protein-containing meals as needed.

GASTROESOPHAGEAL REFLUX AND/OR HIATAL HERNIA

The esophageal sphincter is supposed to keep the stomach contents in place, but if the sphincter relaxes, acid can be pushed back up into the esophagus, causing heartburn. This is not exclusively an adult condition; in fact, gastroesophageal reflux disease (GERD) in children and teenagers is widely under-diagnosed. It has not been well examined in children, but one study estimates that about 3 to 5 percent of children and teenagers experience GERD.

In children, the most common symptoms of GERD are vomiting, chronic cough, and respiratory problems including asthma. Your child may report a painful or burning feeling in the stomach area or chest, or tell you that it hurts to eat, or complain of burping and a sour liquid that comes back into his/her mouth. You may notice that your child has sour breath or a scratchy voice, or is clearing his/her throat a lot. He/she may also complain of stomachache, sore throat, trouble swallowing, or other symptoms.

In a child with GERD, it's important to investigate food allergies and/or sensitivities as a possible cause. A recent study found that allergy to cow's milk alone played a role in the reflux problems of almost 25 percent of the children tested. If you suspect that your child has GERD, the National Institute of Diabetes and Digestive and Kidney Disease recommends eliminating the following foods and food groups from his/her diet to discover which ones contribute to the symptoms:

- Caffeinated drinks
- Chocolate
- Citrus fruits
- Fatty and fried foods
- Garlic and onions
- Mint flavorings
- Spicy foods
- Tomato-based foods like spaghetti sauce, chili, and pizza

Some children with GERD have an infection of *Helicobacter pylori,* the bacteria implicated in stomach and duodenal ulcers. Studies indicate that low stomach hydrochloric acid levels contribute to the indicidence of *H. pylori* infections. Treatment with antibiotics and bismuth-containing supplements or drugs can cure the infection, but research results conflict as to whether eradicating this bacteria will help with gastroesophageal reflux; in a recent study, treating *H. pylori* had no correlation with relieving the children's pain and GERD symptoms. Some researchers feel that *H. pylori* may even be protective.

In many infants and children, GERD is due to a constriction called a hiatal hernia. Hiatal hernia occurs when a portion of the stomach gets pushed through the diaphragm and into the chest cavity; this can happen, for example, during a newborn's passage through the birth canal. It may or may not cause symptoms, but when it does, the most common is heartburn. Chiropractic or osteopathic therapy may be useful to correct a hiatal hernia. GERD is also found in infants and children who have neurological problems that interfere with muscle contraction and relaxation. Genetics probably play a role as well, as children of parents with GERD are more likely to experience it.

Functional Laboratory Testing for Children with Gastroesophageal Reflux and/or Hiatal Hernia

Testing for specific food allergies and sensitivities is recommended. See Appendix A for details on testing including:

1. Food allergy tests (modified RAST) for IgE antibodies

2. Food sensitivity tests by ELISA for IgE, IgG, and possibly IgM and IgA antibodies

3. *H. pylori* test

Healing Options for Children with Gastroesophageal Reflux and/or Hiatal Hernia

Investigate possible food intolerances and try physical manipulation therapies before resorting to medications. If blood and scratch tests show that sensitivities or allergies are contributing to the problem, eliminate the culprits from your child's diet for at least two weeks; if his/her symptoms improve, continue to avoid those foods and food groups for at least four months; then, retest.

Currently, the medications most frequently used for GERD are protein pump inhibitors (PPIs) that block acid production in the stomach. Stomach acid, however, is needed for proper absorption of minerals such as calcium, magnesium, iron, copper, and zinc. Long-term use of PPIs has been associated with anemia.

There is also concern about bacterial overgrowth in the small intestine and over-secretion of the protein-splitting enzyme gastrin by the stomach; high amounts of gastrin (hypergastrinemia) are found in 10 percent of people with autoimmune illnesses.

F. Batmanghelidj, M.D., author of *Your Body's Many Cries for Water* (Falls Church, VA: Global Health Solutions, 1995), suggests that heartburn and GERD can be treated easily by drinking more water. While a prisoner in an Iranian jail, Dr. Batmanghelidj had very few tools available to help fellow inmates, and he found that simply having them drink more water could cure many conditions including ulcers and heartburn.

Although the use of glutamine for treating heartburn is unstudied so far, it makes theoretical sense, as glutamine is effective in healing stomach ulcers, irritable bowel syndrome, and ulcerative bowel diseases. See Appendix B for more details on the following nutrients, herbs, and supplements.

Osteopathic or Chiropractic Adjustment—to put a hiatal hernia back in place. One or two gentle cranial-sacral adjustments can often solve the problem, especially in children.

Hydrate—by having your child drink more water. It's easy, nontoxic, and worth trying.

Consider Food Sensitivity/Allergy—see Chapter 11. This is often overlooked, but may be the source of the problem.

Try HCI—give your child some betaine HCI with a protein-containing meal. Low stomach HCI can be the cause of GERD. If your child experiences a warm or burning sensation, he/she has adequate HCI levels. If not, add more HCI until that occurs. Correct dosage is the highest amount that does not cause "burning." The burning can be neutralized with milk or ½ teaspoon baking soda in water.

Dietary Changes—to emphasize healthful foods and avoid problematic foods. Increase fruits, vegetables, grains, beans, and high-fiber foods. Acidic drinks and foods like tomato and citrus are more likely to cause heartburn, and you may discover that your child has additional "trigger foods." Caffeinated beverages and soft drinks often worsen GERD.

Elevate the Head of Your Child's Bed—to alleviate nighttime heartburn symptoms. Although you might expect the slant to feel strange, it's barely noticeable, and it helps.

Consider Helicobacter pylori Infection—although it is unclear whether curing this infection will help with GERD symptoms (see page 140).

Deglycyrrhized Licorice—to soothe and heal esophageal and stomach inflammation, and also to inhibit the growth of *H. pylori.* Dosage for children: one to six chewable tablets or capsules daily before meals, according to child's size and age.

Cabbage Juice—to help cure heartburn. Its high glutamine content (see below) is probably the key to its success. Dosage for children: 1–2 ounces daily. *Note:* Cabbage juice has a strong flavor, so dilute with other vegetable juices or your child won't drink it.

Glutamine—to heal the GI tract. Dosage for children: 1–8 grams daily, according to child's age.

Slippery Elm—to soothe mucous membranes. Drink as a tea, chew on the bark, or suck on lozenges as needed. Large amounts can be used without harm.

Lobelia—to promote relaxation and soothe pain. Dosage for children: internally, one to three drops tincture as needed; externally, massage tincture onto the painful area as needed.

Ginger Tea—to provide temporary relief. Dosage for children: drink regularly and freely (hot or cold).

Meadowsweet Tea—to soothe inflamed mucous membranes. Dosage for children: 3 cups daily.

NAUSEA AND VOMITING

Kids generally vomit more than adults do. A single incidence of nausea or vomiting isn't cause for much concern. Usually, a vomiting child is sick, perhaps with a bacterial or viral infection, and may also have diarrhea and fever. Vomiting and diarrhea could easily be due to food poisoning, which usually won't induce fever. If your child isn't sick, explore the possibility of accidental poisoning, as kids are curious and often eat and drink poisonous things. Prolonged or chronic nausea or vomiting, of course, is something to investigate. In infants, the first thing to look at is formula, as vomiting may be due to food intolerance, and sometimes changing the type of formula will solve the problem. Toddlers and children can also vomit or experience nausea for emotional reasons such as overexcitement, nervousness, or fear; they react with their tummies to things they don't fully understand or can't express. Talking or counseling can help dramatically.

Healing Options for Children with Nausea and Vomiting

It's important to increase fluids so your child doesn't get dehydrated from repeated vomiting. With an infant, in some cases, you may want to increase fluids rectally by giving a fleet enema. If vomiting persists for more than six hours, if there is blood in the vomit, or if your child's condition seems to worsen, call his/her doctor. (See also "Projectile Vomiting" on page 123.) See Appendix B for more details on the following nutrients, herbs, and supplements.

Hydrate—with sips of water, ginger-ale, or ginger tea (see Ginger, below). You might find that your child likes sucking on ice chips. Give clear chicken, beef, or vegetable broths. If you are breast-feeding, feed often. You'll know your child is on the mend when he/she drinks heartily.

Liquid Diet, then Bland Diet—to settle the stomach. Give your child only liquids for a few hours, and then ask if he/she would like something to eat. Kids usually know when they are ready. Bland foods such as toast, oatmeal, banana, yogurt, and applesauce are all very easy to digest, and as your child feels better, he/she will eat more.

Ginger—to prevent and ease nausea. If your child is sick, ginger tea is best. Dosage for children: 4 cups daily. If nausea is chronic, small pieces of candied ginger may be useful. Candied ginger is also great to keep around for motion-sickness.

Umeboshi Plum—to soothe the stomach and alkalize the body. Dosage for children: up to 3 cups tea daily; older children may prefer to eat the plums whole.

Curing Pills—for nausea, vomiting, and upset stomach. This is a traditional Chinese remedy. Dosage for children: varies according to child's age; use as directed on label.

Honey—to settle the stomach. Dosage for children: 1 teaspoon raw honey (but remember, no honey for babies under the age of one year).

Slippery Elm—to soothe the stomach. Drink as tea, chew the bark, or suck on lozenges. Dosage for children: 1–3 cups tea daily (can be sweetened with honey); other forms as needed.

Lactobacillus acidophilus and Bifidobacteria infantis—to calm the digestive system by restoring its ecological balance, and to speed healing. Dosage for children: one or two capsules, or $\frac{1}{4}$–$\frac{1}{2}$ teaspoon powder, twice daily. If you are breast-feeding, take some yourself as well to pass through your breast-milk.

Deglycyrrhized Licorice—to soothe the stomach. Dosage for children: 1 cup tea three times daily; older children can also suck on a licorice root.

CHAPTER 15

Issues of the Small Intestine

The most common symptoms of small intestinal problems are gas, bloating, and cramping. There are, however, many other health issues that occur in the small intestine. This organ has a dual function: to allow for absorption of nutrients while keeping out any harmful substances. When the intestinal barrier gets "leaky," a wide variety of health problems can occur. Celiac disease is one result of a breach in gut barrier function.

CELIAC DISEASE/SPRUE/GLUTEN INTOLERANCE

An autoimmune illness, celiac disease features an inability to properly digest gluten, which is a protein fraction found in several types of grain (including wheat, rye, barley, oats, millet, and spelt). When people with this disease eat gluten-containing foods, the lining of the small intestine becomes damaged, and the flattening of villi and microvilli makes it difficult to absorb the remaining food. Previously thought to be rare, this condition is now believed to occur in one in 100–200 people, and new studies indicate that many people without obvious symptoms have subclinical celiac disease. Four out of five people with the disease have never been diagnosed, and it is often mistaken for irritable bowel syndrome or other problems. Celiac disease has long been thought to be a digestive disorder. Newer research shows that many people with celiac disease have no digestive symptoms at all. People who have autoimmune diseases, like type 1 diabetes, osteoporosis, lupus, and autoimmune thyroiditis are at greater risk to have celiac disease. Many people also experience joint problems, migraines, failure to gain weight, behavior and learning issues in children, and more. (See the inset "Symptoms of Celiac Disease" on page 147.)

Celiac disease is also called celiac sprue, non-tropical sprue, or gluten-sensitive enteropathy. It occurs about twice as often in women as in men and may affect several family members. It rarely occurs among people of African, Jewish,

Celiac Disease and Autoimmunity: A Protein Connection?

It has recently been shown that the level of a protein called zonulin is elevated during active stages of celiac disease. It appears that this protein may be produced by the body in response to bacteria. Zonulin opens the tight junctions between cells of the gut lining, causing an increased permeability that enables large gluten molecules to enter the bloodstream directly from the intestinal tract. Zonulin has also been implicated in autoimmune conditions including diabetes, multiple sclerosis, and rheumatoid arthritis. This interesting new research may eventually shed light on the etiology and treatment of celiac and other diseases.

Mediterranean, or Asian descent, mainly affecting people of northwestern-European ancestry. The incidence of celiac disease is high in people with autoimmune diseases including lupus, insulin-dependent diabetes, liver disease, rheumatoid arthritis, and Sjogren's syndrome.

Celiac disease is usually recognized early in childhood, but may disappear in adolescence and reappear later in adulthood. Its symptoms are recurring attacks of diarrhea or constipation, abdominal cramping, bloating, gas, failure to grow, and an irritable personality. Infants may show failure to thrive. (Interestingly, breast-feeding delays the development of the disease, and research shows that the longer a baby is breast-fed, the greater the preventive benefit.) In children, the most common symptom is irritability. Celiac disease can also lead to anemia, so a child with chronic anemia should be checked for celiac disease. In a recent study, half of the children tested for anemia were indeed anemic, and a small percentage of those children also had undiagnosed celiac disease.

The disease is incurable, but the great news is that if people with celiac disease avoid gluten, their intestinal lining repairs itself, and improvements begin within the first week or two of gluten avoidance. Untreated celiac disease, however, can lead to long-term complications including lymphoma, adenocarcinoma, osteoporosis, being shorter than you would have been otherwise, seizure disorders, miscarriage, and, in offspring, congenital birth defects such as neural tube defect. Other consequences of celiac disease can be diminished calcium reserves, iron-deficiency anemia, and other mineral deficiencies, as well as poor fat absorption and low levels of fat-soluble nutrients: vitamins A, B_6, D, E, and K, folic acid, zinc, and selenium.

It appears that there are several types of gluten sensitivity with similar symptoms but with different treatments and outcomes:

Symptoms of Celiac Disease

Digestive Symptoms

- Abdominal pain
- Abdominal distention, bloating, gas, indigestion
- Constipation
- Decreased appetite (may also be increased or unchanged)
- Diarrhea
- Nausea and vomiting
- Lactose intolerance (common upon diagnosis; usually resolves following treatment)
- Pale stools
- Stools that float, are foul smelling, bloody, or "fatty"
- Weight loss, unexplained (although people can be overweight or of normal weight upon diagnosis)

Non-Digestive Symptoms

- Anemia
- Asthma
- Behavioral changes
- Bone pain
- Bone disease
- Bruising easily
- Dental enamel defects and discoloration
- Depression
- Developmental delay
- Diabetes, type 1
- Eczema
- Fatigue
- Growth delay in children
- Hair loss
- Hearing loss
- Hypoglycemia (low blood sugar)
- Irregular menstrual cycles
- Irritability
- Joint pain
- Learning disorders
- Malnutrition/Malabsorption
- Migraine headaches
- Mouth ulcers
- Muscle cramps
- Neurological problems
- No symptoms at all
- Nosebleed
- Numbness
- Psoriasis
- Schizophrenia
- Seizures
- Short stature, unexplained
- Shortness of breath (due to anemia)
- Skin disorders (dermatitis herpetiformis)
- Swelling, general or abdominal
- Tingling
- Tooth enamel loss
- Vitamin or mineral deficiency, single or multiple nutrient (for example, iron, folate, vitamin K)
- Weight loss, difficulty gaining weight

- People with celiac disease must avoid gluten-containing foods for life.

- People with tropical sprue, caused by an infection or toxin, are generally treated with antibiotics and, over time, can consume gluten-containing foods without further problems.

- People with gluten sensitivity caused by leaky gut syndrome often find that, after avoiding gluten for four to six months and following a nutritional program to support intestinal healing and friendly flora, they can resume eating grain and gluten-containing products without further problems.

It's not easy to avoid gluten when the standard American diet depends so heavily on wheat and other grains. In addition to the obvious sources, many products contain "hidden" gluten: salad dressings, some hot-dogs, ice cream, bouillon cubes, chocolate, and foods containing hydrolyzed vegetable protein, for a start (see the inset "Foods That May Contain Hidden Gluten" below for more examples). Fortunately, excellent gluten-free breads, pastas, crackers, pancake mixes, cereals, and cookies are now available. A new home test-kit to identify gluten-containing foods may soon be on the market.

Foods That May Contain Hidden Gluten

- Hydrolyzed and/or texturized vegetable protein: may contain wheat

- Barley malt

- Starch (when listed in the ingredient list): if it doesn't say "cornstarch," it may contain gluten

- Desserts: most cakes, cookies, and muffins, and also ice cream that contains gluten stabilizers

- Meats: luncheon meats, hot-dogs, and sausages may contain grains, and self-basting turkeys contain hydrolyzed vegetable protein (see above)

- Cheese and dairy: some processed cheeses contain wheat flour and/or oat gum

- Pasta: most pasta is wheat; semolina wheat contains a high level of gluten

- Miscellaneous (some brands contain gliadin, some don't): curry powder, most white pepper, dry seasoning mixes, gravy mixes and extracts, meat condiments, catsup, chewing gum, pie fillings, baked beans, baking powders, salad dressings, sandwich spreads, muesli, cereals, instant coffee, breadcrumbs, vanilla and other flavorings made with alcohol, and most dips

About half of all people with celiac disease are also lactose intolerant at the time of diagnosis. Because lactase, the enzyme required to split lactose, is produced at the tips of the villi, people with untreated celiac disease and damaged villi can't manufacture lactase. Once a gluten-free diet is adopted and the intestinal lining repairs itself, some of these people will be able to tolerate dairy products. Remember, though, that about 70 percent of people in general are lactose intolerant, so many people with controlled celiac disease will still be affected by dairy products.

Functional Laboratory Testing for Children with Celiac Disease/Sprue/Gluten Intolerance

Traditionally, physicians have diagnosed celiac disease by excluding other possibilities and then performing an endoscopic examination of the small intestine and taking a bit of tissue (biopsy), which is very invasive. The rectal gluten-sensitivity challenge is a newer, less-invasive, and very accurate test, but it is not widely available. New tests for antiendomysial, antigliadin, and transglutaminase antibodies more easily diagnose the disease; the antiendomysial test seems most accurate, but none of these tests is 100-percent accurate, so it would be best to have at least two of them for confirmation.

If celiac disease is suspected, IgE and IgG antibody testing for wheat, oats, rye, barley, gluten, and gliadin are required. Gluten antibodies are positive in people with celiac disease and gluten intolerance, and additional food sensitivities are likely. IgA levels are also higher in people with celiac disease, but a negative result does not always rule out the condition. Celiac disease causes malabsorption, and several labs offer tests to help determine which nutrients should be supplemented. See Appendix A for details on testing. Available tests include:

1. Antiendomysial, antigliaden, and tissue transglutaminase antibody tests

2. Food sensitivity/allergy test(s)

3. Intestinal permeability test

4. Iron status/nutrient status test

5. Comprehensive digestive and stool analysis with parasite screening

6. Lactose intolerance test

7. Vitamin D test

Healing Options for Children with Celiac Disease/Sprue/Gluten Intolerance

For many people, avoiding gluten leads to quick relief in three to four days, although complete healing will take longer. If your child doesn't feel better in four to six weeks, investigate other factors that may be delaying the process.

Supplementation is often necessary to counter the malnutrition that can result from celiac disease. Although no specific research has been conducted on therapeutic use of gut-healing nutrients in celiac disease, clinical experience with celiac and other diarrheal illnesses indicates the utility of these nutrients, and nutritional therapies may speed healing. See Appendix B for more details on the following nutrients, herbs, and supplements.

Avoid Gluten—to stop the irritation and allow the intestinal lining to heal. It is essential to read all food labels carefully and become an expert at reading between the lines. Some children with celiac disease may be able to tolerate oats, whereas others may not be able to eat oats until adulthood; those who can tolerate them often feel better, have better nutritional status, are more satisfied with their diet, and have higher overall fiber and higher nutrient intake. But introduction of oats can cause gas at first, so do it gradually and be patient.

Digestive Enzymes—to enhance digestive function. Dosage for children: one or two capsules with each meal. Specific amylases (starch-digesting enzymes) can be of particular benefit.

Probiotics—to enhance digestive function. Look for lactobacillus and bifidobacteria species; for small children, focus on *Bifidobacteria infantis*. Dosage for children: one capsule, or ¼–½ teaspoon powder, with meals.

Glutamine—to heal the intestinal lining. Dosage for children: powder, 2–20 grams daily, in water or juice.

Gamma-Oryzanol—to heal the intestinal lining. Dosage for children: capsules, 25–100 mg three times daily.

Daily Multivitamin-Mineral Supplement—to counter the nutrient deficiencies often found in people with celiac disease. *Note:* Be sure the supplement is hypoallergenic and contains no grains or dairy.

FLATULENCE/INTESTINAL GAS

It's normal to have gas. In fact, we "pass gas" an average of ten to fifteen times a day. Most of it comes from swallowed air, which we take in by chewing gum, drinking carbonated beverages, and eating whipped foods like egg whites and whipped cream. Babies, of course, swallow a lot of air, and need to be burped after feeding. The gas we pass is mainly nitrogen (up to 90 percent), carbon dioxide, and oxygen, which are odorless, but fermentation of small pieces of food undigested by our intestinal bacteria also produces stinky gases like methane and hydrogen sulfide. Other substances like butyric acid, cadaverine, and putrescine, even in tiny amounts, can give gas a mighty odor.

Although some gas is normal, if your child continually has really stinky gas and lots of it, it's good to explore the possible causes. Intestinal gas can be an uncomfortable sign that something is out of balance. Various foods have different effects on different children; extra gassiness is often a result of being lactose intolerant and eating dairy products, having food sensitivities (especially to wheat and other grains), or switching from a highly processed diet to a more natural, high-fiber diet. Cucumbers, celery, apples, carrots, onions, and garlic are commonly known to cause an abundance of gas, and sulfur-containing foods such as beans, dried sulfured fruits, and vegetables in the cabbage family can produce that rotten-egg odor. Your child's flatulence may also be due to insufficient levels of hydrochloric acid, intestinal flora, or pancreatic enzymes, due to a problematic dysbiosis or parasite.

Functional Laboratory Testing for Children with Flatulence/Intestinal Gas

See Appendix A for details on testing. Available tests include:

1. Small bowel bacterial overgrowth test

2. Comprehensive digestive and stool analysis with parasite screening

3. Food sensitivity/allergy test(s)

4. Lactose intolerance test

Healing Options for Children with Flatulence/Intestinal Gas

See Appendix B for more details on the following nutrients, herbs, and supplements.

Chew Well and Eat Slowly—to promote thorough digestion. No gulping!

Avoid Chewing Gum and Carbonated Beverages—to prevent the swallowing of extra air.

Consider Lactose Intolerance—see Appendix A. Eliminate all dairy products and all foods containing "hidden" dairy products (see page 264) from your child's diet for at least two weeks and see whether he/she improves.

Probiotics—to reestablish intestinal microbial balance and improve digestion. Look for lactobacillus and bifidobacteria species; for small children, focus on *Bifidobacteria infantis*. Dosage for children: one or two capsules or $\frac{1}{4}$–$\frac{1}{2}$ teaspoon powder, two or three times daily on an empty stomach. *Note:* The powder can be mixed with a cold beverage, but a hot liquid will kill the flora in the supplement.

High-Fiber Diet—to help regulate your child's digestion. High-fiber foods include whole grains, beans, and many fruits and vegetables (see Chapter 9). Increasing fiber intake too dramatically or quickly, however, can cause our flora to "go wild" with fermentation, which can produce a lot of gas and discomfort. Increase your child's fiber slowly to avoid this problem.

Consider Food Sensitivity/Allergy—see Chapter 11. Lactose intolerance is the most common food sensitivity, with sugars and grains the other most likely culprits. Use a Food Diary (see page 73) to keep track of your child's flatulence and the foods associated with it. Food sensitivities don't usually exist by themselves, so if your child has several, check for candida and dysbiosis (see pages 60–61).

Digestive Enzymes—enzymes can support your child's digestive process. Give 1–2 digestive enzymes with meals and snacks.

Consider Fermentation Dysbiosis and Candida Infection—see Chapter 6. Excessive fermentation of sugar, fruit, and starch, experienced as gas and bloating, can be caused by candida infection or another dysbiosis.

Avoid Sucralose (Splenda), Sorbitol, and Xylitol—to prevent the gas often caused by consuming even small amounts of these indigestible sugars. Found in most sugarless or low-carbohydrate foods, candy, and gum, these sweeteners are often used by diabetics and dieters.

Consider Parasitic Infection—see pages 152–158. If you have already explored more obvious causes, fill out the parasite questionnaire for your child (see page 153) and follow with a stool test.

Chlorophyll—to help prevent gas. Dosage for children: $\frac{1}{2}$–2 teaspoons liquid, or one capsule, two or three times daily with meals.

Ginger, Fennel, and Anise—to dispel gas (from both ends). Dosage for children: $\frac{1}{4}$–1 cup tea as needed; the seeds of fennel and anise can also be chewed for the same effect.

Other Herbs—to aid digestion. Many digestive herbal tea blends are available. Nearly all common kitchen herbs and spices including basil, oregano, marjoram, parsley, thyme, celery seed, peppermint, spearmint, fennel, bayberry, caraway seed, cardamom seed, catnip, cloves, coriander, lemon balm, and sarsaparilla are beneficial against flatulence/intestinal gas.

PARASITIC INFECTION

Although we usually think of a parasite as something picked up primarily when traveling in other countries, this is a misconception. The U.S. Centers for Disease Control and Prevention found one or more parasites in one out of six randomly selected people. Similarly, Genova Diagnostics in North Carolina finds parasites

Parasite Questionnaire
for Adults, Children, and Infants

Adults, check if yes:

1. Have you ever been to Africa, Asia, Central or South America, China, Europe, Israel, Mexico, or Russia? ☐

2. Have you traveled to the Bahamas, the Caribbean, Hawaii, or other tropical islands? ☐

3. Do you frequently swim in freshwater lakes, ponds, or streams while abroad? ☐

4. Did you serve overseas while in the military? ☐

5. Were you a prisoner of war in World War II, Korea, or Vietnam? ☐

6. Have you had an elevated white blood count, intestinal problems, night-sweats, or unexplained fever during or since traveling abroad? ☐

7. Is your water supply from a mountainous area? ☐

8. Do you drink untested water? ☐

9. Have you ever drunk water from lakes, rivers, or streams on hiking or camping trips without first boiling or filtering it? ☐

10. Do you use plain tap-water to clean your contact lenses? ☐

11. Do you use regular tap-water that is unfiltered for colonics or enemas? ☐

12. Can you trace the onset of symptoms (intermittent constipation and diarrhea, muscle aches and pains, night-sweats, unexplained eye ulcers) to any of the above? ☐

13. Do you regularly eat unpeeled raw fruits and/or raw vegetables in salads? ☐

14. Do you frequently eat in Armenian, Chinese, Ethiopian, Filipino, fish, Greek, Indian, Japanese, Korean, Mexican, Pakistani, Thai, or vegetarian restaurants; in delicatessens, fast-food restaurants, steak houses, or sushi or salad bars? ☐

15. Do you use a microwave oven for cooking (as opposed to reheating) beef, fish, or pork? ☐

16. Do you prefer fish or meat that is undercooked, i.e., rare or medium rare? ☐

17. Do you frequently eat hot dogs made from pork? ☐

18. Do you enjoy raw fish dishes like Dutch green herring, Latin American ceviche, or sushi and sashimi? ☐

19. Do you enjoy raw meat dishes like Italian carpaccio, Middle Eastern kibbe, or steak tartare? ☐

20. At home, do you use the same cutting board for chicken, fish, and meat as you do for vegetables? ☐

21. Do you prepare gefilte fish at home? ☐

22. Can you trace the onset of symptoms (anemia, bloating, distended belly, weight loss) to any of the above? ☐

23. Have you gotten a puppy recently? ☐

24. Have you lived with, or do you currently live with, or frequently handle pets? ☐

25. Do you forget to wash your hands after petting or cleaning up after your animals and before eating? ☐

26. Does your pet sleep with you in bed? ☐

27. Does your pet eat off your plates? ☐

28. Do you clean your cat's litter box? ☐

29. Do you keep your pets in the yard where children play? ☐

30. Can you trace the onset of your symptoms (abdominal pain, distended belly in children, high white blood count, unexplained fever) to any of the above? ☐

31. Do you work in a hospital? ☐

32. Do you work in an experimental laboratory, pet shop, veterinary clinic, or zoo? ☐

33. Do you work with or around animals? ☐

34. Do you work in a daycare center? ☐

35. Do you garden or work in a yard to which cats and dogs have access? ☐

36. Do you work in sanitation? ☐

37. Can you trace the onset of symptoms (gastrointestinal disorders) to any of the above? ☐

38. Do you engage in oral sex? ☐

39. Do you practice anal intercourse without the use of a condom? ☐

40. Have you had sexual relations with a foreign-born individual? ☐

41. Can you trace the onset of symptoms (persistent reproductive organ problems) to any of the above? ☐

Major Symptoms: Please note that although some or all of these major symptoms can occur in any adult, child, or infant with parasite-based illness, these symptoms might instead be the result of one of many other illnesses.

Adults

1. Do you have a bluish cast around your lips? ☐
2. Is your abdomen distended no matter what you eat? ☐
3. Are there dark circles around or under your eyes? ☐
4. Do you have a history of allergy? ☐
5. Do you suffer from intermittent diarrhea and constipation, intermittent loose and hard stools, or chronic constipation? ☐
6. Do you have persistent acne, anal itching, anemia, anorexia, bad breath, bloody stools, chronic fatigue, difficulty in breathing, edema, food sensitivities, itching, open ileocecal valve, pale skin, palpitations, PMS, puffy eyes, ringing of the ears, sinus congestion, skin eruptions, vague abdominal discomfort, or vertigo? ☐
7. Do you grind your teeth? ☐
8. Are you experiencing craving for sugar, depression, disorientation, insomnia, lethargy, loss of appetite, moodiness, or weight loss or gain? ☐

Children

1. Does your child have dark circles under his/her eyes? ☐
2. Is your child hyperactive? ☐
3. Does your child grind or clench his/her teeth at night? ☐
4. Does your child constantly pick his/her nose or scratch his/her behind? ☐
5. Does your child have a habit of eating dirt? ☐
6. Does your child wet his/her bed? ☐
7. Is your child often restless at night? ☐
8. Does your child cry often or for no reason? ☐
9. Does your child tear his/her hair out? ☐
10. Does your child have a limp that orthopedic treatment has not helped? ☐
11. Does your child have a brassy, staccato-type cough? ☐
12. Does your child have convulsions or an abnormal electroencephalogram (EEG)? ☐

13. Does your child have recurring headaches? ☐

14. Is your child unusually sensitive to light and prone to blinking frequently, eyelid twitching, or squinting? ☐

15. Does your child have unusual tendencies to bleed in the gums, the nose, or the rectum? ☐

Infants

1. Does your baby have severe, intermittent colic? ☐
2. Does your baby persistently bang his/her head against the crib? ☐
3. Is your baby a chronic crier? ☐
4. Does your baby show a blotchy rash around the perianal area? ☐

Interpretation of Questionnaire—Adults

1. If you answered "yes" to more than 40 items, you are at high risk for parasites.

2. If you answered "yes" to more than 30 items, you are at moderate risk for parasites.

3. If you answered "yes" to more than 20 items, you are at risk.

Interpretation of Questionnaire—Children and Infants

If your child or infant has two or more of the symptoms listed in the sections for Children and Infants, you may want to have him/her examined by a physician.

Additional Note

If you are not exhibiting any overt symptoms now, remember that many parasitic infections can be dormant and then spring to life when you least expect them. Be aware that symptoms that come and go may still point to an underlying parasitic infection because of reproductive cycles. The various developmental stages of parasites often produce a variety of metabolic toxins and mechanical irritations in several areas of the body—for example, pinworms can stimulate asthmatic attacks because of their movement into the upper respiratory tract.

—adapted with permission from *Guess What Came to Dinner?* (AL Gittleman, Garden City Park, NY: Avery Publishing Group, 1993) in 20 percent of samples tested. More than 130 types of parasites have been found in Americans. My own family contracted giardia in Chicago, and we have absolutely no idea how it happened.

Also contrary to popular myth, having parasites isn't necessarily a reflection of uncleanliness. Most people will meet a parasite at some point in their lives, and parasites are very common in children. Their increased prevalence is attributable to such sources as contaminated water supplies, daycare centers, ease of international travel, imported foods from all over the world, increased immigration, pets, and the sexual revolution.

If your child experiences prolonged digestive symptoms, consider parasites as the possible cause. Common symptoms of parasitic infection are: abdominal pain, allergy, anemia, bloating, bloody stools, chronic fatigue, constipation, coughing, diarrhea, gas, granulomas, irritable bowel syndrome, itching, joint and muscle aches, nervousness, pain, poor immune response, rashes, sleep disturbances, teeth grinding, unexplained fever, and unexplained weight loss. Note that these symptoms can resemble those of other digestive problems. If you suspect that your child might have parasites, fill out the questionnaire on the following pages; if your child's score is 2 or more, see a physician.

Functional Laboratory Testing for Children with Parasitic Infection

A comprehensive digestive and stool analysis with parasite screening is most accurate and is performed by labs that specialize in parasite testing. A simple ova and parasite stool sample is more commonly performed but can be highly inaccurate, so repeated testing is often necessary to obtain definitive results with this method. Because many parasites live further up the digestive tract than the rectum, labs often administer an oral laxative that induces diarrhea in order to detect them. Other parasites are found by using a rectal swab.

Healing Options for Children with Parasitic Infection

A prescription medication may be the most efficient treatment for parasitic infection, leaving your child parasite free within a week or two. These medications, however, can be hard on the liver and disruptive to the intestinal flora, so after using an antiparasitic drug, it's wise to replenish your child's acidophilus and bifidobacteria populations. Many herbal remedies are highly effective against parasites, but they work more slowly, taking about a month. In selecting an approach, take your child's age and health condition into account. If he/she is very ill and dehydrating easily, consider the prescription medication; if he/she is young and not that ill, consider an herbal remedy. You may wish to consult your child's doctor or another healthcare professional for advice.

The most common natural antiparasitic agents include barberry, blackseed, black walnut, boldo, butternut bark, clove, garlic, gentian root, goldenseal, grape-fruit-seed extract, Jerusalem oak/American wormseed, Oregon grape, pumpkin seed, and wormwood/artemisia. Many of these are found in combination products. Acidophilus and bifidobacteria should also be replaced after herbal antiparasitic therapy. See Appendix B for more details on the following nutrients, herbs, and supplements.

Garlic—to treat *Entamoeba histolytica, Giardia lambia,* and pinworm infections. Dosage for children: supplement, as directed on label; fresh garlic, two to four cloves daily.

Goldenseal—to treat amoeba, giardia, and candida infections. Dosage for children: one to three capsules daily.

Wormwood/Artemisia—to treat worms and other parasitic infections. Dosage for children: powder, $\frac{1}{4}$–$\frac{1}{2}$ teaspoon once or twice daily; tea, $\frac{1}{2}$ cup daily, sipped 1 teaspoon at a time. *Caution:* Wormwood is as safe as a tea, powder, or capsule, but pure wormwood oil is poisonous.

Black Walnut—to treat parasitic and fungal infections. Dosage for children: as directed on label.

Dichroea febrifuga/Changshan—to treat malaria, amoeba, and giardia infections. Dosage for children: as directed on label.

Jerusalem Oak/American Wormseed—to expel roundworms, hookworms, and tapeworms. Dosage for children: as directed on label.

CHAPTER 16

Issues of the Large Intestine

The colon's main functions are to absorb nutrients, reabsorb water, and eliminate wastes. Adequate intake of liquids is therefore essential for good colon health. Water, juices, herbal teas, and fresh fruits hydrate the body and the stool. Alcohol and soft drinks, on the other hand, are more diuretic, and increase our need to drink healthful fluids. Proper colon function also requires a high-fiber diet. The large intestine is home to trillions of beneficial flora that ferment dietary fiber, producing the short-chained fatty acids that are the primary fuel of the colonic cells (one of these compounds, butyric acid, has also been shown to stop the growth of colon cancer cells *in vitro* and is used clinically to heal inflamed bowel tissue). Without adequate fiber, the colonic cells starve and the organ weakens.

In addition to inflammatory bowel disease and irritable bowel syndrome (see Chapter 17), common problems of the large intestine include diarrhea, constipation, pruritis ani, and appendicitis.

DIARRHEA

Diarrhea is the body's way of quickly getting rid of something disagreeable like a problematic food, microbe, or toxin. It is a symptom, not a disease. Most diarrhea is self limiting, so if your child has an acute case of diarrhea, just "let it flow" and prevent dehydration by making sure that he/she takes in plenty of liquid. Loss of fluids and minerals through diarrhea can make us disoriented and weak; in infants and small children, dehydration can be dangerous and can happen suddenly. Replace your child's lost fluids with water, diluted fruit and vegetable juices, and/or broth. Infants can also be given a rehydrating fleet enema (an inexpensive enema solution sold in pre-lubricated squeeze-bottles, available at drug stores).

If your child's diarrhea is chronic, it's important to find the underlying cause. Chronic diarrhea can result from many things: foods or beverages that disagree with the child's system, infection, inflammatory bowel disease, celiac disease, irritable bowel syndrome, malabsorption of fats, and more. Diarrhea is a common symptom of food sensitivities and allergies, and lactose intolerance is a common source of diarrhea in children.

Call a doctor if your child's diarrhea has lasted for more than three days, or if he/she has any of these accompanying symptoms:

- Severe abdominal or rectal pain
- Fever of at least 102°F
- Blood in the stool
- Signs of dehydration (dry mouth, anxiety, restlessness, excessive thirst, little or no urination, severe weakness, dizziness, or light-headedness)

Functional Laboratory Testing for Children with Diarrhea

Acute diarrhea usually passes on its own. Prolonged diarrhea, however, warrants thorough investigation. A few of the tests that may yield information about the cause(s) of your child's problem are listed below. See Appendix A for details on testing.

1. Comprehensive digestive and stool analysis with parasite screening

2. Small bowel bacterial overgrowth test

3. Lactose intolerance test

4. Food sensitivity/allergy test(s)

5. Fill out parasite questionnaire (page 153)

Healing Options for Children with Diarrhea

Diarrhea and hunger usually don't go together. Rather than "feeding" the bugs that can be behind a digestive upset, children may instinctively stop eating to get better more quickly. The recommended feeding for people with diarrhea is called the BRAT diet, which stands for bananas, rice, apples, and toast. Other suggested bland and binding foods are soda crackers, chicken, and eggs. Try making a tasty, binding rice pudding from apples, rice, eggs, and cinnamon. A child with chronic diarrhea won't be able to absorb all of the nutrients from foods, so giving him/her easy-to-digest protein powders (with added vitamins and minerals) or shakes is a good way to ensure adequate nutrition during this time. See Appendix B for more details on the following nutrients, herbs, and supplements.

Wash Hands—to reduce the incidence of ongoing diarrhea. In one study, mothers of children with prolonged diarrhea were simply asked to wash their own hands with soap and water before preparing food and eating, and to wash their children's hands before eating and as soon as possible after a bowel movement; this produced an 89-percent reduction in the children's diarrhea.

Saccharomyces boulardii—to prevent and treat post-antibiotic diarrhea. Saccharomyces is often found in combination products with other probiotics (see below). Dosage for children: 250 mg three times daily, as needed.

Probiotics—to normalize bowel function and prevent traveler's diarrhea. For younger children, use *Bifidobacteria infantis;* a breast-feeding mom should take *B. infantis* as well. For older children, use *Lactobacillus acidophilus* and *B. infantis*. Dosage for children: capsules, one to four daily; or powder, ¼–½ teaspoon two or three times daily.

Consider Lactose Intolerance—see Appendix A. Have your child avoid all dairy products (don't forget "hidden" sources of dairy) for two to three weeks to see whether the diarrhea stops.

Zinc—to shorten acute diarrhea by boosting the immune system. Much research has been done on zinc and diarrhea in children. Dosage for children: 20 mg daily, for up to two weeks.

Consider Food Sensitivity/Allergy—see Chapter 11. Try a one-week to two-week elimination/provocahon diet to discover your child's possible food sensitivities and/or allergies.

Cultured Dairy Products—to stop or prevent diarrhea by normalizing bowel flora. Yogurt (which contains active *Lactobacillus thermophilus* and *L. bulgaricus*), buttermilk, or kefir can be helpful for either diarrhea or constipation, as long as your child is not lactose intolerant.

Fiber Supplement—to solidify the stool. Dosage for children: begin with ½ teaspoon daily in at least 8 ounces water, increasing up to 3 teaspoons daily as needed.

Avoid Low-Calorie Sweeteners—to prevent the diarrhea, gas, and bloating often caused by eating nondigestible sugars (sucralose/Splenda, sorbitol, mannitol, and xylitol).

CONSTIPATION

Having one to three easy bowel movements daily, usually right after eating, is normal for many children. A child is considered constipated if he/she has fewer than three bowel movements a week; strains to have a bowel movement; has hard stools, infrequent or incomplete bowel movements, or discomfort; or if there is a perception (parent's or child's) that the child's bowel habits are different from usual. Constipation affects about 3 percent of children and represents one-quarter of all visits to pediatric gastroenterologists. One study of infants and toddlers found that the incidence of constipation was 2.9 percent in the first year of life, but rose to over 10 percent at two years of age. This is probably due to the introduction of so many new foods once a baby has his/her first birthday.

Ninety-five percent of the time, constipation doesn't have a medical reason; rather, it is usually due to poor diet, poor bowel habits, or emotional factors (but see also "Hirschsprung's Disease" on page 132 and Cystic Fibrosis in Chapter 22). Forty percent of Americans, for example, fail to meet the recommended daily allowance for magnesium, and magnesium deficiency contributes to constipation by leading to poor bowel muscle tone. Additionally, people with lactose intolerance sometimes become constipated from eating dairy products.

Toilet-training can be an upsetting time for some children. Kids may feel uncomfortable because having a bowel movement is messy, or because they've been scolded for soiling their clothes. Still others experience pain, so they avoid defecating. *Note:* A bowel movement should never involve pain; if your child experiences pain, it may indicate a structural abnormality, fissure, hemorrhoid, or other problem, and you should take him/her to a physician.

Children often get too engrossed in what they are doing to stop and pay attention to their body's needs. When the urge to defecate is ignored, stool gets dehydrated and small, the rectum gets used to being stretched and fails to respond normally, and feces then back up into the colon, causing discomfort. Some children (and adults!), out of embarrassment, won't have a bowel movement at school or in a public restroom or even at a friend's house, but that attitude needs readjustment—after all, everybody's doing it!

A note about bowel movements in your breast-fed infant: Breast-feeding babies will efficiently utilize much of what they eat, and it is not uncommon for babies who are 100-percent breast-fed to skip having bowel movements for a day or two from time to time. As long as your baby seems comfortable and is not fussing, don't worry about it. If this happens regularly, consider trying probiotic supplements for the baby and also for mom.

Functional Laboratory Testing for Children with Constipation

Most cases of constipation resolve with changes in diet, increased fluid consumption, and exercise. Children with chronic constipation that does not respond to fiber, liquids, and activity (see "Healing Options for Children with Constipation" on page 163) should be tested for possible underlying food sensitivity/allergy, dysbiosis, leaky gut, and/or parasitic infection. Available tests include:

1. Lactose intolerance test

2. Comprehensive digestive and stool analysis with parasite screening

3. Food sensitivity/allergy test(s)

4. Intestinal permeability test

Healing Options for Children with Constipation

For most children, a diet high in fluids and fiber solves a constipation problem. Have your child drink plenty of water, juices, and/or herbal teas and eat at least five servings of fruits and vegetables (preferably fresh and organic) each day. Cut back his/her intake of low-fiber foods including candy, dairy products, meats, pastries, soft drinks, and white bread. Make whole grains like amaranth, brown rice, millet, oatmeal, quinoa, rye-berries, and wheat-berries the rule, and processed grains the exception. A high-fiber cereal at breakfast can make a big difference; other fiber-loaded foods include asparagus, Brussels sprouts, cabbage, cauliflower, corn, kale, legumes like peas and beans, parsnips, peas, and potatoes.

Encopresis

Encopresis, or fecal incontinence, is the term used when a child over the age of four years has soiling or involuntary bowel movements in inappropriate places at least once a month for three months. Although it is underdiagnosed, encopresis is common, and still affects about 2 percent of children by the time they enter school; at that age, it is more common in boys than in girls.

Encopresis results from chronic constipation. Constipated children may hold back bowel movements because it hurts or because it's inconvenient to stop whatever else they're doing, and this promotes a cycle of more constipation, leading to impaction, distention, and pain. Eventually, stool behind the impaction leaks out from the rectum. The child has no control of this leakage and may not even be aware that it's happening. Finding "skid-marks" on his/her underwear is a pretty typical sign of encopresis.

The normal treatment for encopresis begins with cleaning out the bowel—but do not give a laxative to a child younger than six years old unless his/her doctor recommends it. Most physicians recommend administering milk of magnesia (1 teaspoon for babies younger than one year, 1½–3 teaspoons for those older than one year) or 1–6 teaspoons of mineral oil daily to make the stool slip out more easily. Taking mineral oil, however, can cause deficiencies of fat-soluble vitamins such as A and D, and over time can cause inflammation of the liver, spleen, and lymph nodes. You can probably achieve the same therapeutic benefit by giving your child nutritional oil such as olive oil instead, and you can easily add 1–2 teaspoons of cod liver oil as well, to prevent any potential vitamin deficit. Physicians also use propylene glycol (Miralax) for encopresis: 1 teaspoon in 4 ounces of water or juice daily, and increase up to 1 tablespoon in 8 ounces of liquid daily. (See also "Healing Options for Children with Constipation" above.)

If you can't get enough fiber into your child's diet, you can give him/her a fiber supplement to add bulk and water to the stool. Although it's not a laxative, psyllium-seed husk can help regulate bowel function, is beneficial for both diarrhea and constipation, and does not cause dependency. Personally, I've found it easier to get a child to eat high-fiber foods than to drink fiber supplements in water.

*I **don't** recommend using laxatives. Chronic use of laxatives, even herbal laxatives, causes the bowels to become lazy, and the muscles become too dependent on the laxatives to function properly on their own. Some laxatives can also damage the nerve cells in the wall of the colon.*

Hypnotherapy, biofeedback treatment, and teaching improved bowel habits have all been used successfully for children with encopresis and chronic constipation. More than a dozen studies have demonstrated that biofeedback effectively trains constipated children to relax their sphincter muscles to have bowel movements appropriately. See Appendix B for more details on the following nutrients, herbs, and supplements.

Dietary Changes—to increase fiber and nutrient intake through a minimum of five servings of fruits and vegetables every day, as well as adding more whole grains and legumes. For a small child, a serving is one-quarter of an apple or a couple of small carrots; for a bigger child, servings are about ½ cup. Make these dietary changes slowly to let your child adapt, as plunging quickly into a high-fiber diet can cause gas and bloating.

Fiber Supplement—to promote easy stool passage. Dosage for children: begin with 1 teaspoon in 4 ounces water or juice daily, building gradually to 1 teaspoon in 8 ounces fluid at each meal. Eventually, with increased dietary fiber, your child will probably no longer need a psyllium supplement.

Hydrate—to help fiber do its work and soften the stool. Make sure that your child drinks plenty of water each day (see Chapter 8). Hot or cold herbal teas with licorice, fennel, and anise have the added benefit of soothing the digestive system. Remember, soft drinks are dehydrating.

Teach Improved Bowel Habits—to help your child recognize when it's time to have a bowel movement and relax about it. If your child learns to go "when nature calls," it'll take just a minute or two. Repetition will help. Have your child sit on the toilet and relax each morning or evening for twenty minutes; sometimes reading or looking at a picture book can help him/her relax the bowel muscles. It's important that kids not feel rushed to have a bowel movement.

Prune Juice—to relax the bowel. Delicious! Dosage for children: ⅓ cup juice diluted in ⅔ cup water. If your child drinks this before bed, it will often have a laxative effect by morning.

Probiotics—to regulate peristalsis. Dosage for children: one capsule or ¼–½ teaspoon powder two or three times daily.

Cultured Dairy Products—to stop or prevent constipation by normalizing bowel flora. Yogurt (which contains active *Lactobacillus thermophilus* and *L. bulgaricus*), buttermilk, or kefir can be helpful for either constipation or diarrhea, as long as your child is not lactose intolerant.

Magnesium—to promote peristalsis. Dosage for children: 100–400 mg or more daily, according to child's size and age. The right dose is easily identified, because when you give your child too much magnesium, he/she will get diarrhea. Magnesium is also found in green leafy vegetables like kale, spinach, and broccoli and in whole grains such as brown rice and barley. *Note:* If your child needs to take large amounts of magnesium for effectiveness, you may want to give ½–1 teaspoon choline citrate per 200 mg magnesium to increase the absorption of magnesium.

Consider Lactose Intolerance—see Appendix A. Have your child avoid milk and dairy-containing foods for two to three weeks and see whether his/her constipation is improved.

Digestive Enzymes—taken with meals, they increase stool bulk and help relieve constipation. Dosage: 1–2 with meals and snacks.

Exercise—"massage" the gut and aid peristalsis. Most of today's children can benefit from more movement! Send them outdoors to play. Encourage them to play outside at recess and to participate after school in a type of movement they enjoy such as sports, dance, or martial arts.

Consider Food Sensitivity/Allergy—see Chapter 11.

Consider Dysbiosis—see Chapter 6.

Consider Leaky Gut Syndrome—see Chapter 12.

Consider Parasitic Infection—see Chapter 15.

Vitamin C—to soften the stool. Dosage for children: varies according to child's need. *Note:* Too much vitamin C will give your child diarrhea.

Biofeedback and/or Hypnotherapy—to treat children who have problems relaxing the pelvic floor muscles.

Consider Hypothyroidism—because a sluggish thyroid gland can slow peristalsis. If your child is still constipated after you've increased fiber, fluids, and magnesium, ask his/her doctor to do a thorough thyroid screening.

PRURITIS ANI/ANAL ITCHING

Pruritis ani is a fancy medical term for itching that is localized right around the anus. It will often be worse at night or right after a bowel movement. The causes are many, and you'll want to rule out the simple before investigating the obscure. The most common causes of anal itching in children are moisture and leaky bowel movements; other contributors are exposure to irritating chemicals in soaps, vitamins, creams, or other items, as well as pinworm or yeast infection and food allergies. Many foods can irritate the gut mucosa (inner lining) around the anus; this irritation often presents itself as itching, and itching means scratching, which leads to more inflammation and more itching. In rare cases, chronic pruritis ani can indicate something more serious like anal fissures, so long-term anal itching should be checked out by a pediatrician.

Healing Options for Children with Pruritis Ani

The general tendency for parents of children with pruritis will be to wash them more vigorously and use more soap and lotions, which can actually aggravate the problem by drying out the skin and/or causing a chemical irritation.

Keep Clean and Dry—by rinsing your child's anus, after a bowel movement, with clean water, wet toilet paper, baby wipes, or a wet washcloth. Use a gentle blotting motion to avoid irritating the skin further. Avoid using soaps, powders, and lotions on the anal area.

Consider Parasitic Infection—see Chapter 15. Just before bedtime, inspect your child's anal area with a flashlight for small, threadlike, white pinworms; alternatively, putting a piece of tape on your child's anus will sometimes pull off a worm or two. If you find pinworms, get an appropriate nonprescription medicine from a pharmacy. Consult a pediatrician if you suspect any other parasite.

Consider Food Sensitivity/Allergy—see Chapter 11. Eliminate possible suspicious foods from your child's diet for at least two weeks and monitor him/her for improvement.

Consider Candida Infection—see Chapter 6. Suspect a yeast infection if the itching is worse on days that your child consumes a lot of sweets. If so, use an over-the-counter antifungal cream (like Monistat), give a probiotic supplement, and eliminate sweets. If these steps don't do the trick, try a more aggressive anti-candida program.

Eliminate Chemical Irritants—see Chapter 2. Use unscented laundry detergents, bath soaps, and toilet paper. Look for other chemicals that could contribute to your child's problem.

APPENDICITIS

The appendix lies on the right side of the belly at the beginning of the cecum. When healthy, this small, fingerlike piece of tissue manufactures antibodies to protect the large intestine. The appendix usually forms a *cul-de-sac* that can easily become infected and inflamed if blocked by food, mucus, or stool. In the United States, appendicitis occurs in about 7 percent of people, mainly from the ages of eleven to twenty years old. It is more common in the winter months and more common in children whose parents have had appendicitis.

In children younger than two years, the most common symptoms of appendicitis are vomiting and a very distended belly. Toddlers may experience appendix pain but not be able to communicate it. In children older than two years, typical symptoms of appendicitis are fever, abdominal pain, and vomiting. The pain, which usually begins near the belly-button and then radiates toward the right side of the body, occurs before nausea and vomiting and can be the tip-off that you are dealing with appendicitis rather than the flu.

Children with appendicitis may also have other symptoms such as diarrhea, difficulty urinating or frequent urination, constipation, and respiratory problems. Your child may be holding his/her belly to protect it. As the infection progresses, a symptom called "rebound tenderness" can occur: that is, if you gently push on your child's abdomen and then release the pressure suddenly, he/she may experience a temporary worsening of the pain. If this happens, take your child to the emergency room or call a doctor right away.

If you suspect that your child may have appendicitis, see a doctor immediately. Blood, urine, and other laboratory tests such as X-ray, ultrasound, or CT scanning will be used to confirm the diagnosis (there is no specific test for appendicitis). Most commonly, surgery to remove the appendix will be performed as soon as possible. If inflammation and infection spread through the appendix wall, it often ruptures, causing systemic infection and high fever; this occurs pretty quickly, usually between forty-eight and seventy-two hours after the first pain, and can be

> *IF YOU SUSPECT APPENDICITIS, SEE A DOCTOR IMMEDIATELY!*
> *The longer you wait, the more likely the appendix can rupture and cause a systemic infection. It's better to see the doctor and find out it's a false alarm than to risk the consequences of a ruptured appendix. Sometimes surgery is even preventable if the infection is caught early.*

life threatening. In cases of rupture, an appendectomy will be done immediately and your child will be given antibiotics to prevent the infection from spreading. Hospital stays for a routine appendectomy are usually two to three days.

Although there is no sure way to prevent appendicitis, Dr. Dennis Burkitt found it to be exceedingly rare in areas where people ate a high-fiber diet, and subsequent studies confirmed a reduced incidence of appendicitis in children eating higher-fiber diets. It was originally suggested that increased stool bulk provides the benefit, and subsequently posited that fiber's support of beneficial flora in the colon keeps children healthier; either way, it appears that eating more fiber can help prevent appendicitis.

Naturopathic physicians and practitioners of integrated medicine may try to control an appendix infection without surgery, and this can be a viable option depending on how early the infection is caught.

Post-Surgical Healing Options for Children with Appendicitis

After an appendectomy, your child may not be hungry, and he/she will not be able to eat solid foods until his/her bowels begin to work again. Begin slowly with broths, diluted juices, and herbal teas, then slowly reintroduce well-cooked foods such as soups and stews (with lots of greens added for minerals and other nutrients) and unsweetened applesauce. See Appendix B for more details on the following nutrients, herbs, and supplements.

Rest—to support the body's healing. It is imperative that your child rest a lot, and it is normal for him/her to need more rest than usual even a month after surgery.

Probiotics—to restore the gut flora altered by antibiotic therapy. Dosage for children: one or two capsules or ¼–½ teaspoon powder twice daily, for at least three weeks after surgery.

Glutamine—to speed the colon's self-repair process. Dosage for children: 500–2,000 mg three times daily, for at least two to three weeks after surgery.

Zinc—to assist in wound repair. Dosage for children: 10–50 mg daily, according to child's size and age, for three weeks after surgery. *Note:* Too much zinc causes nausea.

Multivitamin-Mineral Supplement—to speed self-healing. Dosage for children: as directed on label.

Echinacea and Goldenseal—to prevent wound infection. Dosage for children: tincture or tablets as directed on label, for several days after surgery.

Vitamin E—to promote the scar's healing. Dosage for children: after all risk of infection has passed and the wound has closed, gently apply vitamin E cream or oil to the scar twice daily until it has healed well; you can also give your child supplemental vitamin E internally, at 100–400 international units mixed tocopherols or d-alpha tocopherol daily.

CHAPTER 17

Inflamed or Irritable Bowels

nflammatory bowel disease (IBD) is considered an autoimmune condition in which the body attacks itself. The causes are multifactoral and have produced much debate. Ulcerative colitis and Crohn's disease are the most common IBDs. Irritable bowel syndrome (IBS) is a more common but less serious illness. IBS is characterized as a "functional bowel disease" because if you actually looked inside the colon, you wouldn't see any inflammation or structural changes.

INFLAMMATORY BOWEL DISEASE

Affecting half a million Americans, IBD tends to run in families and is more prevalent among people of Jewish descent. About one-third of people with IBD will be diagnosed as children, and the rest typically by the age of forty years old. Ulcerative colitis and Crohn's disease, though similar, have certain distinguishing characteristics; in all forms of IBD, however, the inflammation inside the digestive tract causes cramping, diarrhea, and often bloody or mucus-filled stool. If your child has these symptoms, take him/her to see a physician. Accompanying symptoms may also be fever, rectal bleeding, abdominal tenderness, abscesses, constipation, weight loss, awakening during the night with diarrhea, and poor growth (weight and height) in children. About half of the people with IBD have only mild symptoms. Symptoms come and go, and remission can occur for months or years. Remission is the goal, and there is hope: Many people who had serious bouts with IBD as teenagers have remained completely in remission.

Ulcerative Colitis versus Crohn's Disease

Ulcerative colitis entails inflammation and ulcers (sores), which are very irritated, in the colon and rectum. Along with bloody diarrhea, pain, and cramping, a child with this condition can feel great urgency when it's time to have a bowel movement and can fear not making it to the bathroom in time. Those symptoms may be accompanied by fevers, abdominal pain, diarrhea, and weight loss. Some children with ulcerative colitis also have pain in their knees, ankles, and other joints.

Twenty to 25 percent of people with ulcerative colitis eventually require surgery because of massive bleeding, chronic illness, perforated colon, or risk of colon cancer. Colon cancer ultimately does develop in 5 percent of people with ulcerative colitis. The degree of illness correlates with the likelihood of developing colon cancer. Ulcerative colitis is generally milder and easier to treat if localized in the rectum, and colitis limited to the rectum is also associated with the same colon cancer rate as that of people without ulcerative colitis.

Crohn's disease can occur anywhere along the digestive tract from mouth to rectum, but is most common in the colon and ileum near the ileocecal valve. Along with bloody diarrhea, pain, and cramping, children with this condition may also develop mouth sores, clubbed fingernails, or arthritis-like joint pains. Because it's hard for children with Crohn's disease to absorb nutrients efficiently, they may show delayed growth and maturation that is probably due to undernutrition.

Unlike ulcerative colitis, the inflammation in Crohn's disease develops in a "skip pattern" (a little here and a little there) and goes more deeply into the tissues. The lining of the gastrointestinal tract may thicken in the affected areas, causing constrictions and blockage. In serious cases, the lining can form abscesses and fistulas, which are little canals that lead to other organs or form tiny caves; if these become serious, surgery may be recommended.

Causes and Consequences

Current theories suggest that a genetic component underlying both Crohn's disease and ulcerative colitis is triggered to a greater or a lesser extent by infection, hypersensitivity to antigens in the gut wall, ischemia (a lack of blood supply to the tissues) caused by inflammation of blood vessels, and/or food sensitivities. The first gene linked with Crohn's disease, called NOD2, apparently causes a rapid immune system response to gut bacteria and/or their toxic byproducts, leading to the overproduction of substances (NF-kappaB and cytokines) that stimulate intestinal inflammation and irritation. The NOD2 gene, however, is found in only 10 to 15 percent of people with Crohn's disease, so it is obviously not the only source of the problem.

Although many microbes including mycobacteria, yersinia, campylobacter, clostridium, chlamidia, herpes, measles, and rotovirus have been suspected in IBD, especially Crohn's disease, none have been found to be the exclusive issue. One study found that infections were evident 10.5 percent of the time, however, in IBD relapses; the infective agents were *Clostridium difficile* in about half of the cases, and infections in the rest included campylobacter, *Entamoeba histolytica,* salmonella, *Plesiomonas shiegelloides, Strongyloides stercoralis,* and *Blastocystis hominis.* There is little research on the yeast-IBD connection, but clinicians often find antifungal measures to be helpful. Many studies have shown the usefulness of probiotics in IBD, and populations of beneficial intestinal bacteria have been shown to be dramatically imbalanced in people with IBD, so using probiotic supplements of lactobacilli and bifidobacteria is highly recommended for people with inflamed bowels.

The role of the measles virus in IBD has been well studied with varying results; some researchers insist on a significant connection, whereas others find none. It appears that measles is not typically associated with IBD but may be a factor in some cases. Swedish researchers found a high incidence of IBD in people who had been exposed to measles *in utero,* and British researchers found the virus in diseased parts of the colon, implicating measles as a possible cause of Crohn's disease. Another study in England showed that people who had received live measles vaccine had a threefold increase of Crohn's disease, and that incidence of ulcerative colitis subsequent to live measles vaccination rose by two-and-a-half times (the demonstrated correlation, however, does not prove that measles actually caused the IBD).

The seasonal cycle of flare-ups in some people with Crohn's disease suggests an allergic component to the illness. A survey of people with IBD found that 70 percent of them reported additional, probably allergic symptoms, leading researcher J. Siegel to comment in 1981 that "inflammatory bowel disease is just another possible facet of allergy." Food sensitivities play a significant role in ulcerative colitis and Crohn's disease, occurring approximately half the time. Grains and dairy products often aggravate IBD, and one study found that 13 percent of children with IBD were allergic to cow's milk during infancy.

In cultures where people eat a "native diet," IBD is rare, but its incidence is growing rapidly in Western countries, and diet plays an important role. People who eat a low-fiber diet and large amounts of sugars have a higher incidence of IBD. The condition is also correlated with smoking cigarettes and eating fast foods; one study found that the frequency of ulcerative colitis flare-ups increased almost fourfold when fast foods were eaten twice a week. Nearly any food can cause bowel irritation and inflammation, and various studies have implicated citrus, pineapple, dairy, coffee, tomatoes, cheese, bananas, sugar, additives, preservatives, spices, bread, beverages other than water, and so forth.

People with IBD often develop complications including arthritis, colon cancer, kidney stones, liver disease, osteoporosis, osteopenia, and skin or eye inflammation. It is unclear whether the bone loss often found in Crohn's disease and ulcerative colitis is only correlated with the use of steroid medication. Increasing intake of all bone nutrients is advisable for children with IBD, as is regular exercise; one study of low-impact exercise for people with Crohn's disease showed a significant increase in bone density.

Inflammatory bowel disease is not caused by emotional illness or psychiatric disorder, but the condition's chronic nature, painful episodes, and lifestyle limitations may lead to emotional problems. Like all children with chronic illness, children with IBD have specific psychological issues, so individual and even family counseling can be of great benefit.

Treatment for Inflammatory Bowel Disease

Medical treatment for IBD consists of anti-inflammatory drugs, steroids, immune modulators, and sometimes antibiotics. Although these medications relieve symptoms and are often necessary, they carry their own risks. Prolonged treatment with steroids can cause side effects of depression, psychotic episodes, mania or euphoria, and bone loss. Using sulphasalazine (Asulfadine) causes folic acid deficiency. A new drug called Infliximab, which helps reduce inflammation in people with severe Crohn's disease by attacking a substance called tumor necrosis factor (TNF-alpha), is now available; it may enable children to stop taking steroid medications and increase their quality of life, but we don't yet know the long-term implications of its use.

Complementary therapies can reduce the need for medication, thereby minimizing side effects and maximizing efficacy. As mentioned earlier, the key to successful IBD treatment appears to be getting people into remission, for which a combination of medication and supplements may be best; once a flare-up dies down, natural therapies that address the disease's underlying factors and heal the bowel are highly effective in preventing recurrence. It's also really important to teach your child good self-care. Practicing stress-management techniques can help reduce the number and severity of flare-ups. Make sure that your child gets regular exercise to prevent bone loss later in life.

If your child ultimately requires surgery for Crohn's disease, it is important to know which part of the intestine is removed and which nutrients may therefore be inadequately digested. See Figure 3.1 on page 30.

Diet

No single diet helps all people with IBD, but many report significant improvement with a three-week elimination/provocation diet, after which specific foods are gradually reintroduced to see which ones provoke bloating, pain, diarrhea, bleeding, or other symptoms. If your child reacts to a specific food, it's good to keep it out of his/her diet for six months; then, reintroduce it as a test to see whether your child can tolerate it. Some foods such as grains or dairy products may necessitate long-term elimination, but it's good to re-check a food from time to time to determine whether your child needs to continue avoiding it.

Studies have shown reduced IBD symptoms and inflammation in people who adhere to a hypoallergenic diet. The Elemental Diet, a synthetic food product that can be consumed as a beverage or administered through a tube, reduces intestinal permeability and was shown to be as good as steroid medication at reducing inflammation in a flare-up of Crohn's disease. Unfortunately, many children find the Elemental Diet unpalatable and won't drink it, but newer, tastier products are now coming on the market.

Many people with digestive issues are unable to split disaccharide sugars (lactose, sucrose, maltose, and isomaltose) into single-molecule sugars. This may explain, in part, why a program called the Specific Carbohydrate Diet is so successful in treating Crohn's disease, because it eliminates all simple sugars as well as the foods that most commonly cause sensitivities (all grains and most dairy products), and it helps restore intestinal balance. Allowed foods are beef, lamb, pork, poultry, fish, eggs, natural cheeses, vegetables, homemade yogurt, fruits, nuts, pure fruit juices, weak coffee, weak non-herbal tea, and peppermint and spearmint tea, as well as corn oil, soy oil, safflower oil, sunflower oil, and olive oil—no grains, dairy products other than yogurt, legumes, potatoes, yams, parsnips, sugars, or alcoholic beverages. The Specific Carbohydrate Diet is even more effective when used in conjunction with food sensitivity/allergy testing. For more details (and delicious recipes), read Elaine Gottschall's book *Breaking the Vicious Cycle* (Kirkton Press, 1994).

Studies have shown that people with IBD have greater than normal amounts of sulfur-eating bacteria. Perhaps for this reason, a low-sulfur diet may be of ben-

Juicing, Vegetarian Diets, and IBD

Several of my clients were diagnosed with Crohn's disease or ulcerative colitis in their teens and went through horrible bleeding, weight loss, even hospitalizations. Long before coming to me, they sought help from other healthcare practitioners who recommended vegetarianism and drinking lots of fresh vegetable juices. Miraculously, decades later, these clients consider their IBD to be their "old" medical history, rather than a continual problem. A specific vegetarian program that seems to work well is called the Natural Hygiene Diet. Despite hundreds of testimonials from people who have been "cured" through this approach, I have found no scientific studies on it. If my child had IBD, however, I would certainly try it!

efit in Crohn's disease. In one study, people were advised to avoid high-sulfur foods including eggs, cheese, whole milk, ice cream, mayonnaise, soy milk, mineral water, sulfite-containing drinks (including wine), nuts, and cruciferous vegetables (broccoli, cabbage, cauliflower, Brussels sprouts); to reintroduce red meats; and to obtain protein from milk, fish, and chicken as well. Although the expected relapse rate was 22.6 percent, the four participants had no relapses or attacks while on the low-sulfur diet, suffered no adverse effects from the diet itself, and experienced improvements such as cessation of steroid medication along with reduced flare-ups, daily bowel movements, and inflammation.

Probiotics

Dysbiosis is believed to be a primary cause in many cases of IBD. An imbalance of our normal friendly flora allows pathogenic microbes such as candida, bacteroides, and citrobacter to proliferate. Probiotics like *Lactobacillus acidophilus,* bifidobacteria, and the Nissle strain of *Escherichia coli* compete with other microbes and push them out; they also stimulate our immune response, increase beneficial antibodies such as secretory IgA, IgM, and IgG, balance pH, and enhance tight-junction integrity. These commensal bacteria are therefore a promising treatment for IBD. Numerous studies have shown that probiotic supplements help maintain remission of flare-ups in Crohn's disease, ulcerative colitis, and pouchitis (an infection that can occur after bowel surgery). Probiotic therapy with Nissle-strain *E. coli* was found to be as effective as a standard medication in keeping ulcerative colitis at bay for a year.

You won't believe this twist on probiotic therapy: For five consecutive days, researchers administered colonic enemas consisting of the bowel movements of healthy people to people with ulcerative colitis. Four of the six participants had total remission of their symptoms within four months, and thirteen years later, they were still completely well and without need of any medications.

Supplements and Herbs

Poor absorption of many nutrients is often found in people with IBD, and many studies have shown an increased need for antioxidants such as vitamins A, C, E, and K, selenium, calcium, iron, zinc, glutathione, and superoxide dismutase. Prolonged bleeding can cause deficiencies of copper, zinc, iron, folic acid, and vitamin B_{12}, which are vital to the body's self-repair, so malabsorption and deficiency become a worsening cycle.

Many people with IBD who have surgery to remove part of the colon are left with chronic diarrhea, a condition called short bowel syndrome. Douglas Wilmore, M.D., former medical director at the Life Restart Center, helps normalize bowel function in these patients with a high-fiber diet, short-term use of growth hormones, and high doses of glutamine. Glutamine, the primary nutrient for intestinal cells, is effective in healing stomach and bowel ulcers and irritable bowel syndrome. It is also the precursor of glutathione, a nutrient shown to be reduced in the colon cells of people with IBD. Another nutrient, folic acid, has been shown to produce beneficial changes in cells of the rectum. As mentioned previously, the medication Asulfadine causes a 30 percent loss of folic acid, but even those who don't take Asulfadine may benefit greatly from daily folic acid supplementation. In my clinical experience, I've found that a combination of glutamine and folic acid can help rapidly reduce inflammation and irritation in active bowel disease.

People with IBD have a higher level of leukotrienes, innately produced substances that increase pain and inflammation. In adults with ulcerative colitis, the omega-3 fatty acid EPA is well studied and has been shown to be quite effective at reducing inflammation by reducing leukotriene production. A recent study also found EPA beneficial for children with ulcerative colitis in remission.

Aloe vera juice has long been used as a folk-remedy for people with IBD, and its value was confirmed by two recent studies showing the herb to be more helpful than a placebo in reducing inflammation and levels of inflammatory markers. Wheatgrass juice may be useful for reducing overall disease activity and lessening the severity of rectal bleeding in active ulcerative colitis, as indicated by a recent Israeli study. Natural inhibitors of the NOD2 gene, such as boswellia and curcumin, can also be of great benefit against IBD. The anti-inflammatory herb boswellia, for example, has been well tested and found effective. Research on the anti-inflammatory herbal extract curcumin is ongoing in mice.

The Future?

Testing of a protease inhibitor called BBI, derived from soybeans and naturally found in all legumes, is in the initial stages. Someone with IBD would need to eat huge amounts of soy foods and/or other legumes to obtain the same effects as with concentrated BBI, but you might find these foods helpful for your child. Another promising natural approach to IBD involves photophoresis, a process that exposes blood to light and in one study reduced patients' need for steroid medications.

Functional Laboratory Testing for Children with Inflammatory Bowel Disease

Increased levels of the inflammatory marker calprotectin are seen in people with IBD, gastrointestinal infections, and inflammatory arthritis. A new lab test for calprotectin can distinguish IBD from IBS; it can also be used to monitor treatment effectiveness and determine the likeliness of a disease flare-up. See Appendix A for details on testing. Available tests include:

1. Comprehensive digestive and stool analysis (CDSA) with parasite screening
2. Lactose intolerance test
3. Food sensitivity/allergy test(s)
4. Calprotectin test (often included in a CDSA)
5. Intestinal permeability test
6. Immune genetic test
7. Nutritional analysis
8. Vitamin D test

Healing Options for Children with Inflammatory Bowel Disease

See Appendix B for more details on the following nutrients, herbs, and supplements.

Dietary Changes—to avoid gastrointestinal irritation. Eliminate simple sugars, alcohol, fast foods, grains, and dairy products.

Natural Hygiene Diet—to avoid gastrointestinal irritation (see page 173 for details). Many people with IBD have helped themselves through an alkalizing, totally vegetarian diet including vegetable juicing.

Wheatgrass Juice—to reduce disease severity and rectal bleeding. Dosage in children: ½–3½ ounces juice daily, according to child's size.

Specific Carbohydrate Diet—see page 173.

Consider Lactose Intolerance—see Appendix A. To assess whether lactose intolerance contributes to your child's illness, eliminate all dairy products from his/her diet for at least one month. Definitely eliminate dairy during any flare-up.

Consider Food Sensitivity/Allergy—see Chapter 11. The most common offenders are dairy products, grains, and yeast, followed in frequency by egg, potato, rye, coffee, apples, mushrooms, oats, and chocolate. Some people are sensitive to more than one food. An elimination/provocation diet is a simple way to restrict your child's eating to foods that are less likely to trigger symptoms.

Aloe vera Juice—to reduce inflammation and prevent flare-ups. Dosage for children: begin with 1–2 ounces twice daily; 3½ ounces twice daily was used in one study, but less is probably advisable for small children. *Note:* Make sure it's food-grade *Aloe vera* juice.

Glutamine—to heal the bowel, promote the synthesis of glutathione, and increase muscle mass. Dosage for children: 8–20 grams (g) daily for four weeks; then, use more during a flare-up and less on a maintenance basis. *Note:* Glutamine can be constipating, so decrease the dose if your child becomes constipated.

Folic Acid—to repair bowel epithelial tissue and prevent diarrhea. Dosage for children: 5–15 g daily. (Try Folixor from Emerson Ecologics; see Resources.)

Omega-3 Fatty Acids—to reduce inflammation in the gut. Dosage for children: 1.8 milligrams (mg) EPA oil daily. Eating salmon, mackerel, herring, tuna, sardines, and halibut several times a week also supplies these essential fats. *Caution:* Brown and red seaweeds provide generous amounts of omega-3 oil, but the seaweed extract carrageenan may increase colon inflammation and can induce IBD in animals (its effect in humans is unclear).

Quercetin—to reduce pain and inflammatory responses, help heal leaky gut, and control allergies. Dosage for children: 250–1,000 mg three or four times daily.

Probiotics—to rebalance intestinal flora and combat dysbiosis. Dosage for children: one or two capsules three times daily of acidophilus, bifidobacteria, Nissle-strain *Escherichia coli,* or *Saccharomyces boulardii.* Remember to begin with a smaller dosage and increase slowly. Your child will probably need this daily "medicine" for life. (A probiotic preparation containing Nissle *E. coli* plus eight other species is available from VSL Pharmaceuticals; see Resources.)

Boswellia—to reduce inflammation. Dosage for children: begin with 100–200 mg three times daily for small children; 350 mg three times daily has been used with adults and is appropriate for teenagers.

Demulcent Herbs—to soothe intestinal membranes and stimulate mucus production. Acacia, chickweed, comfrey, marshmallow, mullein, plantain, and slippery elm are gentle enough for children. Dosage for children: capsules or tinctures, as directed on label; tea or throat lozenges, as needed. (Other herbs used for bowel disease include agrimony, *Aloe vera,* American cranesbill, bayberry, cabbage, chamomile, echinacea, feverfew, ginger, ginkgo, goldenseal, hawthorne, milk thistle, neem, peppermint, purple cornflower, St. John's wort, valerian, wild indigo, and wild yam.)

Multivitamin-Mineral-Antioxidant Supplement—to counter malabsorption, poor dietary habits, and oxidative damage. A supplement free of food ingredients, herbs, and common allergens is best. Dosage for children: as directed on label.

IRRITABLE BOWEL SYNDROME/RECURRENT ABDOMINAL PAIN

Recurrent abdominal pain, the most common symptom of IBS in children, may also be accompanied by spasms, bloating, gas, and abnormal bowel movements with alternating diarrhea and constipation. Although IBS is extremely common in children, affecting at least 17 percent of high-school students and 8 percent of middle-school students in North America, it is often underdiagnosed, and there are no good studies on smaller children with the condition. Because the syndrome is multifactoral, it is important to look for its underlying causes rather than simply accepting the diagnosis as an endpoint.

Predominant triggers of IBS are stress, food sensitivities/allergies, repeated antibiotic use, parasites, insufficient beneficial gut bacteria, and hormonal changes. It is estimated, for example, that 10 to 17 percent of cases start with a bacterial, viral, or parasitic infection. One study found the parasite *Blastocystis hominis* in 18 percent of people with IBS. In another study, 9 percent tested positive for giardia; oddly enough, an additional 15 percent responded to treatment with the antiparasitic drug metronidazole or tinidazole, even *without* a positive diagnosis of giardia, suggesting another parasitic or bacterial infection.

Children with IBS often have a leaky gut. In a study of seventeen children with IBS, lactulose-mannitol testing showed increased intestinal permeability in nine, and symptoms disappeared in seven of the nine when foods that increased intestinal permeability were excluded from their diet. Virtually any other food can play a role in a child's IBS.

Children who can't tolerate lactose (milk sugar) often complain of stomachaches and cramping. In fact, various studies have found undiagnosed lactose intolerance in 24 to 68 percent of people with IBS. With the elimination of dairy products and lactose-containing foods, 43.6 percent achieved total remission of symptoms and an additional 40 percent had moderate improvements. Other sugars such as sorbitol, mannitol, and artificial sweeteners may be problematic for some children as well.

Does your child drink a lot of juice? A recent study assessed sugar digestion in children with symptoms of IBS, diarrhea, and RAP who drank more than 6 ounces daily of apple juice or pear nectar; one-third were unable to digest lactose and one-half were unable to digest the sugars in apple juice adequately. When apple and pear juices were eliminated for one month, 46 percent of the children experienced improvement, with those who'd been drinking the most juice improving the most. When all of the children then switched to white grape juice for one year, those who'd initially improved continued to be well, half of the other children became symptom free, and by the end of the year, 71 percent of the entire group were symptom free. It seems well worth trying white grape juice for a year to see whether your child's IBS disappears!

Functional Laboratory Testing for Children with Irritable Bowel Syndrome

A child suspected of having IBS should be tested for celiac disease, as the two conditions can have similar symptoms. See Appendix A for details on testing. Available tests include:

1. Comprehensive digestive and stool analysis with parasite screening

2. Intestinal permeability test

3. Food sensitivity/allergy test(s)

4. Lactose intolerance test

Healing Options for Children with Irritable Bowel Syndrome

See Appendix B for more details on the following nutrients, herbs, and supplements.

Consider Food Sensitivity/Allergy—see Chapter 11. If your child has pain and cramping, dairy and/or other foods are very possibly the cause. First, eliminate all dairy products as well as apple juice and pear juice. Any food, however, could be an offender.

Consider Bacterial, Fungal, and/or Parasitic Infection—see Chapters 6 and 15.

Consider Lactose Intolerance—see Appendix A. Having your child avoid all dairy products for at least two weeks is a valuable way to discover whether he/she would benefit from a lactose-free diet.

Fiber—to normalize bowel function. Increased dietary fiber plus a fiber supplement, or a fiber supplement combined with pectins, has been found useful. Use ground flaxseeds, psyllium-seed husks (the fiber in Metamucil) or try Citrucel or a more natural fiber supplements. Dosage for children: begin with ½–1 teaspoon with at least 8 ounces water daily; increase as desired up to 2 tablespoons daily along with an appropriate increase in water. *Caution:* Wheat bran is *not* a recommended fiber source, and made 55 percent of people with IBS worse.

Probiotics—to dramatically reduce diarrhea, alternating diarrhea/constipation, and other symptoms. In children younger than seven years of age, use *Bifidobacteria infantis*. In children whose predominant symptom is diarrhea, try *Saccharomyces boulardii*. Dosage for children: *Lactobacillus acidophilus* with or without *B. infantis*, one or two capsules or ¼–½ teaspoon powder one to three times daily, according to child's size and age; *S. boulardii*, 250 mg one to three times daily. Initially, your child may experience bloating and gas, so begin with a lower dose and increase slowly.

Peppermint Oil—to relieve cramping and spasm. *Note:* Use enteric-coated capsules to convey the oil intact to the colon. Dosage for children: one or two capsules daily, between meals.

Ginger—to relieve gas pains. Also shown to increase levels of the enzymes that digest fats and sugars. Dosage for children: tea or crystallized (candied) ginger, as needed.

Stress Management—to lessen the emotional stress that is an important factor in IBS. Look at the stressors in your child's life and talk with him/her about them. Studies have shown that hypnotherapy, biofeedback, and counseling can be very helpful.

Herbs—to relieve gas, strengthen the stomach, and soothe pain. Antispasmodic herbs include chamomile, lemon balm, rosemary, and valerian; valerian can be found in combination products with other calming herbs like hops, skullcap, and passionflower. Dosage for children: as directed on label.

PART FOUR

Additional Conditions That Benefit from a Healthy Gut

CHAPTER 18

Arthritis

A rthritis refers to more than a hundred diseases causing joint inflammation. Although we usually think of it as a condition affecting the elderly, it can afflict children and teenagers as well. About 300,000 of our children have arthritis. Rheumatoid arthritis (RA), the most devastating type, affects 70,000–75,000 children. For some, juvenile arthritis (JA) is outgrown by puberty, whereas for others it becomes a life-long illness. Juvenile arthritic disease varies widely in severity and expression, as detailed in the inset on page 184.

The many causes and triggers of arthritis include genetic predisposition, infection, physical injury, nutritional deficiency, allergy, metabolic or immune disorder, stress, pollutants, and toxins. Tests for parasites, metals, candidiasis, intestinal permeability, and the like often point to an underlying condition. Some children with JA have been found to have a leaky gut; in one study, 39 percent had gastrointestinal problems. Leaky gut could be due to medications. Increased intestinal permeability, in turn, allows more food particles to cross the intestinal mucosa, triggering a greater food sensitivity response (more about this on page 185).

GENE, MEET MICROORGANISM

Rheumatoid arthritis (RA) often runs in families. The illness is triggered when predisposing genes are stimulated by certain environmental factors, but it's not a one-to-one correlation: Many genes may be involved and many environmental factors, including various kinds of infections. Once triggered, arthritis and joint inflammation are difficult to halt.

A recent study of specific HLA genes examined which alleles (gene pairs that are responsible for various differentiating characteristics) were associated with a greater risk of JA. Half of the children with HLA-A2, DR8, DR5, or DPB_1*0201 alleles developed JA before their third birthday, and children with more than one of these alleles developed JA at an earlier age.

The Major Types of Juvenile Arthritis

Doctors categorize juvenile arthritis according to the number of swollen and painful joints and also according to the absence or presence of rheumatoid arthritis antibodies (RA factor) or antinuclear antibodies (ANA).

Pauciarticular ("Few-Joints") Disease

Pauciarticular disease occurs in just a few joints, usually four or less. Pain is typically asymmetrical (that is, not on both sides of the body or in the same places). Most commonly involves large joints (knees, hips, shoulders, ankles). Two forms.

• Type I Pauciarticular Disease: Accounts for 30 to 40 percent of JA. Onset early in life, usually before age of four years. Mainly in girls. Elevated ANA in 80 percent of Type I. About one-third of children with Type I develop eye complications, must see ophthalmologist every three to four months for first several years of disease.

• Type II Pauciarticular Disease: Accounts for 10 to 15 percent of JA. Mainly in boys. Typically involves hip. Eye complications may be associated. When in spine, often has genetic component involving HLA $B_2 7$ gene (HLA $B_2 7$ is also involved in adult type of arthritis called ankylosing spondylitis).

Polyarticular ("Many-Joint") Disease

Polyarticular disease occurs in many joints, often including hands. Pain is usually symmetrical (on both sides of body in same places). Accounts for 35 percent of JA. Mainly in girls. Two forms.

• Rheumatoid-Factor-Positive Polyarticular Disease: More-severe form. Onset most frequently in late childhood or early teens. Lumpy nodules often occur at joints. Positive blood test for RA factor. About 25 percent of RA-positive children will have persistent arthritic problems through life.

• Non-Rheumatoid-Factor-Positive Polyarticular Disease: Less-severe form. Onset can occur during childhood or teen years. Negative blood test for RA factor. Stiff and painful joints, especially in morning and after inactivity.

Systemic JRA

In both boys and girls, systemic JRA accounts for 10 to 20 percent of JA. Typically begins with high fever and brief, salmon-colored rash; joint pain may accompany fever or may not occur until much later. About 25 percent of children with systemic JRA will have persistent arthritic problems through life.

The common intestinal bacterium *Proteus mirabilis* typically doesn't cause illness; in someone with the gene allele HLA-DR4, however, the presence of proteus may set off an autoimmune response that leads to RA. In a recent study of children with arthritis and accompanying vision complications, proteus was found in nearly 15 percent, and primarily in children with RA; when proteus infection was present, eye disease progressed much more quickly. In another interesting study, adults placed on vegetarian diets (long known to benefit people with RA) showed a decrease in antibodies to proteus.

Researchers are looking for microbes that may trigger JA. Some cases are associated with infections of influenza virus type AH2N2 or parvovirus B19. One study found at least one viral infection in 92 percent of children with RA (primarily Coxsackie A13 virus, rubella, and adenoviruses) and found mixed infections in 80 percent. Why infections move to the joints or cause joint pain is unknown, but the phenomenon is well documented.

THE ROLE OF FOOD SENSITIVITY

The connection of food sensitivity to RA was first noted in 1949 by Michael Zeller, who found that adding and eliminating various foods showed a direct cause and effect between diet and the disease. Dr. Zeller's colleague Theron Randolph, the "father of clinical ecology" (a field of medicine concerning how our environment affects our health), found that people with RA who were not reacting to foods were sensitive to at least one environmental chemical. Dr. Randolph sent questionnaires to more than 200 of his patients with osteoarthritis and/or RA to assess treatment effectiveness, and found that they experienced a significant reduction in arthritic symptoms when they avoided environmental and food allergens.

More recently, in a study of children with JRA, 43 percent reported aggravation of their disease after eating certain foods, and 26 percent reported having tried specific diets to reduce their symptoms; of the children who'd tried diets, 46 percent reported having less pain and stiffness and 36 percent reported having less joint swelling as a result. In a study of adults with rheumatic diseases, two-thirds reported that fasting produced symptom improvement. A few studies have looked at the role in JRA of specific food sensitivities such as dairy or wheat, but children can be sensitive to any number of unstudied foods. The only way to know for certain what your child reacts to is to do specific food allergy testing.

Wheat allergens like gliaden do pose problems for many people, and the presence of antigliaden antibodies in people with RA is of great interest to clinical researchers. Many adults with RA have high levels of antigliaden antibodies in their blood despite having no symptoms of celiac disease. In one study of adults with RA, nearly 50 percent had elevated levels of IgG antibody to gliadin, and 86 percent of that subgroup was RA-factor positive. In another, fifteen of the twenty-four participants had elevated levels of IgA, RA factor, and wheat-protein IgG; six of the wheat-positive and one of the wheat-negative people showed intestinal brush border damage, which the researchers felt played an important role in RA's progression.

CONVENTIONAL DRUG TREATMENT

Conventional JA treatment focuses on use of medications to reduce inflammation and pain. A drug, however, can be a two-edged sword: We want our children to feel well, but medication may have long-term negative effects.

Treatment for JA typically begins with nonsteroidal anti-inflammatory drugs (NSAIDs) such as ibuprofen, but these are tough on the stomach and intestinal lining, and by blocking production of the prostaglandins that normally stimulate repair of that lining, NSAID use also increases the likelihood of developing leaky gut syndrome. A study of children using NSAIDs for RA showed that more than 75 percent had gastric erosions or ulcers; the more NSAIDs taken, the leakier the gut wall becomes, and the more pain and inflammation follows, setting up an escalating problem. Making arthritic matters worse, many NSAIDs block the body's ability to repair and regenerate cartilage because they lower levels of healing prostaglandins, glucosaminoglycans, and hyaluronan, and raise levels of inflammatory leukotrienes.

The medication picture for JA doesn't get any better aside from NSAIDs. Steroids such as prednisone are often used in the short term to reduce inflammation and pain, but cannot be used on a long-term basis because they negatively affect growth, thin the bones, and cause weight gain and early cataracts. Disease-

Herbal Medicines for Rheumatoid Arthritis

Because DMARDs and NSAIDs can be so damaging to the body, researchers are seeking alternatives among traditional medicines. Two anti-inflammatory Chinese herbs are being investigated for potential benefits in adults with RA. In a recent study, 60 percent of the participants who took 180 milligrams (mg) daily of *Tripterygium wilfordii* Hook F showed improvement, as did eight of the ten who took more than 360 mg daily, and one patient even went into remission. Another study of this herb also showed favorable results. (Its main side effect? Diarrhea.) Tetrandrine, extracted from the herb Han-Fang Chi and historically used to suppress the immune system and lower inflammatory markers, is being studied as well. In China, these two medicines are often taken in combination for greater effectiveness.

modifying antirheumatic drugs (DMARDs) may be prescribed for a child with inflammation in many joints, but DMARDs can take up to six months to work and their possible side effects are even more serious. For example, cyclosporin blocks pain but suppresses the immune system, making your child vulnerable to infection. Methotrexate is another commonly used arthritis medication. In addition to suppressing the immune system, it also interferes with DNA synthesis and folic acid metabolism. Gold appears to slow the production of proteins and antibodies, thereby decreasing joint pain, but can easily become toxic. Drugs like Ethanercept, Infliximab, and adalimumab help with JA by reducing inflammation and lowering levels of tumor necrosis factor-alpha (TNF-alpha, a cytokine molecule that causes inflammation in response to a challenge such as an infection), but their many possible side effects include infection, rash, cough, nausea, abdominal pain, headache, and more.

SUPPLEMENTARY TREATMENTS

Natural therapies can be astonishingly effective. They can serve as a valuable adjunct to medical intervention or even, in some cases, as a replacement. By reducing the need for medications, natural therapies for arthritis also reduce the accompanying side effects. Many of the supplementary treatments described in this section have antioxidant properties. Anyone with increased inflammation has an increased need for antioxidant nutrients, which are found in fruits, vegetables, nuts, seeds, and whole grains, as well as in supplements. Think of inflammation as a fire: Antioxidants help put out the fires of arthritis.

Minerals

Children with JA commonly lose minerals from bone and have many other nutritional deficiencies as well, so it's essential to feed them healthful foods and also give them supplements to compensate. All children with RA lose bone calcium, especially those who take corticosteroid drugs like prednisone; supplemental calcium and vitamin D are useful for most of these children.

People with RA often have marginal levels of copper, a metal involved in collagen formation, tissue repair, and anti-inflammatory processes. Traditionally, copper bracelets have been worn to reduce arthritic symptoms. W. Ray Walker found that sweat dissolves about 13 mg of bracelet copper per month, much of which is presumably absorbed through the skin. In an interesting test with forty people who had previously benefited from wearing copper bracelets, Dr. Walker had them wear copper-colored bracelets (actually made of aluminum in this case) for two months; more than 50 percent reported that their arthritis had worsened, and fourteen participants deteriorated too much to finish the two-month test.

Oils and Herbs

The general health benefits of omega-3 fatty acids in fish oil were introduced in Chapter 8. Fish oil lowers TNF-alpha levels, and daily dosages from eight to twenty capsules have produced moderate but definite improvement in arthritic diseases. Compared to placebo, supplemental fish oil enabled a group of children with RA to reduce their ibuprofen use, and omega-3 fatty acid supplementation in children with RA has been shown to lower levels of the inflammatory marker C-reactive protein (CRP).

Oils containing gamma-linolenic acid (GLA) are also useful in arthritis treatment. In one study of patients with RA, 1.4 grams (g) daily of GLA from borage oil significantly reduced symptoms of swollen joints by 36 percent, tenderness by 45 percent, swollen joint count by 28 percent, and swollen joint score by 41 percent; some people improved in more than one area. In another study, oil of evening primrose and olive oil (both contain GLA) helped reduce pain and morning stiffness in both test groups of adults with RA. Several participants were able to reduce their use of NSAIDs, but none were able to stop taking them entirely.

Here is a sampling of the plentiful research on herbal arthritis remedies:

- Turmeric has the ability to block inflammatory and pain-producing leukotrienes and arachadonic acid. Turmeric's active pain-relieving agent, curcumin, lowers TNF-alpha levels.

- Boswellia, traditionally used for arthritis, pain, and inflammation, has been shown to moderate inflammatory markers. When a boswellia preparation called H-15 was given to 260 people with RA, 50 to 60 percent of them achieved good results.

- Ginger reduced pain and swelling in 75 percent of people with RA and/or osteoarthritis, with no reported side effects for three months to two-and-a-half years of use.

- Yucca is a rich source of anti-inflammatory compounds called saponins. Studies have shown significant improvement in 56 to 66 percent of adults with RA and/or osteoarthritis who tried yucca, with no reported negative side effects for one-and-a-half years of use.

- Devil's claw, commonly used for arthritis, has been shown in several studies to work as well as the NSAID phenylbutazone at reducing pain and inflammation.

- Cayenne pepper is well studied for temporary relief of arthritis pain. Topical creams containing the cayenne derivative capsicum work by blocking the formation of inflammatory leukotrienes, arachadonic acid, and substance P.

Probiotics

Research is still lacking on the use of probiotics in JA. In one study giving Lacto-bacillus GG, a species of lactobacillus, to adults with RA, the group receiving the probiotic had much greater improvement in symptoms and sense of well-being than the placebo group did, even though their blood tests were similar.

Enzymes

An animal study found that rabbits receiving supplemental enzymes did not develop arthritis while rabbits without the supplements did develop arthritis; high doses of the enzymes produced the best results. Research on enzyme supplementation for human arthritis looks promising as well. In a study of 156 adults with RA, the group treated with enzymes reported less morning stiffness and pain than did the group treated conventionally with NSAIDs and methotrexate. In the enzyme group, a few participants had the undesired side effect of frequent bowel movements, but none had any of the drug-group's side effects, which included low white blood cell count, nerve damage, and liver toxicity. In a study of forty adults with ankylosing spondylitis, the group treated for six months with enzymes experienced more lasting and sustainable improvement in pain than did the group treated for six months with the common NSAID indomethacin.

Other Nutrients

Children with JA have been found to have low levels of superoxide dismutase (SOD), another important anti-inflammatory and antioxidant enzyme. Although most people who try it for arthritis experience benefits, there is little human research to date. Veterinarians, however, have obtained excellent results using wheat-grass extracts of SOD on arthritic animals.

More supplements of interest for arthritis treatment:

- Quercetin, a bioflavonoid, appears to lower levels of TNF-alpha and inflammatory cytokines in adults with RA. Bioflavonoids also help maintain and strengthen collagen, a fibrous protein that forms robust connective tissue necessary for strong bones, cartilage, joints, and muscles.

- The naturally occurring substance methylsulfonylmethane (MSM) has been shown in animal studies to be an anti-inflammatory antioxidant. MSM provides the body with sulfur compounds necessary to build cartilage and collagen and help with methylation pathways, and it is now being used for arthritis and pain management, but there are no studies on MSM for JA.

- S-adenosylmethionine (SAMe), a chemical found naturally in every living cell, is a recent arrival on the anti-inflammatory scene. SAMe has been shown to be as potent as indomethacin and other NSAIDs, but with fewer negative side effects.

- The amino acid DL-phenylalanine (DLPA) is effective for treating RA and osteoarthritis pain. DLPA appears to inhibit the breakdown of our body's natural pain relievers, the endorphins.

FUNCTIONAL LABORATORY TESTING FOR CHILDREN WITH ARTHRITIS

Examine your child's ability to detoxify. Ask your child's pediatrician to look for possible infectious triggers including rubella, Coxsackie, parvovirus, influenza AH2N2, candida, Lyme, chlamydia, klebsiella, salmonella, or other organisms. See Appendix A for details on testing. Available tests include:

1. Food sensitivity/allergy test(s)
2. Genetic tests for inflammatory markers
3. Intestinal permeability test (Note: stop use of NSAIDs for three weeks prior to test)
4. Liver detoxification function test
5. Screening for viral, fungal, and bacterial infection

HEALING OPTIONS FOR CHILDREN WITH ARTHRITIS

Treating JA calls for an integrated approach. Some of the suggestions herein may help significantly, and others may not help at all. Be patient and give whatever you try some time to work. You might want to try one or two ideas at a time until you come up with a program that suits your child. (It is unlikely that you will need to use every suggested option.)

It is essential to dampen your child's inflammatory processes by addressing any food and/or environmental sensitivities as well as acid-alkaline balance. Along with beneficial flora and supplements, changes in diet and lifestyle can be recommended according to his/her needs. Vegetable-based diets balance pH, provide an abundance of antioxidants and natural anti-inflammatory factors as well as vitamins, minerals, and phytonutrients, and tend to be hypoallergenic. Numerous studies have shown vegetarian, vegan, and raw-food diets to reduce RA symptoms in adults. Work with a clinical nutritionist to make certain that any diet your child undertakes is nutritionally balanced.

Exercise and stretching are useful for all types of arthritic conditions. Walking, swimming, physical therapy, and massage therapy may all play a role in symptom reduction. Yoga has been found helpful for range of motion, pain, stiffness, and joint tenderness. Movement is *not* optional! Even small amounts can give great relief. See Appendix B for more details on the following nutrients, herbs, and supplements.

Alkalizing Diet—to conserve bone and reduce inflammation and pain. An alkalizing diet may be the single most useful anti-arthritis idea. See Chapter 7 for details.

Elimination/Provocation Diet and Food-Sensitivity Testing—to reduce inflammation, pain, and stiffness, and increase mobility. See Chapter 11 for instructions. For best results, work with a nutritionist or physician familiar with food-sensitivity protocols. Blood testing aids this process significantly by identifying specific foods to which your child is sensitive. After four to six months, your child will be able to tolerate most of the formerly troublesome foods; repeat blood testing at that time is advised.

Exercise and Physical Therapy—to help keep your child's joints flexible. It's important to move the body gently as much as possible without aggravating the joints. Yoga, walking, swimming, water exercises, physical therapy, massage, and acupressure massage may all be helpful. Encourage your child to do some type of movement that he/she enjoys nearly every day.

Enzymes—to reduce inflammation, pain, and swelling, increase flexibility, boost natural immune response, and support complete digestion. In adult studies, results are typically seen in about six weeks. Dosage for children: digestive enzymes, one capsule with each meal; proteolytic enzymes, one to three capsules two or three times daily on an empty stomach (good times are upon arising and at bedtime), varying dosage according to intensity of pain.

Vitamin C—to reduce pain, inflammation, and swelling. Vital for formation of cartilage and collagen, this antiviral antioxidant is an essential nutrient for every anti-arthritis program. Dosage for children: 500 mg–3 g daily.

Multivitamin-Mineral Supplement—to compensate for nutrient deficiencies. Dosage for children: as directed on label. Make sure that your child also gets additional calcium (250–1,000 mg) and magnesium (100–500 mg) daily.

Omega-3 Fatty Acids/Fish Oils—to reduce morning stiffness and joint tenderness. Dosage for children: begin with 1,000 mg daily and build slowly to as much as 10,000 mg daily according to child's size, age, and response. Similar results can be obtained by eating high-EPA/DHA fish two to four times a week. *Caution:* Because fish oils increase blood-clotting time, they should not be used by people who have hemophilia or who regularly take anticoagulant medicines or aspirin.

Gamma-Linolenic Acid—to reduce inflammation and pain. Dosage for children: 700–1,400 mg daily, according to child's size, weight, and response.

Probiotics—to prevent infection, manufacture needed vitamins, reduce inflammation, and normalize gastrointestinal function. Choose lactobacillus and bifidobacteria species; for infants and small children, use *Bifidobacteria infantis.* Dosage for children: powder, ⅛–½ teaspoon two or three times daily; capsules, one or two, two or three times daily.

Quercetin—to reduce inflammation and pain, control allergic responses, and maintain joint tissue. Dosage for children: 500–2,000 mg daily.

Turmeric/Curcumin—to reduce inflammation. Dosage for children: turmeric is effective at 10–60 g daily; curcumin can be taken in much smaller doses of 500 mg three times daily.

Boswellia—to reduce inflammation. Boswellia is taken as a long-term treatment for RA, not specifically for immediate pain. Dosage for children: 600–1,200 mg two or three times daily.

Ginger—to reduce pain and swelling. Dosage for children: fresh root, 2 ounces daily; powder, 3,000–7,000 mg daily. Candied ginger or ginger tea can also be used.

Superoxide Dismutase—for antioxidant effects. Dosage for children: 500–2,000 mg daily. (See also Copper, below.)

Yucca—to alleviate pain and improve digestion. Dosage for children: 1,000–2,000 mg daily.

Methylsulfonylmethane—to reduce pain, inflammation, and allergic response, and build cartilage and collagen. Dosage for children: 500–5,000 mg daily. *Note:* Best taken with an equal amount of vitamin C for proper absorption.

S-Adenosylmethionine (SAME)—to reduce inflammation. Dosage for children: 200–400 mg twice daily, adjusting up or down as needed. If your child's symptoms do not respond, try a higher dose; if your child's symptoms respond well, try a bit less to see whether symptom reduction is sustained. *Note:* Should be taken concurrently with a good multivitamin containing B-complex vitamins.

Bromelain—to reduce inflammation. Dosage for children: 500–1,000 mg two or three times daily between meals.

Devil's Claw—to reduce pain and inflammation. Dosage for children: 250–750 mg three times daily.

Capsicum—to block inflammation and temporarily relieve joint pain. Best used topically. Capsicum often appears on ingredients lists as capsaicin (one of the active ingredients). Dosage for children: as directed on label.

DL-Phenylalanine—to reduce pain. Dosage for children: 200–500 mg three times daily.

Copper—to support collagen formation, tissue repair, and anti-inflammatory processes, and increase levels of SOD. Dosage for children: 1–2 mg daily, or have your child wear a copper bracelet. In consultation with a physician, you may temporarily add a supplement of copper salicylate or sebacate until copper level returns to normal. *Note:* Supplemental copper can interfere with zinc absorption, so give 5–10 mg zinc daily as well to prevent zinc deficiency. You may be able to find the necessary amounts of both copper and zinc within a multivitamin-mineral or mineral supplement.

CHAPTER 19

Asthma

A sthma's technical name is reversible obstructive pulmonary disease (ROPD). It can be a chronic or occasional problem. Asthma attacks can come on suddenly or build over several hours or days; symptoms include trouble breathing, wheezing, chest tightness, chest pain, and coughing. The condition is more common in children and in people of African descent, and childhood asthma is more common in boys than in girls.

Asthma affects 7.3 percent of American children under the age of eighteen—that's more than five million children! The incidence of asthma in the United States has been rising at an alarming rate: Between 1980 and 1993–1994, it increased 75 percent overall, 74 percent in children aged five to fourteen years, and an astonishing 160 percent in children up to the age of four years. This epidemic continues to grow, which is truly sad, because much asthma is preventable. Many children outgrow their asthma during puberty. According to the Centers for Disease Control, asthmatic children lose 14 million school days each year, asthma is the third most common reason children under fifteen are hospitalized, and the number of children and teens dying from asthma has nearly tripled from 1979 to 1996.

A MULTIFACTORAL DISEASE

Interplay among genetic predisposition, environmental stimuli, and gut ecology appears to be basic to the condition. Triggers of asthma attacks include stress, poor air quality, grasses, molds, smoke, chemicals, bacterial infections, colds, viruses, pollens, dust, and sensitivity to cockroaches and pets. Increasing ozone levels, sulfur dioxide, and particulate matter in the air outside are all directly correlated with increased hospital admissions for asthma. Asthma attacks are increased significantly in households where family members smoke.

During an asthma attack, the lungs begin to produce more mucus than normal; it's very thick and sticky, and tends to clog the breathing tubes. These tubes become inflamed, swollen, and narrowed, and breathing becomes difficult. The oxygen supply to the body is limited, carbon dioxide builds up, and the entire body becomes more acidic. On a biochemical level, exposure to allergens can precipitate an asthma attack by stimulating the activity of mast cells (specialized white blood cells that break apart, flooding the body with histamines) and the production of inflammatory cytokines and interleukins, all of which play a central role in initiating and sustaining the inflammation associated with asthma. You may recognize the names of these substances for their association with allergic reactions.

Although the symptoms of asthma are felt in the lungs, it is believed that people with asthma have problems with their mucous membranes in general, and that exposure to allergens leads to inflammation in their digestive tract, causing a leaky gut. Poor gut integrity, in turn, increases all childhood atopic illnesses including asthma, eczema, and allergies. Most children with asthma also have allergies. Interestingly, for children born into "allergic" families, antibiotic use during the first year of life increases their risk of asthma. A 2004 study from the University of Iowa reported that children living on hog farms have higher asthma rates than other children do, and that on farms where antibiotics are used, asthma rates are even higher.

Candida and other fungal infections have been linked with asthma. Candida overgrowth is often caused by use of antibiotics and other medications, which is why the hog farm findings above are not much of a surprise. A recent study of sixty-four people with asthma found fungal infections in fifty-two of them. Ironically, the increased risk of candida infection in asthmatics may be partially due to steroid medications and inhalers, as steroid inhalers promote candida growth in the gut and lungs of children who use them for asthma. Other studies, however, also report a high incidence of candida in asthmatics who don't use steroids. In my clinical practice, I often find that when candida overgrowth in the gut is tamed, breathing becomes easier and attacks less frequent.

One consequence of asthma is a deficiency of the secretory IgA (sIgA) normally found in mucous membranes throughout the body. Acting as sentries, sIgA antibodies alert the immune system to mobilize an attack on a foreign substance. When our sIgA is low, we are vulnerable to allergies and infections of all types.

NATURAL ASTHMA-REDUCING TECHNIQUES

Medical treatment for asthma utilizes medications such as steroids, inhalers, allergy shots, and peak-flow meters that help the sufferer breathe. Asthma responds best, however, to lifestyle changes and stress-management techniques. Learning to develop emotional hardiness and a relaxed manner in stressful situations can greatly reduce the incidence and severity of asthma attacks. Exercise usually benefits people with asthma as well (though there is one type of asthma that only occurs post-exercise).

Cleaning up the diet is essential. Sensitivity to foods is usually a major problem in asthma. In children, the most common food allergens are fruits, eggs, dairy products, and nuts, but virtually any food can be a problem. Some studies, surprisingly, have shown dairy products to be protective against asthma instead of contributing to it. It's important to test for your child's specific food sensitivities and allergies, and then have him/her avoid those foods. Because the effects of asthma on the body's gases produce a generally acidic condition, pH testing and an alkaline diet can be of great benefit.

Allergic reactions of all sorts occur when the body is overloaded with stressors. Imagine your child's body as a glass filled with water; add a little pollen, a little dust, a little emotional stress, a little food sensitivity, and eventually the glass overflows. If you can keep your child's total stress level below the top of the glass, he/she will stay symptom free, so your objective in fighting his/her asthma is to reduce whatever stress you can.

Asthma responds to adrenal support, so corticosteroid drugs like prednisone and cortisone that mimic the body's natural adrenal hormones are often used in asthma. The downside of such drugs is that they can stunt bone development and suppress the immune system. Natural supplements may be useful for supporting your child's adrenal glands and enhancing his/her own steroid production. The herb lobelia, for example, promotes the adrenals' production of hormones that relax the bronchial muscles, and has been used for centuries to treat asthma in Europe.

Fish oils rich in healthful omega-3 fatty acids are well known to reduce levels of inflammatory leukotrienes, cytokines, and arachadonic acid. Research on fish oils for asthma has been extensive, but results have been mixed: some children benefit tremendously, others don't. Research does, however, clearly document an increased need for the antioxidants glutathione peroxidase and vitamins C and E in

Mother's Milk

When a child is born to an asthmatic parent, it's advised to breast-feed for at least four months. This reduces the risk that the child will develop asthma by 30 to 50 percent. The exact mechanisms behind this aren't fully understood, but we do know that breast-feeding increases a child's natural immunity to disease. It is also known that babies are often allergic to dairy-based or soy-based formulas, which sets up the potential passage of antigens through a leaky gut.

people with asthma, and magnesium deficiency is common in asthmatic children. A powerful muscle relaxant and bronchodilator, magnesium can prevent and reduce the severity of asthma attacks.

Vitamin B_6 and B_{12} levels have also been found to be lower in asthmatics. Jonathan Wright, M.D., tells of a 1931 study showing that 80 percent of asthmatic children had digestive problems: specifically, low HCl and pepsin secretion in the stomach. When given daily B_{12} injections for one month, about half of the children's asthma symptoms disappeared. (Today, vitamin B_{12} can be taken sublingually in the well-absorbed form of hydroxycobalamine.) In a recent study of asthmatic children allergic to sulfite preservatives, four of the five did not have an asthma attack in response to sulfites after being given vitamin B_{12}.

Children with asthma can benefit from herbs and other nutrients that promote the health of mucous membranes in the lungs and gut. A study of ginkgo for asthma showed improvement in symptoms and lung function, as well as reduced airway hyper-reactivity. Astragalus strengthens the lungs over time. The natural antihistamine quercetin inhibits mast cell activity. Vitamin C is well documented to protect lung responsiveness and function and reduce asthma symptoms. Taking probiotic bacteria helps build and restore a child's gut ecology when it's been disrupted by antibiotic use, and supplemental probiotics given to children confer a protective effect against developing asthma. The herb *Coleus forskohli* has bronchodilation effects and has been shown to be beneficial for asthma (but is not yet studied in children). It stimulates the production of cyclic AMP; impaired cyclic AMP production is believed to be an underlying cause of asthma.

A great deal of anecdotal evidence indicates that proteolytic (protein-splitting) enzymes can help reduce asthma's severity and frequency, although this effect is not yet corroborated by clinical research. These enzymes work throughout the body to break down proteins into amino acids. Antigens are the substances that produce an allergic response. They are proteins floating around in the bloodstream. Proteolytic enzymes can reduce inflammatory cytokines and allergic reactions by activating the immune system to scavenge for antigens.

One study looked at the benefits of bee propolis, a natural resin with antibiotic and antifungal properties, for adults with asthma; after two months of taking propolis, night-time attacks decreased in number and severity, pulmonary function tests improved, and inflammatory cytokines decreased. Another study gave the homeopathic product Traumeel S to adult asthmatics who continued to use corticosteroid medications; after twenty weeks of taking Traumeel S, average daily medication use decreased from 4.6 to 2.6 milligrams (mg), symptoms improved significantly, serum IgE levels dropped substantially, infection frequency decreased, and sense of well-being increased.

FUNCTIONAL LABORATORY TESTING FOR CHILDREN WITH ASTHMA

Testing can be useful in finding underlying issues associated with breathing problems. Fortifying your child's overall health can significantly reduce the incidence and severity of his/her asthma. See Appendix A for details on testing. Available tests include:

1. Food sensitivity/allergy test(s)

2. Intestinal permeability test

3. Candida antibodies test

4. Organic acid test

PROTECTIVE OPTIONS FOR CHILDREN WITH ASTHMA

See Appendix B for more details on the following nutrients, herbs, and supplements. (It is unlikely that you will need to use every suggested protective option.)

Improve the Indoor Environment—by keeping it as clean as possible. Do your best to eliminate the mold often found in basements, bathrooms, closets, and shower curtains. Using high-quality air-filtration systems and efficient vacuum cleaners can be effective in preventing attacks. Make your child's bedroom a hypoallergenic oasis by keeping it scrupulously clean and uncluttered, laundering bedding in hot water, and removing carpeting, stuffed animals, curtains, and anything soft that can collect dust. Keep pets out of the bedroom (keep them outdoors, if possible). Be aware of your child's outdoor environment, too.

Balance pH—see Chapter 7. Bringing your child's pH into the desirable range with urine testing and an alkalizing diet can be the one most useful thing you do for his/her asthma.

Dietary Changes—to quickly reduce your child's asthmatic symptoms. Eliminate sugar, processed foods, and additives from your child's diet. Focus on fresh fruits and vegetables and natural foods (organic, when possible).

Consider Food Sensitivity/Allergy—see Chapter 11. Test potential food allergens (starting with fruits, dairy, eggs, and nuts or any other foods you may suspect), have your child avoid all foods to which he/she is reactive, and then slowly reintroduce them after four to six months.

Probiotics—to rebalance your child's gut and reduce fungal overgrowth. *Lactobacillus acidophilus* and bifidobacteria species are recommended, with *B. infantis* for small children and babies. Dosage for children: powder, $\frac{1}{4}$–$\frac{1}{2}$ teaspoon two or three times daily, according to child's age; or capsules, one or two twice daily, according to child's age.

Omega-3 Fatty Acids/Fish Oil—to reduce inflammation in the lungs. Cod liver oil may be particularly beneficial because it also contains vitamin A, which protects the lung mucosa. Dosage for children: 1,000–10,000 mg daily, according to child's age. There's nothing to lose from a month-long trial. Alternatively or additionally, have him/her eat high-EPA/DHA fish at least twice per week.

Multivitamin-Antioxidant Supplement—to quench free radicals caused by lung irritation and inflammation. Antioxidants include glutathione peroxidase, n-acetyl cysteine, selenium, and vitamins B_6, B_{12}, C, and E. Dosage for children: as directed on label; for a small child, use a children's chewable multivitamin.

Magnesium—to prevent asthma attacks and reduce their severity. Dosage for children: 100–800 mg daily; increase the dosage from 100 mg in 100-mg increments until your child gets diarrhea, then decrease it to the lowest effective amount. *Note:* If more than 1,000 mg is needed for magnesium to take effect, your child may benefit from 1 teaspoon of choline citrate daily for each 200 mg of magnesium to increase magnesium absorption.

Digestive Enzymes—to promote complete and efficient digestion. Dosage for children: one capsule with each meal.

Astragalus—to strengthen the lungs. Dosage for children: one or two capsules, or ten to fifty drops tincture, daily for six months.

Vitamin C—to reduce asthma symptoms. Dosage for children: 200–1,000 mg or more, up to your child's bowel tolerance (you'll know you've reached this when your child gets diarrhea).

Proteolytic Enzymes—to reduce asthma symptoms. Dosage: one to two capsules two to three times daily between meals. Take with 8 ounces of water.

HEALING OPTIONS FOR CHILDREN WITH ASTHMA

Many children are able to use the below-listed therapies regularly and use medications with less frequency. See Appendix 2 for more details on the following nutrients, herbs, and supplements. (It is unlikely that you will need to use every suggested healing option.)

Lobelia—to open up the lungs. Dosage for children: three to twenty drops tincture three times daily, according to child's size.

Vitamin B_{12}—to counteract possible deficiency caused by low HCl levels. Dosage for children: 2,000–6,000 micrograms daily under the tongue.

Heal Mucous Membranes—to fight leaky gut and strengthen lungs. Vitamin A, glutamine, n-acetyl glucosamine, n-acetyl cysteine, and folic acid are often combined in a single supplement designed to help with leaky gut syndrome. Dosage for children: as instructed on bottle.

Quercetin—to reduce allergic reactions and protect the gut lining. Dosage for children: 150–1,000 mg as needed, at first sign of lung tightness and throughout the duration of the attack. (*Author's note:* As far as I know, there is no toxic dose.)

Eucalyptus and Peppermint Oil Steam—to open the lungs. Take 5 drops each of eucalyptus and peppermint oils and place in a bowl of boiling water. Put a towel over your child's head and have him/her breathe the steamy vapors. Dosage: as needed up to 4 times daily.

Ginkgo—to reduce asthma symptoms and aid lung function. Use a standardized extract. Dosage for children: toddlers, 30–60 mg daily; young children, 75–100 mg daily; older pre-pubertal children, 100–150 mg daily; teenagers, 180–240 mg daily. *Note:* It may take up to twelve weeks to see improvement.

Bee Propolis—to reduce asthma symptoms and attacks. Dosage for children: teenagers, 1,000 mg daily; small children, 200–500 mg daily. *Caution:* If your child is allergic to bee stings and/or bee products, *don't use* bee propolis.

Traumeel S—to reduce need for medication and symptoms and increase general well-being. Dosage for children: one ampoule injected into the skin every five to seven days.

Coleus forskohli/Forskolin—to open and relax air passages in the lungs. Dosage for children: 20–100 mg *Coleus forskohli* daily, according to child's size and age. Look for a supplement that lists Forskolin content between 10 and 18 percent.

Adrenal Support—to promote resilience to stress and environmental allergens. Options include adrenal glandulars, pantothenic acid, Siberian ginseng, real licorice candy or licorice root, tea, tincture, or capsules. Dosage for children: as directed on label. *Caution:* Too much licorice may raise blood pressure, so if you are using licorice root, check your child's blood pressure regularly. *Note:* Most licorice candy does not contain any actual licorice, but Panda and some gourmet brands do.

Meyer's Cocktail—to revitalize your child's nutrient status quickly. This intravenous combination of magnesium, calcium, pantothenic acid, and vitamins B_6, B_{12}, and C has been used successfully in people with a variety of ailments. I'd try Meyer's cocktail with an older child, or a child with severe asthma. Intravenous nutrients, given by a physician, can be administered and absorbed at higher concentrations than oral supplements can. Dosage for children: as determined by physician.

CHAPTER 20

Attention Deficit Disorder

ttention deficit disorder (ADD) and attention deficit hyperactivity disorder (ADHD) affect from 3 to 6 percent of our children (depending on the studies you look at), and an estimated 17 million Americans total. Attention deficit disorders are three to ten times more prevalent in boys than girls.

In children, ADD is characterized by patterns of inattention and impulsive behavior in home, social, and school settings. Children with ADD often fail to complete tasks, have difficulty staying organized and keeping track of things, make careless mistakes, get easily overwhelmed, and are easily distracted. ADHD has the additional characteristic of hyperactivity, which can appear as fidgeting, excessive movement or talking, impatience, difficulty waiting or taking turns, or blurting out answers. The main symptom in girls with ADD/ADHD, however, is usually inattentiveness, rather than the hyperactivity that's usually seen in boys. Children with inattentiveness seem to daydream and be "spaced out," and their problem often goes undiagnosed.

ADD/ADHD has been called a "reward deficiency syndrome" because dopamine activity is reduced. Dopamine is the brain neurotransmitter that is associated with reward mechanisms. Dopamine deficiencies are implicated in addictive behaviors including alcohol abuse, drug abuse, smoking, and addictions to food, gambling, and sex. ADD/ADHD may also involve deficits in other neurotransmitters such as acetylcholine and serotonin.

Children with ADD/ADHD aren't trying to misbehave; in fact, they are trying their hardest much of the time. Their brain biochemistry is different from that of the average child. They are easily overstimulated, and either shut down or hype up in reaction to feeling overwhelmed. When children with ADD/ADHD become teenagers, their problems can continue, and the incidences of drug addiction, poor grades, dropping out of school, and crime increase—all the more reason to be

Adult Attention Deficiency

Children with ADD/ADHD often have parents with ADD/ADHD. If the description for the disorder in children sounds like you as a child and you are still experiencing such problems, you may have adult attention deficiency. In adults, some of the signs are difficulty being organized, difficulty wrapping up projects or tasks, difficulty remembering appointments or obligations, being easily bored, an internal sense of restlessness, getting easily overwhelmed or frustrated, lack of attention to detail, procrastination and avoidance of new projects, hyperactivity, fidgeting a lot, and inefficiency at work. These symptoms interfere with relationships at home and on the job.

proactive in figuring out how your child's biochemistry is contributing to his/her problems, and what you can do to help.

The causes of ADD and ADHD are many. It is imperative to consider the uniqueness of each child's case and perform functional tests to consider the condition's many and varied triggers including environmental toxins, recurrent antibiotic use, imbalances in essential fatty acids or neurotransmitters, hypoglycemia, dysbiosis, nutritional insufficiencies, and genetic predisposition.

DIGESTIVE, INFECTIOUS, AND DIETARY ISSUES

Children with ADD/ADHD often have impaired digestion and leaky gut. In one study, the Institute for Functional Medicine found a 74 percent incidence of increased intestinal permeability in children with ADD/ADHD. In another study, 46 percent of sixty-three children with ADHD were found to have no lactobacilli or bifidobacteria in their stool samples. Still another stool-sample study found dysbiosis to be prevalent in ADHD, with the incidence of candida at 32 percent and protozoa at 41 percent. Supplementing with probiotic bacteria may therefore be useful in children with ADHD.

A higher incidence of ADHD is associated with recurring ear infections, and its severity increases with the number of infections; in one study of children with ADHD, 94 percent had experienced three or more ear infections, and 69 percent had experienced more than ten. Hyperactive children have histories of more ear infections than do children with other learning problems. What's more, children with recurring ear infections usually have food allergies, most commonly to dairy products. Food and environmental allergies are also extremely common among children with ADD/ADHD. A string of coincidences? Not likely.

Various studies have looked at food allergies, reactions to food additives, types of foods, sugar intake, and other dietary factors in ADD/ADHD. One study mapping the brains of fifteen children with ADHD and food-induced ADHD even noted changes in brainwave patterns when the children were given various symptom-provoking foods. Not all children with attention, behavior, and learning problems have food allergies or sensitivities, but most do, and for them, an elimination/provocation diet will produce dramatic improvements. In a study of twenty-six children with ADHD, 73 percent reacted to many foods, dyes, and/or preservatives, and responded favorably to an elimination/provocation diet. Various other studies have shown that the ADD/ADHD symptoms of children placed on a hypoallergenic diet improve significantly.

Because of low blood sugar levels, children with ADD often crave and eat a large amount of sugar and refined carbohydrates. Supplementing with chromium, vanadium, and B-complex vitamins, eliminating refined carbohydrates, emphasizing good-quality protein and fats, and eating small, frequent meals can be helpful to address these cravings. Improved nutrition can be highly beneficial for other reasons too: An interesting recent study compared the efficacy of treating children with ADD/ADHD with the common medication Ritalin *versus* administering essential nutrients including vitamins, minerals, phytonutrients, amino acids, essential fatty acids, phospholipids, and probiotics—and the researchers concluded that the nutritional therapy was equal in effect to Ritalin treatment.

Levels of nutrients such as magnesium, iron, calcium, zinc, and B-complex vitamins are consistently low in children with ADD. Many studies have found zinc deficiency in children with ADD/ADHD. A recent study found a significant improvement in behavior and cognitive learning in children with ADD who received zinc sulfate for twelve weeks. Try an oral zinc sulfate test for your child. The test solution ought to taste bad; if it tastes like water or tastes sweet, your child will likely benefit from zinc supplementation. Interestingly, magnesium-deficiency symptoms look a lot like the symptoms of ADHD; and in a six-month trial giving children 3 milligrams (mg) of magnesium per pound of body weight daily, symptoms associated with ADHD were significantly reduced.

Other nutrients and herbs can be useful as well. A recent study found a 25 to 65 percent improvement in behavior and learning test scores in boys with ADD/ADHD who received eight weeks of supplemental L-carnitine, a natural substance involved in fat burning, heart health, and energy production (it is not known, however, how L-carnitine affects children). Recent research on children with ADD and autism has shown great improvement by use of carnosine, a nutrient often packaged with zinc and vitamin E and commonly used for irritable bowel syndrome and stomach pain. In a study giving American ginseng plus ginkgo for four weeks to thirty-six children with ADHD, one symptom-measuring scale showed a 44-percent improvement and another showed a 74-percent improvement in attention and behavior; side effects, however, caused five children to drop out of the study. Anecdotal evidence for the usefulness of the antioxidant pycnogenol (derived from pine bark or grapeseed extract) in ADHD is widespread on the Internet, although there are no studies at this time to confirm it.

TESTING YOUR METTLE—AND TESTING FOR METAL

Standard treatment for ADD/ADHD relies on pharmaceutical agents to control symptomatic response. The best approach to ADD/ADHD, however, is to find the underlying causes on which to base treatment. This involves more time and effort on the part of the child and parents, but the rewards of normalizing your child's chemistry without the use of drugs can be great. I have had the opportunity to see PET scans of children with ADD/ADHD without medication, with medication,

The Feingold Diet

In 1973, Ben Feingold, M.D., was the first physician to theorize that certain foods and food chemicals could cause ADD/ADHD. I've seen a film from his clinic that shows a child playing and drawing happily; when exposed to a specific food coloring, the child's behavior becomes wild and erratic and she can't continue to draw; antibody-neutralizing drops are given, and within about twenty minutes, the child becomes calm and is able to draw properly again. Dr. Feingold's book *Why Your Child Is Hyperactive* (Random House, 1985) is widely available. The Feingold Diet excludes foods and medications that contain artificial colors, artificial flavors, and chemicals called salicylates. Salicylates are found in aspirin and aspirinlike substances as well as in almonds, apples, apricots, cherries, cucumbers, grapes and grape drinks, nectarines, oranges, peaches, plums, prunes, raisins, and tomatoes.

In a recent six-week trial of the Feingold Diet for fifty-five children with ADD/ADHD, 72.7 percent had improved behavior, and 47.3 percent of these remained improved when their diet was subsequently broadened over a three- to six-month period. Parents of fourteen of the children reported that their child's behavior worsened after he/she ingested specific synthetic food colorings, so eight children were further tested by being put on a strict diet and challenged daily for eighteen weeks with 50 mg of red dye #3 (carmoisine), yellow dye #5 (tartrazine), or placebo, each for two weeks at a time. When given a daily dose of synthetic food coloring, the children experienced symptoms of extreme irritability, restlessness, and sleep disturbance.

and with combined natural therapies; those on medication had reduced symptoms, but their PET scans were highly abnormal, whereas the PET of those using natural therapies were almost normalized. Hearing or visual problems can easily affect a child's behavior and mood, so one of the first things to do is have your child's hearing and vision evaluated. Testing for sensitivities/allergies is another good place to begin.

Amino acid testing is important in ADD/ADHD as well. Normally, amino acids transform from one into another like a waterfall forming pools that run to other pools. Some children, however, have inborn errors in amino acid metabolism, and the result is huge pools of certain amino acids but little or no flow downstream. If these metabolic problems can be identified, supplementing with the missing amino acids can be extremely useful. One study found that in comparison to other children, twenty-eight children with ADD had significantly lower levels of the amino acids phenylalanine, tyrosine, tryptophan, histidine, and isoleucine, all of which are critical to healthy brain function and mood regulation.

The brain and central nervous system also rely on fatty acids to function properly; DHA deficiency, for example, results in increased brain membrane permeability, allowing neurotoxins free access. Imbalanced essential fatty acid profiles are commonly found in ADD/ADHD, especially low levels of arachadonic acid and DHA and high levels of undesirable trans-fatty acids. Testing can determine exactly which fatty acids to increase through diet and/or supplementation. In one study, children with ADD/ADHD given a DHA/EPA fish oil supplement with vitamin E and thyme oil for twelve weeks showed significantly decreased behavioral symptoms compared to children who received an olive oil placebo. In another, either a fish oil supplement or a placebo was given to 117 kids with ADD/ADHD for three months, after which the placebo group was given the fish oil; improvements were seen in reading, spelling, and behavior in both groups. Not all studies, however, have found benefit from giving fish oils to children with learning and behavior problems.

It's important to test your child's detoxification capabilities as well, as research indicates that some children with behavior and learning problems have high levels of lead, mercury, or other heavy metals. When scalp hair from 277 first-graders was examined for lead content and the children's teachers completed an ADHD-rating questionnaire, hair lead levels ranged from less than 1 to 11 parts per million and there were strong correlations between the children's lead levels and their teachers' perceptions of them; the correlation was even stronger for children who had been diagnosed with an attention deficit. A striking relationship between hair lead levels and behavior has been found in many other studies: the higher the lead level, the worse the behavior.

Immunizations containing the preservative thimerosol have a high mercury content that can be damaging to children. The worst-affected experience autistic behavior, but I believe that a wide spectrum of childhood issues including problems with learning, behavior, speech, eosinophilic esophagitis, and allergy are related to mercury toxicity; see Chapter 2. High levels of manganese in hair have also been associated with violent behavior in children. Hair mineral analysis is a confusing screening tool, however, as high levels can indicate either metal toxicity or that your child's body is really good at ridding itself of metals through the hair.

The most accurate test for heavy metals is a provoked urine challenge. In this fairly inexpensive test, your child is given a single dose of a medication that chelates (pulls) metals from his/her body, and then urine is collected for five to six hours and sent back to a laboratory for analysis (stool may be examined in younger children). If your child's test is positive for heavy metals, or if it comes up with no heavy metals at all, you may want to consider chelation therapy. Many children's bodies bind heavy metals so tightly that none show up in the urine or stool until the children have been chelated for several months, and then metals begin to pour out; this is very common in autistic children.

Note: This chapter provides only a brief overview of ADD/ADHD and integrative medicine. Many excellent books on the topic are available at your local library or bookstore.

FUNCTIONAL LABORATORY TESTING FOR CHILDREN WITH ATTENTION DEFICIT DISORDER

Although insurance will probably not cover all of these tests, it's worth obtaining as many of them as you can afford in order to identify the imbalances that may underlie your child's learning and behavioral problems. See Appendix A for details on testing. Available tests include:

1. Organic acids test

2. Amino acids test

3. Fatty acids test

4. Provoked urine test (or stool test, for children in diapers) for heavy metals

5. Intestinal permeability test

6. Food sensitivity/allergy test(s)

7. Comprehensive digestive and stool analysis with parasite screening

8. Liver detoxification profile

HEALING OPTIONS FOR CHILDREN WITH
ATTENTION DEFICIT DISORDER

Each child with ADD/ADHD is different. Base your choice of therapies on your child's test results. (It is unlikely that you will need to use every suggested healing option.) See Appendix B for more details on the following nutrients, herbs, and supplements.

Elimination/Provocation Diet—to test for food intolerances. First, eliminate sugar, dairy, wheat, and all food flavorings and colorings from your child's diet for two to three weeks, and you may notice a huge improvement; if not, you may want to test for specific foods and additives. See Chapter 11.

Feingold Diet—to alleviate learning and behavioral problems. Although this diet won't help all children with ADD/ADHD, it can have profound benefits for those who do respond to it. See the inset "The Feingold Diet" on page 204 for details.

Consider Fatty-Acid Deficiencies—see Chapter 8. If indicated by the fatty acids test results, have your child eat fish high in omega-3 fatty acids at least twice a week and take a fish oil supplement. Dosage for children: 1,000–8,000 mg daily, according to child's size and age.

Magnesium—to reduce symptoms by countering possible deficiency. Dosage for children: begin at 100 mg daily and increase until your child gets diarrhea, then reduce the dose. *Note:* If a high dose of magnesium is required for effectiveness, give choline citrate to help with its absorption. Use 1 teaspoon for every 200 mg of magnesium.

Probiotics—to re-establish healthy gut ecology. Dosage for children: one or two capsules or ⅛–½ teaspoon powder, twice daily.

B-Complex Vitamins—to improve energy, behavior, mood, and cognition. Dosage for children: as directed on label; usually 25–50 mg daily for most of the B-complex vitamins.

Dimethylaminoethanol—to improve brain synthesis of the neurotransmitter acetylcholine. Dosage for children: 100–500 mg daily.

Zinc—to counteract possible zinc deficiency. See page 203 for details on an oral zinc sulfate challenge. Dosage for children: 5–50 mg daily, according to child's size and age.

L-Carnitine—to improve behavior and learning. Dosage for children: 100 mg/kg of body weight, up to 4,000 mg, daily. *Note:* Acetyl L-carnitine is absorbed more effectively, so dosages of this form could be lower.

Carnosine—to improve behavior and learning and support digestive function. Dosage for children: 200–400 mg twice daily.

American Ginseng plus Ginkgo—to improve behavior and learning. Dosage for children: 200 mg American ginseng plus 60 mg ginkgo twice daily.

GABA (gamma-amino-butyric acid)—to calm your child. GABA helps stimulate dopamine production. Dosage: 50–300 mg twice daily.

Pycnogenol—to improve behavior and learning. Dosage for children: as directed on label; typical dosages are 10–100 mg.

Chelation Therapy—to remove accumulated heavy metals. Gentle methods include oral medications, rectal suppositories, skin patches, and clay baths. Work with a qualified healthcare professional who is familiar with chelation in children. While you do this, remember to replenish your child's vitamins and minerals and increase his/her antioxidant intake.

CHAPTER 21

Autism

Autism, a serious disorder of neurological development, is now more commonly called autistic spectrum disorder because it manifests itself with a wide diversity of causes and characteristics in different children. Autism usually becomes evident by the age of three years. Some children exhibit symptoms shortly after birth, whereas many others function normally for a year or two and then have a sudden backslide in their language and social skills; this is often called regression-onset autism. One and a half million Americans are affected by autism, and four out of five of those affected are males. The disorder is equally distributed among all races and economic strata.

Autistic children have poor social interaction and communication skills and trouble relating to the outside world. People with autism are often docile but can also be aggressive and can hurt themselves. They often show repeated body movements such as hand-flapping and rocking and are prone to seizures. In addition to autism's behavioral and social aspects, the disorder also involves immune dysfunction and gut abnormalities.

In the United States, one out of 160 children born in recent years has been diagnosed with autism; in California, this figure is one in 135 children. Autistic disorders have increased in the United States by 544 percent since 1991, reaching epidemic proportions, yet autism has not received the political attention that it warrants.

Asperger's syndrome is often characterized as "a touch of autism." These children may excel at math, science, and computer work but are socially inept. They often fail to make eye contact and don't understand that it is part of normal human interaction. It's difficult for them to understand other people's emotions; they don't know how to empathize and find social customs hard to understand. On the other hand, they can often tell you all about the workings of the furnace in their house or the difference between motors in various cars. It sometimes seems as if they come from another planet with a different way of organizing reality.

Until the 1960s and beyond, autism was believed to be the result of an unloving mother, but this has since been determined to be completely untrue. Autistic spectrum disorders including Asperger's syndrome are biomedical illnesses although in people with high-functioning Asperger's syndrome, it may be seen as a "nerdy" personality type rather than as an illness. High-functioning autistic adults have explained that it's as if there is no filtering of sensory information; it all comes flooding in and is completely overwhelming, and the natural tendency is to completely withdraw as a matter of self-protection. Although a highly ordered environment, behavior-modification techniques, and loving families help autistic children, these do not address the underlying causes of the illness.

Autism is multifactoral, so you'll have to be a persistent detective to find the specific factors that are affecting your child. The rising incidence of autism (see "Once Rare, Now an Epidemic" on page 214) suggests a genetic predisposition that is triggered by an environmental factor. Many parents report, for example, that their child became autistic after a course of antibiotics or after an immunization, which is a matter of ongoing, roaring debate. The great news is that many children are being cured of autism, and many more are being significantly improved, by physicians using integrative therapies.

DIGESTION, INFECTION, AND ANTIBIOTICS

The causes of autism are many and varied. Virtually all autistic children exhibit faulty digestion and an inability to easily detoxify substances with which they come into contact. This faulty digestion can take the form of dysbiosis, leaky gut, candida infection, and parasitic infection.

The work of Bill Shaw, M.D., on urinary metabolites has been pivotal in changing ideas of autism's etiology and treatment. These metabolites, which are fungal in origin, are broken down in the bodies of normal people, but in people with autism, they instead become brain-toxic substances that resemble opiates. When autistic people found to have these metabolites are treated with antifungal drugs, their symptoms improve significantly and their urinary metabolites normalize; interestingly, those who do not respond to antifungal medications often respond to antiparasitic medications. These metabolites are easily identified through laboratory testing.

Many children with autism have a candida infection called yeast overgrowth. The link between dysbiosis and autism was recently examined in a study of ten children who were developing normally and then had a deterioration of skills,

Pioneers in Autism

Many people have been inspired by their own children to work with autistic spectrum disorders:

- Bernard Rimland, M.D., whose son was born with autism in the early 1960s when the condition was rare, has spent his life studying autism. He has written many books including *Vaccines, Autism and Childhood Disorders* (New Atlantean Press, 2003) and *Biological Treatments for Autism and PDD* (Sunflower Publications, 1998). In 1995, he and two other doctors cofounded Defeat Autism Now (DAN) for research and data collection; DAN holds meetings to present integrated and nutritional treatment of autism.

- Victoria Beck's investigation of her autistic son's chronic diarrhea led to the discovery that exposure to the testing agent secretin (see page 212) had dramatically improved his behavior, stimulating further research on the use of secretin for autism treatment.

- Jon Pangborn, Ph.D., a co-founder of DAN (above), was inspired by his own child's disease to pioneer the investigation of amino acid balance in autistic children. He and DAN co-founder Sidney Baker, M.D., who works extensively in clinical practice with autistic children and their families, coauthored *Autism: Effective Biomedical Treatments* (Autism Research Institute, 2005).

- Rashid Buttar, M.D., whose son has been cured of autism, is a physician who works with autistic children in North Carolina. According to Dr. Buttar, a baby's biliary tree (tubelike structures that carry bile to the intestines) does not develop until after the age of one year, and a mature biliary tree is essential for the body's detoxification of mercury.

- Nurse practitioner Lynn Redwood is one of many parents to link her son's autism to vaccinations: "At two months of age, my son had received 62.5 mcg of mercury from three infant vaccines. According to EPA criteria, his allowable dose was only 0.5 mcg based on his weight. He had received 125 times his allowable exposure on that one day." Autism Summit Conference, April 25–26, Mesa, AZ.

- Sallie Bernard, as a spokesperson and bearer of ideas, has made invaluable contributions in the political arena and in parent advocacy to increase awareness of autism issues. She is the mother of an autistic son and the executive director of Safe Minds (www.safeminds.org).

along with chronic diarrhea, after taking antibiotics. Theorizing that the skill regression was due to a change in protective gut flora, researchers gave the children an antibiotic for twelve weeks; they found a marked improvement in mood, behavior, cognitive and social skills, but the benefits didn't last.

I am not surprised that the results of the above-described study weren't long lasting. It would have been interesting, however, to do this study giving probiotics along with the antibiotic or just using probiotic supplements alone. Probiotic supplements may be preferable to antibiotics as a long-term way to combat dysbiosis and rebalance gut flora in autism. Antibiotics affect some children positively and some negatively. Antibiotic use contributes to dysbiosis and leaky gut by changing the balance of intestinal microbes. Most children's bodies can rebalance their own internal flora after a round of antibiotics, but repeated antibiotic use can cause inflammation and immune dysfunction that can "spill over" into the nervous system in a susceptible child.

As mentioned on page 211, gastroenterologists' use of the intestinal neuro-transmitter-hormone secretin to test pancreatic function led fortuitously to its use as an experimental treatment for autism. Secretin may work to heal the gut, and therefore the immune system, of autistic children. Research is ongoing, with disappointingly mixed results so far, but individual children have obtained significant benefit; it appears that gluten-sensitive children respond best to secretin.

SENSITIVITY, DIET, AND SUPPLEMENTS

Autistic children tend to have multiple food sensitivities. Much improvement has been shown in autistic children who follow a specific diet, and many autistic children respond to a diet free of casein (a protein found in milk products) and gluten (a protein fraction found in many grains). It is essential to test autistic children for food and environmental sensitivities in order to find the specific substances causing inflammation and irritation to the gut lining.

Many autistic children are constipated. If your child is constipated, increase fiber in his/her diet, supplement with ground flaxseed to provide fiber and essential fatty acids, and add ascorbate powder (a form of vitamin C) to soften the stool. Normalizing magnesium levels will help correct constipation, and probiotics and digestive enzymes can also be helpful. (See "Constipation" on page 161.)

Autistic children also have specific nutritional needs that can be identified through testing. Abnormalities in fatty acids have been shown in people with autism, and one study found benefit with the omega-3 fatty acids EPA and DHA in autistic children. Supplementation with omega-3 fatty acids may be highly useful, but medical literature on the topic of fatty acid and amino acid imbalance in autism is scant. An impressive twenty-two studies, however, have shown supplemental vitamin B_6 to have positive effects on behavioral symptoms of autism, with marked improvement in 30 to 40 percent of the children. A few children in these studies exhibited minor side effects including irritability, sensitivity to noise, and bedwetting, which are all symptoms common to magnesium deficiency, and cleared when additional magnesium was given. Most autistic children are magnesium deficient.

Structures called G-protein receptors, which sit on the surface of our cells and are responsible for much of cellular communication, are an exciting topic in autism research, as animals that have blocked G-protein receptors show symptoms that are virtually identical to those of autism. Mary Megson, M.D., who sees many children with autism, gives her patients fat-soluble cis-vitamin A in the form of cod liver oil to bypass blocked G-protein receptors and has observed that it significantly helps some children almost immediately. In April 2000, Dr. Megson reported her findings to the House Government Reform Committee on Autism and Vaccines:

> After two months on vitamin A treatment, some of these children, when given a single dose of bethanechol to stimulate pathways in the parasympathetic system in the gut, focus, laugh, concentrate, show a sense of humor, and talk after thirty minutes as if reconnected. This improves cognition, but they are still physically ill. When these children get the MMR vaccine, their vitamin A stores are depleted; they can not compensate for blocked pathways. Lack of vitamin A, which has been called 'the anti-infective agent,' leaves them immunosuppressed. They lack cell-mediated immunity. T cell activation, important for long-term immune memory, requires 14-hydroxy retro-retinol (vitamin A). On cod liver oil, the only natural source of this natural substance, the children get well.

METALS, MERCURY, AND IMMUNIZATIONS

In many autistic children, doctors William Walsh and Anjum Usman have discovered defective functioning of the metallothionine enzyme system that normally enables us to excrete metals from our bodies. This defect impairs brain functioning and makes these children more susceptible to toxic metals and chemicals in their environment.

A standard blood test is not useful for assessing metal accumulation in the body, because these toxins are deeply embedded in the tissues. Urine testing can help you discover whether heavy metals play a role in your child's illness (a stool test is available for children in diapers). A normal child's test shows some excreted mercury and other metals, whereas autistic children often do not excrete any mercury, lead, or cadmium until they have been treated with chelation therapy (methods that pull metals out of the tissues) for several weeks or more. Physicians using chelation therapies to remove heavy metals have achieved great results, with many autistic children improving dramatically and some completely normalizing.

Thimerosol, a preservative used in vaccines, contains ethyl mercury, a known neurotoxin. (The University of Calgary's website features a fascinating video about the effects of low-dose mercury on nerve cells at http://commons.ucalgary.ca/mercury.) In 1987, the number of immunizations recommended by the U.S. Centers for Disease Control increased substantially, and with them came a bigger challenge to a baby's or toddler's developing immune system, along with potentially toxic doses of mercury. Through immunizations alone, American children typically receive 237 micrograms (mcg) of mercury by the age of two years, far exceeding the safe level of 0.1 mcg/kilogram body weight per day as currently defined by the U.S. Environmental Protection Agency (EPA). American children given the normal amount of vaccinations receive more mercury than the EPA recommends during an entire lifetime!

Immunization has saved millions of lives, but vaccines don't require a mercury-laden preservative for effectiveness. Although most children are *not* negatively affected by immunizations, autism or any of a range of other problems may be triggered in children who have poor detoxification abilities. Rises in autism rates coin-

Once Rare, Now an Epidemic

The incidence of autism and autistic spectrum disorders in the United States has risen at alarming rates. In the 1970s, autism was estimated to affect about one in 25,000 people; by the 1980s, one in 2,500; and in the 1990s, one in 250. And since 1993, according to data collected by the U.S. Department of Special Education, the national incidence of autism has risen more than eightfold. Their statistics also show that rates of autism rose over 5,000 percent in seventeen out of the fifty states plus Puerto Rico and Washington D.C. between the time spans of 1992–1993 and 2001–2002.

Dan Burton, chairman of the congressional Subcommittee on Human Rights and Wellness, made the following statement at a 2003 hearing: "Only fifteen years ago, autism was considered a relatively rare disease, affecting roughly one in 10,000 children. Since then, the growing rates of autism are reaching epic proportions in this country. Currently, conservative estimates of autism rates in the United States indicate that one in every 500 children is afflicted with these various spectrum disorders, while scientific studies reported in the *Journal of the American Medical Association* have observed autism rates of one in every 150 children, and the problem just continues to escalate."

cide with the introduction of thimerosol in vaccines in the 1930s and with subsequent increases in the amounts received. The frequent incidence of children becoming autistic between the ages of eighteen months and two years after receiving multiple immunizations is especially noted by parents whose children received the MMR vaccine against measles, mumps, and rubella; but although a British researcher has found a correlation between the MMR vaccine and increased incidence of autism, other researchers have found no evidence of this connection.

If your child is autistic, be very cautious about any more immunizations until he/she is older. Adopt the precautionary principle of "better safe than sorry." All parents can insist that their doctors use only thimerosol-free vaccines, which are finally available for all American vaccine categories.

FUNCTIONAL LABORATORY TESTING FOR CHILDREN WITH AUTISM

You will definitely want to find out more about your child's biochemistry by obtaining some of these tests. See Appendix A for details on testing. Available tests include:

1. Provoked urine test (or stool test, for children in diapers) for heavy metals
2. Comprehensive digestive and stool analysis with parasite screening
3. Amino acids test
4. Food sensitivity/allergy test(s)
5. Organic acids test
7. Fatty acids test
8. Liver function profile
9. Vitamin D test

HEALING OPTIONS FOR CHILDREN WITH AUTISM

Autism is a treatable illness. More and more children with autistic spectrum disorders are becoming healthy again, which was never before believed to be possible. Look for a doctor who is familiar with integrative therapies and who has been trained to treat children with autism. See Appendix B for more details on the following nutrients and supplements. (It is highly unlikely that you will need to use every suggested healing option.)

Consider Food Sensitivity/Allergy—see Chapter 11. Children with autism are commonly sensitive to gluten, gliaden, and casein. Other foods may also trigger reactions. Try testing and an elimination/provocation diet.

Probiotics—to replace beneficial intestinal flora. Dosage for children: ¼ teaspoon powder two or three times daily (acidophilus and bifidobacteria); if the child is being breast-fed, the mother can take the same dosage of *B. infantis.*

Consider Dysbiosis and Candida Infection—see Chapter 6. An alkaline diet and probiotic supplements will rebalance your child's internal environment (see Chapters 5 and 7). Eliminate all refined carbohydrates and sugars. If necessary, treat infection directly with prescription medications or natural products; infection will recur, however, if dietary changes are not made.

Cod Liver Oil—to bypass blocked G-protein receptors, nourish the nervous system, and reduce inflammation. Dosage for children: enough oil to provide 5,000 international units of vitamin A daily; this is typically 1 teaspoon, but read the label.

L-Carnosine—to improve behavior and communication skills. A recent study of carnosine showed significant improvements in autistic behaviors plus increased language comprehension. Dosage for children: 400 milligrams (mg) twice daily.

Vitamin B$_{12}$—to activate ability to detoxify. Dosage: 2,000–10,000 mg sublingually each day.

Vitamin B$_6$ plus Magnesium—to improve behavior and communication skills. Vitamin B$_6$ and magnesium do not cure autism but do improve symptoms significantly. Dosage for children: vitamin B$_6$, 75–800 mg daily; magnesium, 150–300 mg daily. *Caution:* Too much magnesium causes diarrhea.

Omega-3 Fatty Acids—to nourish the nervous system and brain and to reduce inflammation throughout the body. *Note:* Supplements of EPA and DHA from fish oil or algae sources (rather than increased intake of coldwater fish) are recommended for children with autism, because of the high levels of mercury in many fish. Dosage for children: 1,000–5,000 mg daily, according to child's age, weight, and response.

Glutamine—to increase immune and muscle strength, normalize bowel movements, and heal gut mucosa. Dosage for children: 5–15 grams daily. It can be mixed with water or other cool liquids.

Di-Methyl Glycine (DMG)—to promote excretion of heavy metals. Some autistic children begin speaking within days of beginning DMG supplementation. Dosage for children: 125-mg tablets, one to four daily.

Digestive Enzymes—to enhance digestion and minimize food allergy reactions. Dosage for children: one capsule with each meal.

Proteolytic Enzymes—to reduce inflammation and enhance immune system function. Dosage for children: one to three capsules on an empty stomach two or three times daily (best times may be upon rising and before bed).

CHAPTER 22

Cystic Fibrosis

C ystic fibrosis (CF) is caused by the inheritance of a certain faulty gene from both parents. If only one parent has the gene, the child will be a carrier of the disease. Ten million people in the United States are carriers; 30,000 children and adults in the United States and 3,000 in Canada have CF. In 80 percent of cases, it is diagnosed by the age of three years, but 10 percent of people with CF are not diagnosed until they are eighteen years old or older. A multi-organ disease, CF primarily affects the lungs and digestive system, but it can also affect sweat glands and sinuses, and can cause infertility in men.

Children with CF excrete large amounts of sodium through their airways, causing dehydration in the lungs; their chloride secretion, however, is diminished. A proper balance of sodium and chloride is pivotal for healthy functioning of the lungs, pancreas, reproductive tract, sweat glands, and GI tract. When sodium and chloride (that is, salt) are not in balance, thick mucus collects that prevents wastes from being carried easily out of the lungs. Common symptoms of CF are persistent coughing (sometimes with phlegm), salty-tasting skin, inability to gain weight, respiratory and/or sinus infections, wheezing, shortness of breath, gagging, vomiting, and excessive sweating. The disease is diagnosed through a painless and simple sweat test, for which a high salt content confirms CF.

People with CF produce many thick secretions throughout the body, including sweat, tears, and mucus in nose, mouth, sinuses, and lungs. Rather than being fluid, these secretions impede respiration and can be life threatening. Accumulated secretions increase the risk of respiratory infections and lung damage; this can further lead to heart damage because the body is chronically oxygen deprived. Mucus can also obstruct the pancreas, preventing digestive enzymes from reaching the intestines, and block ducts in digestive organs including the pancreas and liver, making it difficult to digest food and absorb nutrients properly. As a result, children with CF may have difficulty gaining weight and are often malnourished.

They often need to eat 20 to 50 percent more calories than other children do, and require supplemental enzymes and nutrients.

DIET, IMMUNE SYSTEM REACTIONS, AND PH BALANCE

Moms whose babies have CF are encouraged to breast-feed, as breast-milk contains immunity-building antibodies that are not present in formula. Mother's milk and infant formulas are both, however, nutrient dense, and provide many of the nutrients that the baby needs. In addition, your physician may recommend a bit of salt, some vitamins, and some pancreatic enzymes. At about six months of age, you'll begin adding solid foods to your baby's diet. I recommend beginning with puréed vegetables such as winter squash, carrots, broccoli, and others. Grains, although usually recommended for babies this age, can be very irritating to the gut mucosa, especially for babies with CF.

Implement an alkalizing diet and test your child's first morning urine to maintain a balanced pH level. Remove mucus-producing foods from your child's diet and increase foods that stimulate bile production and digestion (see page 222). Common mucus-forming foods include dairy products, wheat, processed foods, and high-sugar foods, but nearly any food to which your child is sensitive or allergic can increase his/her mucus secretion. Although children with CF have been consistently found to have increased intestinal permeability (leaky gut syndrome), few studies have looked at allergies and sensitivities in children with CF. Of the children studied, many were found to have true allergies to dust, mold, and pollen; there were also rare instances of food allergies to dairy products and gluten. For children with CF who had chronic diarrhea and poor weight gain, avoidance of dairy products corrected the problem, and one child also needed gluten removed in order to benefit.

In one study evaluating twenty children with CF, diarrhea, and failure to thrive in comparison to twenty relatively healthy children with CF and twenty healthy children, higher levels of IgE, IgA, IgG, and IgM antibodies to foods were found in all of the children with CF, but these levels were three times as high in the severely ill children. When the foods they reacted to were eliminated from their diets, 90 percent of the children improved. When these foods were reintroduced, 78 percent of the children had negative reactions to them.

As your child grows, you may be surprised by the amount of food that he/she can pack away in a day! Remember that a child with CF needs to eat up to one-and-a-half times more than an average child. Fill your home with healthful foods and encourage your child to eat every two to three hours. Trail mix with nuts, seeds, and small amounts of dried fruit is a healthful and portable snack that's loaded with calories. Make sure your child gets plenty of salt; pickles, pretzels,

A High-Sulfur Diet for CF

In a recent conversation, Russell Jaffe, M.D., told me about an anthroposophic protocol being used for CF in Switzerland (anthroposophy, a medical field developed by
Rudolf Steiner, is more commonly practiced in Europe). Staying on a high-sulfur
diet keeps lung secretions more fluid, and debris can be processed and removed
more effectively. Dr. Jaffe recommended a high-sulfur diet including ginger tea, vegetable broths, and mustard-seed sprouts. (Other high-sulfur foods include garlic,
onions, and egg yolks.) He reported that a few people in their thirties and forties
were without CF symptoms as a result of adhering to such a diet; unfortunately, I
was unable to confirm this information from other sources.

chips, and other high-salt foods will be welcomed. You'll need to supplement pancreatic enzymes, vitamins, and minerals (see following section). Some children
and teenagers may need high-protein drinks or even additional tube feeding.

HEALTH-ENHANCING PROBIOTICS AND ENZYMES

Children with CF need all the digestive help they can get. Probiotic bacteria are an
important part of the digestive system as well as the immune system. Although it is
logical to assume that probiotics would greatly benefit children with CF, the use of
probiotic supplements in CF is relatively unstudied. Two studies showed that use of
yogurt and *Lactobacillus casei* prevented pseudomonas infection (which is common in children with CF) in the lungs of mice. Research also shows that probiotics
such as Lactobacillus GG reduce gut inflammation in children with CF. Because
probiotics produce vitamins, protect against infection, prevent diarrhea, and protect the immune system, it makes sense to provide supplemental probiotics in CF.

It is essential that a child with CF take enzyme supplements for digestive support. Pancreatic enzymes have been used for decades in the care of people with
CF, but because the potency and quality of pancreatic products can vary dramatically, the Cystic Fibrosis Foundation has lobbied the U.S. Food and Drug Administration for testing; by 2008 every pancreatic enzyme on the market will have
been adequately tested for effectiveness in people with pancreatic diseases. Children using pancreatic enzymes occasionally develop an intolerance to them or
develop a leaky gut, so plant-based enzymes are preferable. A couple of studies
looking at digestive enzymes from *Aspergillis oryzae* and *Rhizopus arrhizus* have
found them comparable to pancreatic enzymes. They also function within a wider
pH range, so they can help with digestion in the stomach, where pancreatic
enzymes fail to work.

Proteolytic (protein-splitting) enzymes taken on an empty stomach may be very useful as well. Although there is no published research on their use in CF, they are known to have anti-inflammatory properties and to help regulate immune system function. Perhaps of particular importance in CF, proteolytic enzymes scavenge oxidized proteins and debris in the bloodstream, enhancing the blood's ability to flow. I believe proteolytic enzymes would also help liquefy lung mucus, but I couldn't find any research on that.

FATS AND OTHER NUTRIENTS FOR CF

Children with CF have a difficult time maintaining a healthy weight. A relatively high-fat diet can help them gain weight and grow more normally—but make sure to give your child healthful fats, not just deep-fried foods or restructured hydrogenated fats. High-quality fats are found in coldwater fish, whole grains, flaxseed meal, nuts, and seeds. Levels of essential fatty acids are typically low in children with CF, and studies have shown that supplementing with medium-chain triglycerides (MCTs) in cod liver, fish, and other oils and linoleic acid-rich foods such as nuts, seeds, and whole grains can normalize these levels. Many studies have shown the benefits of fish oil in CF: better growth, reduced bronchial inflammation, lowered IgG antibody levels, and fewer days of antibiotic treatment for infections.

Children with CF are typically deficient in many nutrients. Infants and children with CF have high needs for zinc and vitamins A, B_2, C, E, and K; some children require extra iron; and some of the medications used for CF can cause magnesium loss. Studies show that children with CF also have an increased need for antioxidant nutrients like carotenoids, vitamins C and E, lipoic acid, n-acetyl cysteine, and selenium. What's more, increased intake of essential fatty acids also requires an increased intake of antioxidants. Low acetyl-carnitine levels in CF may be due to faulty fatty acid metabolism. Carnitine and taurine, both of which help with fat metabolism and heart function plus dozens of other metabolic processes, have been extensively studied for use in CF. And when children with CF were supplemented with whey protein twice daily, their levels of the important antioxidant glutathione rose significantly.

Glutamine is a useful nutrient for people with increased intestinal permeability. Two studies looked specifically at glutamine for children with CF, but the supplement was only given for four days, and the researchers concluded that it probably wouldn't be effective at increasing muscle mass in these children; by contrast, studies on using glutamine to build muscle mass in people with HIV and other chronic illnesses have been conducted over months or years. Glutamine has, however, been shown in hundreds of studies in non-CF populations to reduce muscle loss, build muscle, reduce risk of infection, and restore gut mucosal health.

Current animal studies on bioflavonoids for CF look promising. Although there have only been a few studies on quercetin, and none in children, it offers a safe and nontoxic way to reduce inflammation in your child's body and lungs. In mice, trials using the bioflavonoid curcumin (a constituent of the spice turmeric), which is a natural antioxidant and anti-inflammatory, normalized the gene that is most commonly mutated in CF. This research is far from being validated in humans, but curcumin is very safe and even in large doses has been shown not to have any side effects.

FUNCTIONAL LABORATORY TESTING FOR CHILDREN WITH CYSTIC FIBROSIS

Although food sensitivities and allergies have not been well-studied in children with CF, it is reasonable to assume that many would benefit from identification of their antibodies to food. Children with CF are known to have increased intestinal permeability, and other children with a leaky gut are known to have increased antibodies to specific foods, so testing your child for antibodies to foods is advisable. Pancreatic elastase, an enzyme found in stool, is used by commercial laboratories to measure pancreatic function in children with CF. See Appendix A for details on testing. Available tests include:

1. Intestinal permeability test
2. Food sensitivity/allergy test(s)
3. Comprehensive digestive and stool analysis with pancreatic elastase
4. Fatty acids test
5. Organic acids test
6. Vitamin D test

Healing Options for Children with Cystic Fibrosis

There is much yet left to be studied in terms of integrated and functional medicine and CF. If your child has CF, you would be wise to consult a nutritionist regularly about his/her many special needs. See Appendix B for more details on the following nutrients, herbs, and supplements. (It is unlikely that you will need to use every suggested healing option.)

Alkalizing Diet—to maintain a balanced pH level, in conjunction with testing your child's first morning urinary pH. See Chapter 7 for details.

Dietary Changes—to eliminate mucus-producing foods and increase bile-stimulating foods. Remove sugar and dairy products; other common mucus-producing foods include bananas, barley, egg whites, oats, oranges, rye, and wheat. Foods that stimulate bile production and digestion include celery, daikon radish, garlic, horseradish, lemon, lime, mustard, onion, parsley, umeboshi plum, watercress, and good-quality oils.

High-Sulfur Diet—to thin lung secretions and promote debris removal. See the inset "A High Sulfur Diet for CF" on page 219.

Hydrate—to dilute thick, sticky mucus. Water is our best natural solvent. Make sure that your child drinks plenty of clean water each day. Try for 1 ounce daily per each kilogram (kg, 2.2 pounds) of your child's body weight.

Pancreatic or Plant-Based Digestive Enzymes—to support complete digestion. If your child's doctor recommends a specific product, use that one; otherwise, look for products with high enzyme activity levels listed on the label. I prefer plant-based enzymes to pancreatic enzymes because they work in the stomach as well as in the intestines. Dosage for children: one or two capsules with each meal.

Multivitamin-Mineral Supplement—to counteract poor nutrient absorption. Make sure that your child gets plenty of calcium and magnesium to build strong bones and prevent bone loss later in life. Dosage for children: as directed on label. *Note:* Liquid, powdered, and chewable supplements may be better absorbed than other forms.

Fish Oil—to reduce inflammation and help with weight gain. Use cod liver oil or fish oil in liquid or capsules. Dosage for children: 1–4 teaspoons or 1,000–5,000 international units daily.

Medium-Chain Triglycerides and Linoleic Acid—to normalize fatty acid levels. Dosage for children: 1–1.25 grams (g) per kg of your child's body weight daily.

Taurine plus Carnitine—to increase fat absorption. Dosage for children: 200–2,000 milligrams (mg) of each daily.

Whey Protein—to increase glutathione levels. This quick and easy addition to your child's food also provides extra calories and protein, and it tastes good too. Dosage for children: 10 g twice daily.

Antioxidants—to protect mucous membranes and restore deficiencies. Foods highest in antioxidants are colored beans (like black or red) and fruits and vegetables. Fresh vegetable juices flood your child with antioxidants and alkalize at the same time. Supplement with an extra-antioxidant formula containing carotenoids, vitamins C and E, and selenium; it may also contain other antioxidants including reduced glutathione, zinc, n-acetyl cysteine, lipoic acid, and superoxide dismutase. Dosage for children: as directed on label.

Probiotics—to support the digestive system and reduce gut inflammation. Dosage for children: bifidobacteria and lactobacilli, one or two capsules or ⅛–½ teaspoons powder two or three times daily.

Glutamine—to reduce risk of infection, promote weight gain, and build muscle. Try giving glutamine if your child is growing poorly or has leaky gut, poor muscle tone, diarrhea, and/or lung infections. Dosage for children: 5–20 g daily.

Curcumin/Turmeric—to normalize gene function. Dosage for children: curcumin, 500–1,000 mg daily; fresh turmeric juice, 2–6 ounces daily.

Quercetin—to reduce inflammation in the body and lungs. Dosage for children: 250–500 mg two to four times daily.

CHAPTER 23

Diabetes

D iabetes is a disorder of overly elevated blood glucose levels. You may recall that glucose (a form of sugar) is the main energy source for most of our cells. When blood glucose levels rise, the pancreas normally secretes the hormone insulin, which acts as a transporter, allowing glucose and amino acids to leave the bloodstream and be taken into the cells for use. This process, however, can go awry. Diabetes occurs when the body doesn't produce insulin, or makes insufficient amounts of insulin, or is resistant to insulin. Symptoms are listed in the following inset "Symptoms of Diabetes" on page 225.

Diabetes is a common chronic illness that runs in families, so children with parents or grandparents who have diabetes are more likely to develop diabetes than other children are. Diabetes affects about 150,000 children and adolescents in the United States.

TYPES AND COMPLICATIONS

Type I diabetes, which used to be called juvenile diabetes, is more specifically termed insulin-dependent diabetes mellitus (IDDM). This form is a chronic autoimmune disease and is diagnosed in about 13,000 children in the United States each year. Its onset is usually sudden and can occur at any time during childhood. Type I diabetes is often triggered by an infection, typically a virus; the body's immune system mounts an attack on the infection, and also mistakenly attacks and destroys the insulin-secreting beta cells in the pancreas. Allergy to milk has also been implicated as a possible trigger. Children with type I diabetes require injections to replace the insulin that their bodies can no longer produce. These children are usually thin, and they may complain of thirst.

Type II diabetes, which used to be called adult diabetes, is more specifically termed non-insulin dependent diabetes mellitus (NIDDM). When it occurs in children, type II diabetes is first diagnosed between the ages of ten and nineteen years.

The hormonal changes around the time of puberty seem to be an important trigger. It is most common in children with close relatives who have diabetes; 45 to 80 percent of children with type II diabetes have a diabetic parent. Rates of type II diabetes are highest in Native American populations (by far the highest in the Puma Indian Tribe) and are also high in Asians, Hispanics, and Blacks. The incidence of this form of diabetes in the general public, however, is fairly low, so pediatricians do not routinely test for it in children. Children with type II diabetes are commonly overweight but typically have no other symptoms until they are diagnosed. In fact, according to the U.S. Centers for Disease Control, almost 30 percent of diabetics in the United States remain undiagnosed.

Until recently, nearly all children with diabetes had type I, and type II was usually found in people over the age of forty years. Nowadays, type II is on the rise and constitutes 8 to 45 percent of diabetes in children and teenagers. About 90 percent of diabetic children have shiny, darkened, or velvety-looking skin around the neck, in the armpits, and/or around fingers or toes. Glucose is often found in the urine of children with diabetes; this can be detected using a simple dip-stick. High blood pressure and/or high cholesterol are additional signs that a child should be screened for diabetes.

If your child is diagnosed with diabetes, a hemoglobin A1C test is a simple way to monitor his/her blood sugar levels. The test shows a three-month average of the amount of sugar found on the outside of your child's red blood cells. Imagine that red blood cells look like gumdrops coated with sugar crystals; the more sugar crystals on the outside, the more damaging they are to your child's blood

Symptoms of Diabetes

Symptoms of diabetes may include:

- Behavioral problems
- Blurred vision
- Dark, velvety-looking skin in the armpit or on the back of the neck
- Dry mouth
- Fatigue
- Headaches
- Impotence (in adults)

- Increased hunger
- Increased thirst
- Increased urination
- Irritability
- Numbness of the hands or feet
- Tummy pains
- Unexplained weight loss

vessels, heart, eyes, and kidneys, and the greater risk exists of long-term health issues related to the diabetes. Studies show that hemoglobin A1C levels of 5 to 6 percent are optimal for normal, healthy children. Many children with both types of diabetes have levels of 10 to 11 percent upon diagnosis. An initial target level is 7 percent, and ideally, with treatment, hemoglobin A1C levels return to normal. Uncontrolled diabetes, however, can lead to serious complications later in life. High blood glucose is the most significant risk factor for developing heart and vascular disease. Diabetes is the leading cause of kidney failure and adult blindness. Careful blood sugar control is essential for preventing these and other complications including nerve problems and gum disease.

Fortunately, type II diabetes is largely preventable. Most children with type II diabetes make enough insulin, but their body's cells are inefficient at utilizing it properly. This condition, called insulin resistance, is associated with obesity, lack of exercise, poor eating habits, and insufficiencies of key nutrients such as B-complex vitamins, chromium, and magnesium. Weight loss and regular exercise can reduce or eliminate the need for medications in type II diabetes, and improvements in diet and lifestyle can sometimes normalize blood sugar levels completely.

New Ideas about Underlying Causes

Accumulating findings suggest that the gut immune system plays an important role in type I diabetes. A study of 141 children with type I diabetes, for example, found elevated antigliaden antibodies in more than 8 percent and found celiac disease (gluten intolerance) in almost 3 percent, which is ten times the average incidence. New research into type I indicates that these children's immune systems are overwhelmed, and also that they have increased intestinal permeability (leaky gut syndrome) compared to nondiabetic children. The leakier the gut, the more variability in blood sugar fluctuation, and antibody reactions to specific foods occur. Continuing to eat these foods further aggravates the condition, creating a vicious cycle.

Food allergy may play a role as well. A considerable amount of research has shown a link between infant allergy to cow's milk and development of type I diabetes. In a similar vein, an epidemiological study in forty countries found that the incidence of type I in children was highest in the countries with the highest consumption of dairy and other animal foods, whereas children eating a mainly vegetarian diet had a lowered incidence of type II diabetes.

Identifying your child's food sensitivities and/or allergies may help in stabilizing his/her blood sugar levels and ultimately reduce the need for medications. A recent study looked at diet and food intolerance in twenty-six adults with type I diabetes; the control group ate their regular diabetic diet and followed their usual lifestyle program, whereas the test group ate a dairy-free diet, removed any additional foods that provoked antibody reactions, and were given specific nutritional supplements. After six months, the test group showed significantly greater improvement in blood glucose and hemoglobin A1C levels than the control group. In an unpublished case study, clinical nutritionist Jayashree Mani reports that by working with an allergen-free and alkalizing diet, she was able to lower blood glucose levels by half in a type I diabetic teenage boy, while also reducing his insulin needs by more than a third.

A protein molecule called zonulin increases intestinal permeability and has been implicated in type I diabetes and celiac disease (see the inset "Celiac Disease and Autoimmunity" on page 146). Animal study shows that if zonulin is blocked, destruction of the pancreatic beta cells can be prevented. Although this research is new, it will be interesting to watch for further developments.

Minerals, Vitamins, Supplements, and Herbs

Studies have shown that nutrient inadequacies play a role in both types of diabetes in children, and that supplementation may benefit children with type I. It is suggested, for example, that magnesium deficiency may underlie the initial development of insulin resistance. Many studies show magnesium deficiency in adult diabetics, and others show decreased magnesium levels in children with insulin resistance, indicating a great need for supplemental magnesium and magnesium-rich foods in diabetes. An interesting British study found that children whose drinking water supply contained higher concentrations of zinc and magnesium experienced lower rates of type I diabetes.

Other minerals, chromium and vanadium, actually have insulin-like effects. They have been shown to help regulate blood sugar levels and reduce insulin resistance, and can reduce diabetics' needs for oral antidiabetes medications and insulin. Foods containing trivalent chromium (an easily utilized form of the mineral) include egg yolks, whole-grain products, high-bran breakfast cereals, coffee, nuts, green beans, broccoli, meat, brewer's yeast, and some brands of wine and beer. Chromium supplementation up to 1,000 micrograms (mcg) daily has been used in glucose-regulation research with adults. Begin with supplemental chromium at 200 mcg daily and watch your child's glucose levels carefully, especially if he/she uses insulin or antidiabetes medications. When the chromium effect kicks in, the appropriate medication dosage can be significantly reduced, which can cause temporary low blood sugar—and that can be a scary event.

The antioxidant alpha lipoic acid has been shown to be protective of liver function in diabetic adults, and research shows an increased need for antioxidants in children with both types of diabetes. If begun early after the diagnosis of type I, antioxidant supplementation leads to more frequent remissions and reduced insulin demand, particularly in the first months. The B-complex vitamins have been shown to be particularly protective for diabetic children. Thiamine (vitamin B_1) protects beta cells in all children with type I and helps prevent their damage in children with long-standing type I. In a case report of two children with mega-loblastic anemia (more common in children with type I) who were given thiamine, their blood glucose levels remained normal for seven and ten years respectively, until they reached puberty, when they needed oral medications and finally insulin injections. Nicotinamide (a form of vitamin B_3) can slow the progression of the disease in children newly diagnosed with type I. Thought to work by preventing free radical toxicity, nicotinamide can put some children into remission, improve glucose control, and help preserve some beta cell function. A study in children with type I showed that daily supplementation with folic acid (another B-vitamin) helped protect blood vessels from damage, which is essential for preventing long-term heart disease.

Good prenatal nutrition for pregnant mothers can reduce the incidence of dia-betes in their children. Diabetic mothers who get extra vitamin D from food during pregnancy reduce the risk of their child developing type I; the same result can be obtained with prenatal cod liver oil supplements containing both vitamins A and D. We can also increase vitamin D levels by spending time in the sun. Vitamin D is also important in the later lives of children who do have type I, because they are at greater risk for bone loss. One study supplementing with daily vitamin D for one year strengthened the children's bone and reduced their risk of osteopenia.

Other natural treatments for diabetes offer a promising avenue of exploration. There is only one really good study on the use of corosolic acid, but it showed a significant decrease in blood glucose levels in adults with type II. I have success-fully used corosolic acid in my clinical practice. Research supports the use of herbs to enhance insulin's utilization and decrease insulin resistance. Gymnema, for example, can be helpful in both types of diabetes by improving the body's abil-ity to use insulin effectively; in type II, by stimulating insulin production; and in one study of type I diabetics, by significantly lowering insulin needs and hemoglo-bin A1C levels. Bitter melon is used in the Philippines to regulate glucose levels in type II. Other herbs and foods found to be useful in lowering blood sugar levels include fenugreek, cinnamon, holy basil, and prickly pear cactus.

Special Needs of Diabetic Children and Teenagers

Children with diabetes have increased needs for nearly every nutrient and must eat a carefully controlled diet. The American Dietetic Association's current favorite diet-control method is carbohydrate counting, and children with type I may do best with a restricted-carbohydrate diet, but some other diets work equally well. I was recently at a medical meeting where studies were presented showing the benefits in diabetes of high-complex-carbohydrate/high-fiber diets, Paleolithic or "caveman" diets, and low-carbohydrate diets. It's important to figure out what works best for your own child; frequently checking blood glucose levels will help with this.

The restrictions imposed on diet, exercise, and social activities can be daunting for a diabetic child or teenager. Unlike other kids, they can't just be casual about cookies and milk or birthday cake. They have to be more responsible more continuously than other children their age. This often seems unfair, and they may experience emotional or social difficulties as well. Engaging the support of friends and relatives is important for success in living with diabetes. Children with diabetes do best when the whole family supports them; consider changing the whole family's diet. Your child may benefit from going to a camp for diabetic children or being in a support group (mom and dad may benefit from a support group as well). As a parent, you also need to learn what's important to your child's health and teach it to any people who help tend your child (such as teachers and healthcare professionals). Once you are thoroughly familiar with your child's specific needs, you'll be his/her best expert.

Many diabetic children and teenagers require oral diabetes medications or insulin injections. If a child with diabetes gets sick, his/her blood sugar levels must be watched carefully because the corresponding appropriate medication dosage may change suddenly. *Note:* Cautioning against cigarettes, marijuana, and alcohol is especially important with teenage diabetics. Smoking increases their already heightened risk of heart disease, and alcohol and marijuana dramatically change blood glucose levels.

Functional Laboratory Testing for Children with Diabetes

If your child is diagnosed with diabetes, taking blood glucose readings at home with a glucometer (which measures the glucose level in a drop of blood) will be essential. This is typically done once or twice daily, although initially you may need to take more frequent readings. Your child's doctor will use the readings to determine the most appropriate treatment plan, and will also order hemoglobin A1C testing on a regular basis.

Additional tests can help assess other underlying issues and help reduce the need for medications. Doctors specializing in environmental medicine can identify their patients' food sensitivities by measuring blood sugar levels and pulse; these often rise significantly within thirty to sixty minutes after an offending food is eaten. I have seen foods produce such blood glucose spikes even when only a couple of bites were eaten. See Appendix A for details on testing. Available tests include:

1. Intestinal permeability test

2. Food sensitivity/allergy test(s)

3. Antiendomysial, antigliaden, and tissue transglutaminase antibody tests for celiac disease (antiendomysial is the most accurate and should be done first; if negative, get one of the others to make sure; biopsy is the most certain test)

4. In type I, test for antibodies to thyroid, adrenal, endomysial, and parietal cells

5. Lactose intolerance test

6. Vitamin D test

Healing Options for Children with Either Type of Diabetes

If your child is prescribed antidiabetes medication, it is critical to use it *consistently and exactly as prescribed.* If your child needs an insulin pump, you'll need specific instructions on its use from his/her physician or diabetes educator.

Historically, people worldwide have used various natural remedies to control blood sugar levels: glucomannan fiber, young barley shoots, prickly pear cactus juice, fenugreek—the list is long. As we integrate this sort of information, many more options may become available. See Appendix B for more details on the following nutrients, herbs, and supplements. (It is unlikely that you will need to use every suggested healing option.)

Regular Blood Glucose Reading—to keep blood glucose levels regulated and prevent long-term complications. You must learn how to check your child's blood glucose; if your child is older, he/she can easily master this task. With regular checking, you'll find that specific foods keep his/her blood glucose down and should be eaten often, whereas other foods may spike it with a single bite and should be avoided.

Regular Exercise—to lower blood glucose levels, reduce medication needs, and help with mood and behavior. It is essential that your child find some type of exercise he/she enjoys and can do nearly daily. In type II, exercise can often make oral medications unnecessary.

Psychological Support—to help manage the times when your child just can't cope or rebels against treatment because he/she wants to be "normal." Counseling provides nurturing and insightful support and can also help with issues of family dynamics. Chronic disease puts a strain on everyone in the family; individual and/or family counseling may be needed from time to time.

Multivitamin-Mineral Supplement—to counteract inadequacies in basic nutrients. Dosage for children: as directed on label.

Antioxidant Supplement plus Lipoic Acid—to reduce inflammation and prevent free-radical damage throughout the body. An antioxidant supplement will likely contain carotenoids, vitamin E, selenium, and glutathione or n-acetyl cysteine, and may also contain additional nutrients. Dosage for children: a good supplement, as directed on label; lipoic acid, 100–600 milligrams (mg) daily.

Magnesium—to counteract insulin resistance and probable magnesium deficiency. Along with supplements, give magnesium-rich foods such as green leafy vegetables (like kale, broccoli, spinach, chard, and collards) and whole grains. Dosage for children: start with 100 mg daily, increase in increments of 100–200 mg until your child gets diarrhea, then reduce in increments of 100–200 mg until his/her bowel movements are normal. *Note:* If the necessary magnesium dosage is higher than 1,000 mg daily, 1–2 teaspoons of choline citrate daily can help with absorption and allow the dosage to be reduced.

Chromium—to reduce insulin resistance and improve blood sugar regulation. Dosage for children: 100–1,000 mcg daily, either from a supplement or nutritional yeast. *Note:* Increase dosage slowly, especially if your child takes medication or insulin, because blood sugar levels can drop suddenly.

Gymnema—to lower hemoglobin A1C levels, stimulate insulin production, and/or promote the body's ability to use insulin more effectively. Look for a product standardized to 25% gymnemic acids. Dosage for children: 200–400 mg daily in divided doses.

Healing Options for Children with Type I Diabetes

The treatment goal for children with type I diabetes is to minimize the amount of insulin needed and prevent long-term complications by prolonging pancreatic beta cell function, maintaining good glucose control, and maximizing helpful lifestyle changes. See Appendix B for more details on the following nutrients, herbs, and supplements. (It is unlikely that you will need to use every suggested healing option.)

Develop a Specific Diet—to help control blood glucose levels and reduce long-term risks. Limiting carbohydrates is a standard dietary strategy for children with type I. Particular food intolerances may cause your child's insulin and blood glucose levels to spike, so it's important to monitor his/her blood glucose to determine which foods evoke the best and worst responses. Work closely with a nutritionist to develop the correct diet for your child's needs.

Consider Autoimmunity—because adults with type I diabetes often have autoantibodies against the thyroid, parietal cells, adrenal glands, and endomysium. If autoantibodies are found to be high, you'll know to be more aggressive about allergen reduction in your child's environment and foods so that damage to organs and glands may be prevented.

Consider Sensitivity/Allergy—see Chapter 11. Testing for antibodies to foods and environmental chemicals and implementing a program to avoid these allergens could be very helpful in lowering insulin needs and preventing long-term health problems in children with type I.

Nicotinamide—to slow/reduce progression of the disease in newly diagnosed children. It can put some children into remission, improve glucose control, and help preserve some beta cell function. Dosage for children: 25 mg per kilogram (kg; 2.2 pounds) body weight daily.

Carnitine—to counteract possible deficiency. Dosage for children: 500–2,000 mg daily (your child's doctor can perform a free-carnitine blood test to determine need).

Folic Acid—to protect against vascular damage. Dosage for children: 5 mg daily. (The high-dose brand Folixor is available through Emerson Ecologics; see the Resources section.)

Thiamine—to reduce numbness and tingling, protect beta cells, and help normalize megaloblastic anemia. Dosage for children: 50–200 mg daily.

Digestive Enzymes—to compensate for lack of pancreatic enzymes and enhance digestion. Dosage for children: one capsule with each meal or snack.

Healing Options for Children with Type II Diabetes

The treatment goal in type II diabetes is to maximize lifestyle changes and minimize medication use. Although there has been much research in adults, type II in children and adolescents is relatively new and little-researched. Most of the studies mentioned in this chapter involved children with type I, but it is likely that the needs and benefits identified by those results bear a good resemblance to the needs and benefits for children with type II. In highly motivated adults with diabetes, I have seen all symptoms and blood tests completely normalize with a healthful diet, weight loss, and regular exercise. Although these adults still have a tendency for diabetes, their illness is kept completely at bay. This can also be accomplished in children, but it takes great motivation and support from the child, family, and extended family. See Appendix B for more details on the following nutrients, herbs, and supplements. (It is unlikely that you will need to use every suggested healing option.)

Develop a Specific Diet—to control your child's glucose levels and reduce his/her need for medication. Various studies have shown benefits with several types of diets. Vegetarian diets, which are richer in fiber, antioxidants, and minerals than meat-based diets are, can help reduce the incidence of type II in children and adults. Doctor James Anderson has researched adult type II for decades, and a diet high in fiber and complex carbohydrates has proven to be of great benefit to his patients. Others recommend carbohydrate counting, which limits carbohydrate-containing foods. By monitoring your child's glucose level frequently, you can find out what works best for him/her.

High-Fiber Diet—to regulate blood glucose levels. See Chapter 8 and see Table 8.1 on page 80. Research shows that eating a high-fiber diet slows the release of glucose into the bloodstream over time. Peas and beans, fruits, vegetables, and whole grains, especially high-fiber cereals containing 9 or more grams of fiber per serving, can be extremely useful.

Glucose-Control Supplement—to regulate blood glucose levels with a combination of vitamins, minerals, and herbs. These products commonly contain B-complex vitamins, chromium, vanadium, bitter melon, and gymnema; they may also contain biotin, vitamins C and E, magnesium, CoQ_{10}, lipoic acid, and/or carnitine. Ask at your local health food store for recommendations. Dosage for children: as directed on label.

Holy Basil—to help regulate blood glucose levels. (*Author's note:* When I lived in Hawaii, my diabetic clients swore that eating three leaves of holy basil daily helped normalize their blood glucose without medication. Hairy basil seed has also been used for the same purpose.) Nontoxic and tasty—you can even make pesto out of it. Dosage for children: 2–3 leaves or more daily.

Corosolic Acid—to normalize blood glucose. Dosage for children: 25–150 mg daily, according to child's size, age, and blood glucose levels.

Bitter Melon—to help regulate blood glucose levels. Can be eaten as food, but tea or supplement may be preferable. Dosage for children: tea, 1–2 cups daily; capsule, as directed on label.

Cinnamon—to help regulate blood glucose levels. Use in and on foods. It is being added to many glucose-regulating supplements as well. Dosage: ½ tsp or more daily.

CHAPTER 24

Down's Syndrome

Down's syndrome (DS) occurs in one out of 800–1,000 births and affects 350,000 Americans. Most people with DS have a third chromosome 21 (trisomy 21) rather than the normal pair, and the presence of an extra chromosome in every cell of the body results in the syndrome's specific characteristics. The risk of this genetic anomaly, a result of faulty cell division during pregnancy, is higher in children born of mothers older than thirty-five years. New research suggests that folic acid deficiencies in the pregnant mother may be one of the causes of DS. The syndrome varies in severity but usually involves some form of mental and developmental delay, characteristic facial features that are relatively flatter than average, and head size that is smaller than average.

Children with DS have an increased risk of respiratory infections and colds, and also have higher incidences of leukemia, heart disease, celiac disease, hypothyroidism, visual and hearing problems, and health problems in general. Some have surgery early in life to correct heart, gastrointestinal, vision, or hearing problems. Babies with DS should be screened for hearing loss by the age of six months, and they should have regular vision testing. People with DS are at greater risk of developing Alzheimer's disease later in life. In addition, studies show a high incidence of decreased thyroid gland function and actual hypothyroidism in children with DS. Some researchers report that up to half of all children with DS whose thyroid function seems normal may actually have subclinical hyperthyroidism, perhaps even compensating for this by producing higher levels of thyroid-stimulating hormone, and would benefit from treatment with thyroid hormones.

Children with DS can do everything that other children can do—walk, talk, get potty-trained, draw, and the like; typically, they just do it a bit later. Their mental delays are usually mild to moderate and can be helped with early interventions, love, and teaching. Special educational programs are available, but many children with DS are integrated into regular classrooms and do quite well there. As adults, many people with DS have jobs, some marry, and many can live independently or semi-independently.

DIGESTIVE ISSUES

Most people with DS have special digestive needs. With investigation and patience, you can discover the underlying digestive conditions that influence your child's DS. Using the natural treatment ideas in this chapter may also reduce or eliminate his/her need for medication. Remember that two-thirds of the immune system is located in the digestive tract; keeping the gut healthy can keep your child healthy.

Some clinicians have found that elimination/provocation diets can make a profound difference for patients with DS. But although it is widely known that children with DS often suffer from food allergies and malabsorption problems, there have been only a few studies on this topic. Increased IgA antibodies to foods have been documented, as well as a high incidence of antibodies to dairy products, and studies show that 3 to 12 percent of children with DS test positive for IgG or IgA antibodies to gluten and gliaden. The incidence of celiac disease (gluten intolerance) in children with DS is also higher than the average. In a recent study surveying parents, more parents of children with DS than parents of children without DS thought that their children were sensitive to specific foods. When these children were then put on an elimination diet, 66 percent of them improved—and yet their physicians had not previously tested them for food allergies.

Many digestive issues in DS aren't yet represented in the medical literature. I was unable to find any published studies that screened children with DS for leaky gut syndrome; given the known problems of malabsorption and food allergy in DS, however, increased intestinal permeability is highly likely to play a role in these children's lives. Although levels of fatty acids may be abnormal in DS, and although it is also common for parents to give digestive enzymes and probiotics to children with DS, I found no published research on these topics either.

NUTRIENT ISSUES

As a result of metabolic variations found in the syndrome, children with DS may have nutrient deficiencies or excesses. Levels of the antioxidant minerals selenium and zinc have been found to be low in people with DS, and numerous studies have shown an increased need for other antioxidants like lipoic acid and vitamins A, C, and E. Interestingly, the thyroid gland requires antioxidants to function properly. Lower levels of carnitine, carnosine, choline, folate, magnesium, manganese, selenium, vitamins A, B_1, B_{12}, and C, zinc, and possibly serine have also been noted; by contrast, higher-than-normal levels of copper and the antioxidant superoxide-dismutase have been found. Testing for nutritional status can be helpful, and children with DS can benefit from supplementation with folic acid, methionine, vitamins B_6 and B_{12}, and zinc.

Amino acid abnormalities are seen in people with DS as well. One study found adults with DS to have decreased levels of amino acids including glutathione (an antioxidant), homocysteine, methionine, S-adenosylhomocysteine, and S-adenosylmethione, but elevated levels of cystathione and cysteine; other

Pioneers in DS Nutrition

More than forty years ago, Henry Turkel, M.D., of Michigan treated more than 600 children with DS by giving them vitamins, minerals, and thyroid hormone supplements. In many cases, the results were extraordinary, including changes in facial features and improvements in learning and motor skills; some of the children went on to finish college.

In 1981, long-time nutrient researcher Ruth Harrell, Ph.D., conducted a nutritional supplement study with sixteen mentally retarded children at John's Hopkins Hospital, two of whom had DS. All of the children showed increases in IQ levels, averaging ten points the first month and sixteen points after four months. Some children made huge gains, beginning to talk and read; others had small gains. This is Dr. Harrell's formula:

- Calcium—410 milligrams (mg)
- Copper—1.75 mg
- Folic acid—0.4 mg
- Iodide—0.15 mg
- Iron—7.5 mg (Caution: Using iron is not advised unless you are sure your child is anemic.)
- Magnesium—300 mg
- Manganese—3 mg
- Niacinamide (vitamin B3)—750 mg
- Pantothenate—450 mg

- Phosphorus—9 mg
- Pyridoxine (vitamin B6)—350 mg
- Riboflavin (vitamin B2)—200 mg
- Thiamin (vitamin B1)—300 mg
- Vitamin A—15,000 international units (IU)
- Vitamin B12—1,000 micrograms
- Vitamin C—1,500 mg
- Vitamin D—300 IU
- Vitamin E—600 IU
- Zinc—30 mg

studies have also found higher-than-normal levels of cysteine and phenylalanine in DS. In healthy people without DS, these amino acid levels can typically be normalized with the help of nutrients including betaine, folic acid, and vitamins B_6 and B_{12}. Adding methionine, folinic acid, methyl B_{12}, thymidine, or dimethylglycine improves these levels in cell cultures. Specific amino acid testing can greatly benefit a child with DS.

FUNCTIONAL LABORATORY TESTING FOR CHILDREN WITH DOWN'S SYNDROME

See Appendix A for details on testing. Available tests include:

1. Vitamin and mineral test(s) (a white blood cell analysis more closely approximates tissue status than a standard blood test does; hair analysis can be useful in detection of some excess or deficient minerals)

2. Complete thyroid panel

3. Amino acids test

4. Anti-endomysial, antigliaden, and tissue transglutaminase antibody tests for celiac disease

5. Organic acids test

6. Food sensitivity/allergy test(s)

7. Lactose intolerance test

HEALING OPTIONS FOR CHILDREN WITH DOWN'S SYNDROME

If your child has DS, look for a physician who specializes in functional medicine or integrated medical care. Each child has unique needs. Your doctor can help you wade through the huge number of possible treatment plans that may substantially improve your child's quality of life. See Appendix B for more details on the following supplements. (It is unlikely that you will need to use every suggested healing option.)

Consider Food Sensitivity/Allergy and an Elimination/Provocation Diet—see Chapter 11. Your child may benefit significantly from testing for and the elimination of offending foods.

Consider Celiac Disease—see Chapter 15. Rates of celiac disease are high in children with DS.

Antioxidant Supplement—to meet higher-than-normal needs for these compounds. The supplement may contain lipoic acid, milk thistle, reduced glutathione or

N-acetyl cysteine, vitamins C and E, and selenium, among other nutrients. Dosage for children: as directed on label.

Multivitamin-Mineral Supplement—to counter probable nutrient deficiencies. Look for a supplement that contains a wide variety of nutrients; everything your child needs may not be contained in a one-a-day, as minerals are bulky. Dosage for children: as directed on label.

Consider Additional Testing—to uncover your child's unique digestive and health issues. Look at essential fatty acids, amino acids, heavy metals, antioxidant status, stool analysis, and more.

Alkaline Diet—to prevent infections. See Chapter 7.

CHAPTER 25

Influenza

In general, people use the term "flu" loosely for any bout of fever, diarrhea, vomiting, extreme fatigue, and weakness, or some combination of those, no matter what the actual cause may be; perhaps it's really food poisoning or another type of bacterial or viral infection, and those types of flu-like illnesses are technically gastroenteritis—but to us, it feels like the flu. Real flu, however, is caused by an infection of one of the many influenza viruses. It is more common during the winter months. The flu usually starts suddenly, is worst the first two or three days, and then subsides. Symptoms vary but can include:

- Body aches
- Cough
- Diarrhea and vomiting
- Fatigue

- Fever
- Headache
- Runny or stuffy nose
- Sore throat

Once your child improves, he/she can still be quite weak for a week or more, and pushing too hard too soon can lead to a relapse. Most of these symptoms are self-limiting. Although a child can run a very high fever, he/she will usually pull through without any complications. In small children, however, the risk of complications including pneumonia, dehydration, ear infections, and sinus problems is higher. And if your child already has another chronic illness, flu can aggravate the existing condition. *See a doctor immediately if your child has these signs:*

- Bluish skin color
- Fast breathing or trouble breathing
- Fever with a rash
- Irritability to the point that the child does not want to be held

- Flu-like symptoms that improve but then return with fever and worse cough
- Not drinking enough fluids
- Not waking up or unresponsive

239

Influenza passes from person to person through touch and through the air. It can be picked up, for example, from a doorknob or a sneeze. If someone around you is sick, make sure to wash your hands often with soap and water, and keep your hands away from your mouth, nose, and eyes. Children are more likely to get the flu and more likely to pass it on, and it can easily spread through a school in no time. If your child is ill, keep him/her home from school, make sure his/her mouth is covered with a tissue when coughing or sneezing, and keep a wastebasket nearby for tissue disposal. Don't make the mistake I did and sleep in the same room with your sick kids, or you'll catch everything they get—I learned the hard way!

The Flu Shot

The flu is not usually fatal. It is not to the advantage of the virus to kill its host, because then the virus will die too, so it just makes us really sick for a few days while it replicates. Each year, one or more influenza viruses completely recombine into new strains; each year, scientists try to outguess the flu by making a combination vaccine to protect against the possible new strains that may appear; and each year, vaccine manufacturers hope that this season's flu mutations will be similar to last year's viruses. Many scientists are concerned, however, that widespread use of flu vaccine helps to make the surviving viruses more virulent. The U.S. Centers for Disease Control and Prevention (CDC) report that 10 to 20 percent of us get sick from the flu each year, and that 20,000 people in the United States die of it annually, but those statistics are not accurate, as they lump the flu and pneumonia together. Upon closer examination, it looks like the flu is actually responsible for about 300 deaths per year and pneumonia for the other 19,700.

According to the CDC, if you have a healthy child over the age of two years, there is no need to vaccinate that child against the flu.

Do you need to vaccinate your child against influenza? The CDC's position is that small children are as vulnerable to the flu as the elderly are; therefore, the CDC recommends a flu shot for all children aged six to twenty-three months, for all children two years and older who have chronic underlying illnesses, and for all children two years and older who are on chronic aspirin therapy. This means that most children do *not* need flu shots.

If you decide to obtain a flu vaccination for your child, make sure that your physician is using a thimerosol-free vaccine. Keep in mind, though, that even a thimerosol-free vaccine is likely to contain potentially toxic ingredients: formaldehyde (to kill viruses), aluminum (to promote antibody response), and ethylene glycol (also known as antifreeze, used in this case as a disinfectant).

Avian Influenza (Bird Flu)

Most flu epidemics in people originated from birds and are typically passed to pigs and on to humans. A new strain of avian flu called influenza A H5N1, however, killed forty-four people in Thailand and Vietnam in 2004. Symptoms of this flu look like those of any other: chills, fever, muscle aches, and sweating—but the fatality rate for people who contract this strain is 50 percent. Until now, H5N1 hasn't been spread from person to person much, but concern has arisen that if it mutates into a more contagious strain, there will be a risk of a pandemic in which millions of people worldwide may die. Recently a large flock of wild birds in China was found to have H5N1, and millions of birds have been slaughtered in Asia in an effort to prevent the spread of the virus through wild birds and domesticated poultry.

It is now known that a flu pandemic that killed 20–40 million people in 1918 was originally bird flu. This provides insights to researchers currently scrambling to develop vaccines and strategies to prevent another global outbreak. Many existing antiviral medications have no effect on the H5N1 strain. But on a positive note, data from Hannemann Medical College shows that of the 26,000 people treated homeopathically for the 1918 flu, only 1 percent died. Two common homeopathic medicines that are used effectively against influenza are arsenicum album and oscillococcinnum.

Preventive Options

The best defense against the flu is a good offense! Many of us are exposed to influenza but don't come down with the illness thanks to a healthy, strong immune response to the virus. The virus doesn't give us the flu unless being run-down makes us susceptible to it, so the best way to protect your child is to strengthen his/her immune resistance. Do this by making sure that your child gets plenty of sleep, eats well, stays hydrated, and has extra nutrients in the winter. Giving your child a daily dose of vitamin C, garlic, elderberry, or echinacea during the winter months can also reduce your child's risk. Additional anti-flu tips:

- Wash your hands and your child's hands frequently with soap and water.
- Eat plenty of fruits and vegetables.
- Get exercise.
- Avoid sugar.

If your child is exposed to the flu, ramp up the supplements, rest, and healthful foods. And if a large portion of the school is already sick, it's okay to keep your child home from school even when he/she is well.

Preventive Supplements—to boost the immune system. Dosage for children: vitamin C, 100–1,000 milligrams (mg) daily; garlic, liberally as directed on label (Kwai makes a small, easy-to-swallow pill); elderberry extract, ½–1 teaspoon daily; echinacea, three times weekly; colostrum, one to three capsules daily; and astragalus, 100–500 mg three times weekly. I'd also give my child a daily multivitamin-mineral containing selenium and zinc, minerals shown to be protective against viral infections.

Combination Products—to provide antiviral and immune-boosting effects. Many products combining herbs and other nutrients such as Source Natural's Wellness Formula, Nature's Way Ultimate Immunity, Gaia's Herbs Echinacea Supreme, Transformation's TPP Immune Complex, Vital Nutrient's Viracon, and Herb Pharm Immune Defense Tonic are available at local health food stores. Dosage for children: as directed on label.

Arsenicum Album—to prevent flu homeopathically. Doses are 30 C or higher (such as 100 C, 100 X, 200 C, or 200 X). Dosage for children: one dose under tongue weekly. (See also in "Healing Options for Children with the Flu" below.)

Oscillococcinum—to prevent flu homeopathically. Dosage for children: for children older than two years, entire contents of one vial dissolved in mouth, up to three times per day as needed. (See also in "Healing Options for Children with the Flu" below.)

Healing Options for Children with the Flu

At the first sign of the flu, act immediately: fluids, rest, washing hands frequently with soap and water, and pouring immune-enhancing products into your child and the rest of the family. When one of you is sick, it's definitely time to pump up everybody else too! See Appendix B for more details on the following nutrients, herbs, and supplements. (It is unlikely that you will need to use every suggested healing option.)

Elderberry Extract—to shorten duration and lessen severity of flu. Tasty, too! Dosage for children: ½–1 teaspoon, according to child's age, in a little water three or four times daily.

Yin Chiao—to shorten duration and lessen severity of flu. Administer this ancient Chinese remedy consistently to your child for the first day or two that he/she feels symptoms of a cold or flu coming on; if you can catch the sickness early, you can often stop it in its tracks. I always keep this on hand. Dosage for children: as directed on label (varies according to manufacturer). *Note:* Your child has to be able to swallow a pill; you could possibly crush the pills, however, and put them into tea.

Arsenicum Album—to treat flu homeopathically. Doses are 30 C or higher (such as 100 C, 100 X, 200 C, or 200 X). Dosage for children: one dose under tongue as often as every two hours, stopping when symptoms improve and resuming when symptoms worsen.

Oscillococcinum—to shorten duration and decrease severity of the flu. I've found it helpful if I take it at the first sign of the flu, or if someone around me has the flu. Dosage for children: for children older than two years, entire contents of one vial dissolved in mouth over a period of six hours, up to three times per day.

Flu Caps—to shorten duration and lessen severity of flu. See the inset "Joy Gardner's Flu Caps" below. Dosage for children: one or two capsules every two to three hours as needed.

Rest and Fluids—to support the body's self-healing. This may sound trite, but if your child has the flu or a flu-like infection, he/she needs to rest (this probably won't be difficult to enforce) and stay hydrated. Give lots of fluids: water, tea, diluted fruit juices, and flat ginger-ale are good, and many children will like sipping hot tea with lemon and honey (see below). Remind your child to drink often. The smaller the child, the higher the fever, and the greater the possibility of dehydration.

Sage-Lemon-Garlic Tea—to limit flu's effects and reduce fever. To 6 cups boiling water, add 2 tablespoons sage, 2 cloves chopped garlic, half a lemon or more, and honey to taste, and steep five minutes. Dosage for children: up to 1 cup per hour.

Joy Gardner's Flu Caps

About thirty years ago, I studied plant medicines with an amazing herbalist, Joy Gardner. She recommended homemade flu capsules, which I have since used many times with family members and friends. I've never seen them fail. In her book *The New Healing Yourself* (Crossing Press, 1989), Joy says, "The flu usually goes away by itself within twenty-four to forty-eight hours, but a dose of slippery elm, cinnamon, goldenseal, and cayenne almost always works within ten minutes. This is the remedy that makes the most skeptical people say, 'You converted me!'"

Her simple remedy works amazingly well when taken at the first signs of the flu, so prepare these flu caps ahead of time to have on hand. Mix 1 teaspoon each of slippery elm, cinnamon, goldenseal, and cayenne in a small bowl, and fill size-00 capsules (available at health food stores) with the powder, using a chopstick to tamp it down a bit. Take one to two capsules every two to three hours as needed.

Umeboshi Plum—to alkalize the body. Umeboshi is very effective against the flu. Dosage for children: plums, one to four daily; or tea (paste mixed into hot water), several cups daily.

Reduce Fever if Necessary—if the fever is prolonged or over 102°F, or if your child seems really uncomfortable. Lukewarm baths and cool compresses are one way; Tylenol is another. *Caution:* Never give aspirin to your child or teenager without first consulting a physician, because aspirin can cause a viral infection such as influenza to turn into a more serious neurological illness called Reye's syndrome.

CHAPTER 26

Migraine

M ost people get an occasional headache. For some, however, these aren't simply tension headaches but migraines. Five to 10 percent of American children—that's 8 million kids—get migraines and lose about a million days of school as a result. Boys and girls are equally affected until puberty, but thereafter, girls have more than boys do (perhaps because of hormone fluctuations). Twenty percent of children with migraines get them before the age of five years old. If your child gets one migraine headache, he/she will probably have many more.

The pain of a migraine often begins on one side of the head, often behind one or both eyes, and can move to both sides of the head. Your child may vomit, complain of a throbbing head and/or dizziness, and want to be left alone in a darkened room. Some children get stomach cramps. Most children want to sleep their migraine away. Children's migraines are shorter than adults' are: often less than four hours, but can be as brief as ten minutes or as long as forty-eight hours.

Small children with a migraine headache usually look pale, have stomach pain and vomiting, and just want to sleep. They may be especially irritable or prone to crying, rock themselves, or prefer to be in a dark, quiet place. They may not be able to express to you what's going on. Children aged five to ten years experience the same symptoms, but often also have sensitivity to light, sound, and/or smell. They know that sleep will help and usually fall asleep shortly after the migraine begins. Additional symptoms may include dark circles under the eyes, tearing, swollen nasal passages, thirst, swelling, excessive sweating, increased urination, or diarrhea. Migraine headaches in older children may become more intense and more frequent, with symptoms comparable to adult migraine; the one-sided or bilateral behind-the-eyes pain pattern often occurs, and there may be an intense throbbing sensation.

Training yourself and your child to look for the more subtle beginnings of his/her migraine can enable you to stop the headache in its tracks. About 60 percent of people experience symptoms twenty-four hours prior to the actual migraine, and medications and other techniques work best if used at this point. People have reported early warning symptoms such as mood changes, food cravings, repetitive yawning, thirst, fluid retention, stiff neck, irritability, fatigue, numbness or tingling on one side of the body, lack of appetite, diarrhea, constipation, feeling of coldness, lethargy, changes in vision and/or sense of smell, and seeing bright spots. Although these symptoms vary from person to person, they follow a consistent pattern within an individual, so you and your child will soon learn his/her particular migraine warning signs.

FOODS, CHEMICALS, AND MANY OTHER TRIGGERS

Migraine usually comes on in response to a "trigger." Common triggers in children and teenagers include emotional stress (school pressure, vexation, excitement, upset), low blood sugar, lack of sleep or too much sleep, loud noise, bright light, strong odor, being hot or cold, and engaging in sports or exercise. Additional triggers include certain foods and beverages, hormone changes, weather changes, medications such as birth control pills, changes in routine, and food additives—especially monosodium glutamate (MSG), which can provoke asthma, diarrhea, vomiting, and gastric symptoms in addition to migraine. These problems can occur immediately after eating or be delayed up to seventy-two hours, making their relationship to MSG more difficult to discover. In some children, celiac disease (gluten intolerance) presents itself as migraines, so removing gluten-containing grains from the diet can be useful. And caffeine is both a potential trigger and a potential remedy (see the inset "Caffeine: Migraine Friend or Foe?" below).

Caffeine: Migraine Friend or Foe?

Caffeine is an active ingredient in some migraine medications. It significantly reduces migraine number and severity of headaches for some people but triggers them for others. You may need to carefully investigate caffeine's effect on your child's migraines. Begin by examining dietary caffeine intake. If your child regularly drinks caffeinated coffee, tea, or soda, try eliminating these beverages completely for two to three weeks to see whether his/her headaches decrease; alternatively, you may notice an increase in headaches if his/her caffeine intake was helping. If, on the other hand, your child does not regularly consume caffeine, try giving a half cup or full cup of coffee at the early onset of one of his/her migraines to see whether it lessens the headache.

Hormone fluctuations can worsen, improve, or trigger migraine headaches. Many girls and women only experience migraine at specific times in their menstrual cycle. Birth-control pills and other estrogen-containing medications are widely recognized as a trigger in women who are susceptible to migraine; when the medications are stopped, the migraines also stop.

Infection with the yeast candida is another possible contributor to migraine. A recent study of the relationship between candida and migraine found that thirteen of seventeen adult migraine sufferers responded to a three-month program of an anti-candida diet and medication by having fewer and less-severe headaches; blood testing showed reduced candida antibodies as well. (The four people who did not respond well didn't stick to the study's program.)

Of 282 migraine patients studied by British physician Jean Munro, 100 percent had food allergies or sensitivities, with more than 200 of the group sensitive to wheat and/or dairy products; other common trigger foods were tea, oranges, apples, onions, pork, and beef. Surprisingly, foods eaten daily provoked more reactions than chocolate, alcohol, and cheese, which are thought to be the most common food triggers of migraine. Dr. Munro also found that people who eliminated these foods from their diets and cleared their homes of environmental contaminants had the best results in migraine prevention. Cleaning frequently with natural household cleaners and getting rid of gas appliances, bedroom carpets and curtains, and houseplants with molds and fungus resulted in fewer migraines. Although these people were still exposed to smoke, perfume, and other environmental triggers outside the home, changing their home environments and diets lowered their thresholds enough so that they became more tolerant of foods and other environmental allergens in their lives.

John Diamond, M.D., believes that foods high in amines provoke migraine in some people, and the Diamond Headache Clinic in Chicago has used a low-amine diet with patients for more than thirty years. Dietary amines that promote vasoconstriction (constriction of blood vessels) are dopamine, serotonin, tryptamine, and tyramine, and are found in the greatest quantities in aged meats, avocados, bananas, beer, cabbage, canned fish, cheese, eggplant, pineapple, plums, potatoes, tomatoes, wine (especially red), and yeast extracts. These amines are normally broken down by enzymes, but some people with migraine have lower-than-normal amounts of the appropriate enzymes. Research results for the Diamond diet, however, have been very mixed.

In a study of seventeen adult migraine sufferers, ten had cow's milk allergy; five had allergies to flour, cabbage, and eggs; four had allergy reactions to preservatives, cottage cheese, Swiss cheese, and pork; three were sensitive to colorings and chocolate; two had reactions to beef, strawberries, lemons, and butter; and others had allergies to single foods. When the participants were put on individualized elimination diets, their headache symptoms improved substantially, and when they were rechallenged with foods they were sensitive to, a migraine was triggered in all but one of the seventeen people.

Similar results have been obtained in research with children. In a recent study of twelve children with migraine, food allergy testing and a restricted diet led to significant improvement in half of the children and mild improvement in another five. And in a study of ninety-two children who had chronic migraines, forty-nine showed positive skin tests to one or more foods, and forty of that subgroup improved after following an elimination diet for four to six weeks; thirty-one of them were cured of their migraines and remained cured for two years even after those foods were reintroduced (the other nine children also improved). All of the food sensitivity findings in these and many other migraine studies point to the need for individual testing.

NATURAL OPTIONS FROM VITAMINS AND MINERALS TO HERBS AND FATTY ACIDS

Certain B-complex vitamins have been shown to dramatically alleviate migraine in adults. When forty-nine adults with recurrent migraines were given 400 milligrams (mg) of riboflavin (vitamin B_2) daily with breakfast for three months, their migraines diminished in frequency by 67 percent and in severity by 68 percent. In a study of fifty-five adults, 59 percent of the group given 400 mg of riboflavin daily for three months improved migraine symptoms by 50 percent or more; minor side effects of diarrhea or frequent urination were experienced by two of these participants. In a study giving 1 mg vitamin B_{12} daily for three months in a nasal spray to twenty adults with a history of two to eight migraines per month for over one year, half of the participants had a 53-percent average reduction in migraine frequency (from 5.2 to 1.9 attacks per month), but the other half of the group showed virtually no improvement. There is no research on the use of vitamin B_{12} for juvenile migraine either, but B_{12} is completely nontoxic, and it does work quite well for children with asthma, via mechanisms similar to those involved in migraine.

Magnesium supplementation is definitely worth trying. Among its other properties, the mineral relaxes muscles and blood vessels. It is estimated that magnesium deficiency plays a role in at least half of all adults with migraine. Numerous studies have also documented a relationship between low magnesium levels and juvenile migraine.

Many people use the herb feverfew against migraine. It is taken on a daily basis as a preventive measure rather than as a pain-relief medication at migraine onset. Numerous studies have shown feverfew to be effective in preventing and minimizing the severity of migraine, but other studies have found no effectiveness. You can try it for your child and see if it works.

In its natural state, the herb butterbur contains liver toxins, but the patented butterbur product Petadolex lacks these toxins and has been shown to be effective against both hayfever and migraine headache. In a 2004 study of 245 adults given 75 mg of Petadolex, 50 mg of Petadolex, or a placebo twice daily for four months, 48 percent of the 75-mg group experienced fewer migraine attacks; 68 percent of the 75-mg group had a 50-percent or greater reduction in migraine frequency, compared to 49 percent in the placebo group; there was a 36-percent reduction of migraines in the 50-mg group, compared to a 26-percent reduction in the placebo group. The major side effect was burping. In another 2004 study, thirty-three people were given 25 mg of Petadolex twice daily, and their average frequency of migraine decreased from 3.4 to 1.8 after three months; 45 percent of the participants responded really well and accounted for most of the results—perhaps your child will be one of the lucky?

Fish oil, which contains high levels of the essential omega-3 fatty acids DHA and EPA, has been shown in many studies to reduce migraine severity, duration, and frequency in adults. In a recent study of twenty-seven teenagers, those taking fish oil experienced a significant improvement in migraine duration and severity compared to those taking an olive oil placebo. The teenagers taking the olive oil, however, also improved. Therefore, polyunsaturated fats in general may be beneficial against migraine.

A case study at Cincinnati Children's Hospital found that two girls suffering from migraine headaches were deficient in carnitine palmitoyltransferase-2, a nutrient used by the mitochondria in our cells to utilize fats for energy. When the girls were supplemented with carnitine, both had a reduction in headache frequency, suggesting that some children with migraine may benefit from carnitine supplementation. Other natural remedies, though unstudied so far for juvenile migraine, are worth exploring. Quercetin's anti-allergy, gut-healing, and anti-inflammatory effects, for example, are likely to be of benefit. Digestive and proteolytic enzymes are safe and worth trying as well, as it has been clinically observed that they enhance digestion and reduce food sensitivities and environmental allergies.

Functional Laboratory Testing for Children with Migraine

See Appendix A for details on testing. Available tests include:

1. Intracellular magnesium test (red blood cells or lymphocytes)

2. Food and environmental sensitivity/allergy test(s)

3. Intestinal permeability test

4. Organic acids test

5. Fatty acid test

Healing Options for Children with Migraine

In December 2004, the American Academy of Neurology and the Child Neurology Society released new medication guidelines for children with migraine. They recommend simple analgesics such as ibuprofen and acetaminophen for children; if these aren't effective, they also suggest sumatriptan nasal spray. They do *not* recommend using other triptan medications or other common antimigraine medications used in adults, as there is not enough research to support their use in children.

The key to success is finding your child's own triggers and the treatments that work best for him/her. Biofeedback and progressive relaxation techniques have been found very effective for reducing severity and frequency of migraine in children, and should be considered as a first line of treatment. See Appendix B for more details on the following nutrients, herbs, and supplements. (It is unlikely that you will need to use every suggested healing option.)

Regular Eating—to avoid the low blood sugar levels that frequently trigger migraines and other headaches. See Chapter 10 for more about eating regularly; teenagers especially forget to do this, and often skip meals.

Consider Sensitivity/Allergy—see Chapter 11. Test your child for reactions to foods and other allergens; then, eliminate any known or suspected trigger foods and chemicals. Remove all sugars, refined carbohydrates, and caffeine from your child's diet (but see the inset "Caffeine: Migraine Friend or Foe?" on page 246). Use only natural cleaning supplies, remove gas appliances, clean out household mold and mildew, use a dehumidifier, and make your child's bedroom a safe haven from mold and dust by removing unnecessary carpeting and drapery.

Behavioral Techniques—to help control migraine-triggering stressors. Many studies have proven biofeedback, hypnotherapy, and stress-reduction techniques to be helpful for children with migraine (they work even better in children than in adults).

Riboflavin—to reduce migraine frequency and severity. Dosage for children: 75–400 mg, according to child's size and age. Riboflavin's maximum effect is reached after two or three months, so be patient. *Note:* If diarrhea or frequent urination is experienced, decrease the dosage.

Butterbur/Petadolex—to reduce pain-producing inflammatory markers. Dosage for children: 10–25 mg twice daily.

Vitamin B₁₂—to reduce migraine frequency. Dosage for children: 500 micrograms–1 mg daily for three months, sublingually or in a nasal spray. If your child gets good results, continue; over time, the needed dosage may decrease.

Magnesium—to reduce migraine frequency. Dosage for children: 100–600 mg daily for at least three or four months; when your child reaches saturation, he/she will get diarrhea, and you can reduce the dose in 100-mg increments. *Note:* If more than 1,000 mg daily is needed to reach the point of loose stool, add 1 teaspoon choline citrate for each 200 mg of magnesium to facilitate magnesium's absorption.

Fish Oils and Polyunsaturated Fats—to reduce migraine severity, duration, and frequency. Eating high-fat fish twice weekly can be helpful. Polyunsaturated fats are easily obtained by adding nuts, seeds, whole grains, and good-quality oils such as olive, sesame, and safflower to the diet. Fish oil capsules may also be very beneficial. Dosage for children: 1–4 grams daily.

Feverfew—to prevent migraine and minimize severity. Dosage for children: tincture, five to twenty drops twice daily; capsules, one to three daily; or fresh leaves, one to three daily. Adjust dosage according to child's size and age. *Note:* Forms and brands of feverfew may differ in effectiveness; if your child doesn't get relief from one type, try another.

Consider Candida Infection—see Chapter 6. A pediatrician can check your child's stool or blood for candida antibodies; if candida infection is indicated, a low-carbohydrate diet and probiotics will probably do the trick.

Acupuncture—to reduce migraine incidence and severity. Acupuncture has been shown effective for this purpose in some people, but study results vary, and your child may obtain great or no benefit.

Avoid Monosodium Glutamate—to avoid triggering migraine and/or other symptoms. *Note:* Food labels can be misleading about the presence of MSG, as the chemical can be called "natural coloring" or hidden in hydrolyzed vegetable protein.

Quercetin—to reduce pain, inflammation, and allergic response. Dosage for children: as a preventive measure, 100–500 mg daily; at migraine onset, 500–1,000 mg three or four times daily.

Chiropractic and Massage—to lessen muscle tension and normalize blood flow to the brain.

Caffeine—to reduce migraine frequency and severity—or not. See the inset "Caffeine: Migraine Friend or Foe?" on page 246.

Digestive Enzymes—to enhance digestion and decrease food sensitivities. Dosage: 1–2 capsules with meals.

Protective Enzymes—to decrease food sensitivities. Dosage 1–2 capsules, twice daily on an empty stomach.

Conclusion

A s parents, we want our children to be happy, safe, and healthy. We hope they'll grow up to be kind and considerate. We hope they'll acquire the skills and tools to live independent (and interdependent) lives. And we hope they'll find passion and follow their dreams. All of this is harder, though, for children who have health issues. Fortunately, reoccurring health conditions become predictable, and you can often learn to head them off at the pass with natural options. I wrote *Digestive Wellness for Children* to help you learn about what you can do to build up your child's digestive and immune systems naturally: beginning with the food they eat, the love you share with them, and the exercise and rest they require, and continuing with nutritional supplements, herbs, stress-management tools, and appropriate laboratory tests.

Although the idea of self-care may initially seem foreign, remember that parents have always been the first line of health care for their children. When caring for a first baby, it all seems complicated and daunting. But we soon learn that most of our children's needs are not life threatening, so we calm down and learn how to tend them. We consult our families and friends, read books to increase our knowledge and skills, and as necessary, we seek professional help. Don't hesitate to take this book along to appointments with your pediatrician or family doctor; because it is science- and research-based, you can use it to brainstorm with the doctor about your child's best treatment options.

I hope you've found *Digestive Wellness for Children* useful and inspiring and that what you've learned helps you feel more empowered as parents. "Thinking outside the box" can renew our belief in what is possible and restore our hopes for our children's health and happiness.

Wishing you the best,

Liz Lipski

Resources

WEBSITES

Botanical.com, *A Modern Herbal,*
www.botanical.com

Family Doctor, www.familydoctor.org

Pediatrician Alan Greene, M.D.,
www.drgreene.com

HealthWorld online, www.healthy.net

Kids' Health for Parents,
www.kidshealth.org

Life Extension Foundation,
www.lef.org

Mayo Clinic,
www.mayoclinic.com

Joseph Mercola, D.O.,
www.mercola.com

Whole Health M.D.,
www.wholehealthmd.com

PROFESSIONAL REFERRALS

For a referral to a physician, nutritionist, or other healthcare professional in your area, contact the following organizations. They usually have referral lists on their websites or at their offices. Most laboratories (see Appendix A) also have lists of doctors who utilize their tests.

**American Academy of
Environmental Medicine**
American Financial Center
7701 East Kellogg, Suite 625
Wichita, KS 67207
316-684-5500
www.aaem.com

**American Association of
Naturopathic Physicians**
3201 New Mexico Avenue, NW,
Suite 350
Washington, DC 20016
866-538-2267, 202-895-1392
www.naturopathic.org

American Botanical Council
6200 Manor Road
Austin, TX 78723
512-926-4900
www.herbalgram.org

American Chiropractic Association
1701 Clarendon Boulevard
Arlington, VA 22209
800-986-4636, 703-276-8800
www.amerchiro.org

**American College of Advancement
 in Medicine**
23121 Verdugo Drive, Suite 204
Laguna Hills, CA 92653
800-532-3688, 949-583-7666
www.acam.org

American Herbalists Guild
1931 Gaddis Road
Canton, GA 30115
770-751-7472
www.americanherbalistsguild.com

**American Holistic Medical
 Association**
12101 Menaul Boulevard, NE, Suite C
Albuquerque, NM 87112
505-292-7788
www.holisticmedicine.org

**Association for Network
 Chiropractic**
444 Main Street
Longmont, CO 80501
303-678-8101, fax 303-678-8089
www.associationfornetworkcare.com

**Clinical Nutrition Certification
 Board**
15280 Addison Road, Suite 130
Addison, TX 75001
972-250-2829, fax 972-250-0233
www.cncb.org

**The Institute for Functional
 Medicine**
P.O. Box 1697
Gig Harbor, WA 98335
800-228-0622
www.functionalmedicine.org

**International and American
 Associations of Clinical
 Nutritionists**
15280 Addison Road, Suite 130
Addison, TX 75001
972-407-9089, fax 972-250-0233
www.iaacn.org

NUTRITIONAL AND HERBAL PRODUCTS

You may be able to find all of the products mentioned in this book at your local health food store, through local healthcare professionals, or online. The following is a partial list of the many excellent companies that manufacture nutritional and herbal products. Not all products may be available in stores. Companies that sell only to healthcare professionals are indicated with an asterisk; However, many of the products can be ordered through my website, www.innovativehealing.com. I have made arrangements enabling my clients and readers to order from several of these companies, as noted below. Most of those feature full lines of nutritional supplements and herbs; for those with more limited offerings, specific products are mentioned.

Ann Louise Gittleman and
Uni Key Health Systems
181 West Commerce Drive
Hayden Lake, ID 83835
800-888-4353
www.annlouise.
com, www.unikeyhealth.com
Parasite products Verma Key and Verma Plus.

Biotics Research Corporation*
6801 Biotics Research Drive
Rosenberg, TX 77471
281-344-0909, 800-231-5777
www.bioticsresearch.com

Emerson Ecologics
18 Lomar Park
Pepperell, MA 01463
800-654-4432, fax 800-718-7238
www.emersonecologics.com
A distributor for dozens of high-quality professional supplement manufacturers and health books. Mention Digestive Wellness for Children *and receive a discount on all purchases. Companies include Allergy Research, AMNI, Designs for Health, Douglas Labs, Folixor, Gaia Herbs, Karuna, Metabolic Maintenance,*

MMS-Pro, NF, Perque, Phytopharmica, Pure Encapsulations, Seacure, Tyler, Vital Nutrients, and dozens more.

Integrative Therapeutics*
9775 SW Commerce Circle, C5
Wilsonville, OR 97070
800-931-1709, 503-582-0467
www.integrativeinc.com
Tyler Encapsulations, NF Formulas, Phytopharmica, and Vitaline. I've made special purchase arrangements for readers of Digestive Wellness for Children. *These products are also available through Emerson Ecologics.*

Metagenics*/Ethical Nutrients
971 Calle Negocio
San Clemente, CA 92673
Metagenics sells to professionals; Ethical Nutrients is the health food store line. Nutritional, herbal, and UltraClear products.

Perque*
14 Pidgeon Hill Road
Sterling, VA 20165
800-525-7372, 703-450-2990
www.perque.com

Nutritional and hypoallergenic products. My favorite for people with autoimmune or complicated illnesses, but great for everyone. Perque products can also be purchased through Emerson Ecologics and Thinking of You.

Premier Research Labs*
2000 N. Mays St., Suite 120
Round Rock, TX 78664
800-325-7734
info@prlabs.com
www.prlabs.com

High Tech Health, Inc.
800-794-5355,
    international +1-300-413-8500
www.quantronic.com/products.htm
Far-infrared saunas, alkalizing water purifiers.

Thorne Research, Inc.*
P.O. Box 25
Dover, ID 83825
800-228-1966, 208-263-1337
www.thorne.com

Vital Nutrients*
45 Kenneth Dooley Dr.
Middletown, CT 06457
888-328-9992
www.vitalnutrients.net
These products are also available through Emerson Ecologics. I've made special purchase arrangements for readers of Digestive Wellness for Children; *use customer #12514.*

ASSOCIATIONS AND INFORMATION

American Celiac Society—Dietary Support Coalition
59 Crystal Avenue
West Orange, NJ 07052
504-737-3293
amerceliacsoc@netscape.net

American Diabetes Association
1701 North Beauregard Street
Alexandria, VA 22311
800-342-2383
www.diabetes.org

American Juvenile Arthritis Foundation
1330 West Peachtree Street
Atlanta, GA 30309
800-283-7800, 404-872-7100

American Liver Foundation
75 Maiden Lane, Suite 603
New York, NY 10038
800-GO-LIVER (800-465-4837)
www.liverfoundation.org

American Pseudo-Obstruction and Hirschsprung's Disease Society
Pull-Thru Network
Bonnie McElroy, President
2312 Savoy Street
Hoover, AL 35226-1528
205-978-2930
www.pullthrough.org/Hirschsprungs.html
A great consumer site on Hirschsprung's disease, with information, discussion groups, and more.

Arthritis Foundation
P.O. Box 7669
Atlanta, GA 30357-0669
800-568-4045
www.arthritis.org

**Autism Research Institute/Defeat
Autism Now (DAN)**
4182 Adams Avenue
San Diego, CA 92116
Fax 619-563-6840
www.autism.com

Celiac Disease Foundation
13251 Ventura Boulevard, #1
Studio City, CA 91604
818-990-2354
www.celiac.org

Celiac Sprue Association/USA, Inc.
P.O. Box 31700
Omaha, NE 68131-0700
877-CSA-4CSA, 402-558-0600,
    fax 402-558-1347
www.csaceliacs.org

**Crohn's and Colitis Foundation
of America**
386 Park Avenue South
New York, NY 10016
800-932-2423, 212-685-3440
www.ccfa.org

Cystic Fibrosis Foundation
6931 Arlington Road
Bethesda, MD 20814
800-344-4823
www.cff.org

**Digestive Disease National
Coalition**
507 Capitol Court NE, Suite 200
Washington, DC 20002
202-544-7497
www.ddnc.org

E-Medicine
www.e-medicine.com
*A wealth of information about all sorts
of topics, very well researched and
documented.*

Environmental Working Group
1436 U Street NW, Suite 100
Washington, DC 20009
www.ewg.org
*A great consumer watchdog group with
a wealth of articles and resources.
Check out information on pesticide
residues and the database of common
household chemicals.*

GERD for Kids
www.kidsacidreflux.org
Good explanations of GERD for kids.

Home Environmental Check List
www.pbs.org/now/quiz/quiz5.html
*A questionnaire for determining your
home's "environmental score."*

**International Foundation for
Functional Gastrointestinal
Disorders**
P.O. Box 170864
Milwaukee, IL 53217
414-964-1799
www.iffgd.org, www.aboutkidsgi.org

Intestinal Disease Foundation, Inc.
100 West Station Square Drive
Pittsburgh, PA 15219
412-261-5888
www.intestinaldiseasefoundation.org

Juvenile Diabetes Foundation
International
120 Wall Street, 19th Floor
New York, NY 10005
800-223-1138
www.jdf.org

Kid's Health
www.kidshealth.org
Good articles for parents, children,
and teenagers, and also in Spanish.

Mastocytosis.org
www.mastokids.org
A parents' support group and information
site for children with systemic
mastocytosis.

Moms Against Mercury
55 Carson's Trail
Leicester, NC 28748
828-776-0082
www.momsagainstmercury.com
Current information on mercury in our
children and in vaccines. You can get
involved.

National Diabetes Education
Program
1 Diabetes Way
Bethesda, MD 20892-3600
800-438-5383
www.ndep.nih.gov

National Digestive Diseases
Information Clearinghouse
P.O. Box NDDIC
2 Information Way
Bethesda, MD 20892
800-891-5389
www.digestive.niddk.nih.gov
Comprehensive information on all
digestive, diabetes, and kidney issues.

National Down's Syndrome Society
666 Broadway
New York, NY 10012
800-221-4602, fax 212-979-2873
www.ndss.org/content.cfm
A huge amount of information on Down's
sydrome for parents, friends, and people
who have Down's syndrome. Local
support group listings.

National Headache Foundation
820 North Orleans, Suite 217
Chicago, IL 60610
888-NHF-5552 (888-643-5552)
www.headaches.org

National Psoriasis Foundation
6600 SW 92nd Avenue, Suite 300
Portland, OR 97223-7195
800-723-9166, 503-244-7404,
    fax 503-245-0626
www.psoriasis.org

Natural Resources Defense Council
40 West 20th Street
New York, NY 10011
212-727-2700, fax 212-727-1773
www.nrdc.org
Reports on safer alternatives to toxic
chemicals (including pet products).

Pediatric Crohn's and Colitis Association, Inc.
P.O. Box 188
Newton, MA 02468
www.pcca.hypermart.net

Reach Out for Youth with Ileitis and Colitis, Inc.
84 Northgate Circle
Melville, NY 11747
631-293-3102
www.reachoutforyouth.org

Rheumatoid Disease Foundation
7111 Sweetgum Drive SW,
   Suite A
Fairview, TN 37062
615-799-1002
www.telalink.net/~taf

Safe Minds
14 Commerce Drive, 3rd Floor
Cranford, NJ 07016
908-276-8032
www.safeminds.org
Sensible action for ending mercury-induced neurological disorders. Great information on the links between mercury, autism, sleep disorders, and attention deficit disorders.

Trade Secrets
   PBS television documentary
www.pbs.org/tradesecrets
An exposé about the chemical industry. Bill Moyers and Sherry Jones report on the use of thousands of manmade chemicals that have not been tested for effects on public health and safety. Includes a great list of environmental resources.

OTHER NOTEWORTHY RESOURCES

Organic Consumers Association
6771 South Silver Hill Drive
Finland MN 55603
218-226-4164, fax: 218-353-7652
www.organicconsumers.org
This is a wonderful consumer resource with information and resources. You could spend all day reading articles.

Safe-Food/Mothers for Natural Law
P.O. Box 1177
Fairfield, Iowa 52556
www.safe-food.org

The Campaign.org
www.thecampaign.org
This is a consumer group that focuses on legislation to put labeling on foods that contain genetically engineered ingredients.

You'll find many more resources on my website,
www.innovativehealing.com

APPENDIX A

Laboratory Testing and Self-Testing

Many of your children's health problems can be solved without testing, but testing is often indicated or appropriate. The first part of this appendix outlines the functional tests that are most useful for children with digestive health problems. Most are laboratory tests, but a few are self-tests that you can administer to your own child at home. In the second part of this appendix, you will find contact information for some of the many available laboratories and information on which tests they offer.

FUNCTIONAL MEDICINE AND TESTING

Modern medicine typically equates health with the mere absence of disease. People often walk into a doctor's office feeling tired and run-down, receive an exam and a battery of tests, and come back a week later to hear, "Nothing's wrong with you. You're perfectly healthy." Although they may be relieved, they still don't feel well. This is where functional, integrative, and complementary ("alternative") medicine can play a valuable role. Chiropractors, naturopathic physicians, nutritionists, and other holistic practitioners offer a different perspective on health, and ought to be used as the first line of care rather than as a last resort.

Functional medicine recognizes that we each have specific biochemical needs determined by lifestyle, genetic structure, and environment; focuses on restoration of health rather than progression of disease; and works to improve quality of life and maximize the potential for health. Functional laboratory testing is relatively new, and new tests are developed each year to look for specific patterns and biochemical markers. Depending on their points of view and training, healthcare providers may order widely differing lab tests. Although the tests described herein are widely used by doctors who practice integrative medicine, your family doctor may be unfamiliar with them. Any doctor, however, can call the laboratories listed to order test kits. Each lab also has professional staff available to explain how the

262

tests are used and how to interpret the results. *Note:* Some of these tests are covered by medical insurance, but many aren't, so be prepared to pay for them; then submit the claim to your insurance company and see what happens. Your best chance for reimbursement is when an M.D. or D.O. orders the test(s).

Comprehensive Digestive and Stool Analysis

Useful for anyone with digestive problems, comprehensive digestive and stool analysis (CDSA) provides a quick reference for your child's healthcare provider. Order a CDSA in conjunction with comprehensive parasite screening (below).

A CDSA assesses bacterial balance and health, digestive function, and dysbiosis. It identifies the types of bacteria present and measures the levels of beneficial, possibly harmful, and disease-causing microbes (including candida). Any bacteria or fungi found are tested to determine what medications or herbs will be most effective against them. In addition, a CDSA measures the extent of protein, fat, and carbohydrate digestion; the levels of pancreatic enzymes produced; and the amounts of short-chain fatty acids and butyric acid in the colon.

Parasite Screening

If your child has had prolonged digestive symptoms, consider a comprehensive parasite screening. Some symptoms of parasitic infection can resemble those of other digestive problems: abdominal pain, allergy, anemia, bloating, bloody stools, chronic fatigue, constipation, coughing, diarrhea, gas, granulomas, irritable bowel syndrome, itching, joint and muscle aches, nervousness, pain, poor immune response, rashes, sleep disturbances, teeth grinding, unexplained fever, and unexplained weight loss. Use the parasite questionnaire in Chapter 15 (see page 153) to assess whether parasites are a likely cause of your child's symptoms.

The standard random stool testing offered by most physicians can be highly inaccurate, so repeated testing is often necessary for definitive results (for example, in order to rule out giardia with random stool testing, you'd have to do eight tests to be sure). The most accurate stool tests are usually performed by laboratories that specialize in parasitology; one of these, Genova Diagnostics, finds parasites in 22 percent of stool samples. (Some parasites are harmless, whereas others cause illness.) Some labs recommend inducing diarrhea with an oral laxative to detect parasites that live further up the digestive tract. Certain parasites may be found by using a rectal swab rather than a stool sample.

Lactose Intolerance Tests

Lactose intolerance is not milk allergy, which is the inability to digest milk proteins such as casein. Rather, lactose intolerance is caused by a deficiency in lactase, an enzyme that digests lactose, which is a sugar naturally found in milk and milk products. This inability to digest lactose affects about 70 percent of the world's population and is highly prevalent in African Americans, Asian Americans, Caucasian Americans of Mediterranean and Jewish descent, Hispanics, and Native Americans.

Lactose intolerance causes a wide variety of symptoms including abdominal cramping, acne, bloating, diarrhea, gas, eczema, headaches, and nausea. Most people with lactose intolerance, however, fail to recognize the relationship between the food they eat and how they feel. There are two ways to test your child for lactose intolerance: a self-test and a lab test.

Self-Test for Lactose Intolerance

This test requires eliminating your child's intake of all dairy products for at least ten to fourteen days. Although it can be difficult to get an older child to agree to follow a dairy-free protocol for two weeks, many children notice a difference in how they feel within four or five days and stay motivated to continue. Obvious dairy sources are cheese, creamed soup, frozen yogurt, ice cream, milk, powdered milk, whipped cream, and yogurt. Less-obvious or "hidden" sources are bakery items, cookies, hot dogs, lunchmeats, milk chocolate, most "nondairy" creamers, pancakes, protein-powder drinks, ranch dressing, and anything containing casein, caseinate, lactose, sodium caseinate, or whey. If you're not sure what's in a food, have your child avoid it. During the testing period, it's probably easiest to prepare all of your child's food at home and to provide a bag lunch on school-days. Remember also to specify what he/she can and cannot eat at a restaurant or a birthday party during the test.

If lactose intolerance is the source of your child's problems, you will probably notice that his/her symptoms change significantly and that reintroduction of dairy products triggers a return of symptoms. If your child has food sensitivities in addition to lactose intolerance, however, the results of this self-test may be inconclusive, with symptoms changing little or not at all; a laboratory test is then indicated.

Laboratory Test for Lactose Intolerance

This simple, noninvasive, doctor-ordered test determines whether lactose intolerance is causing a digestive problem and/or contributing to another health problem. It is ideal for people who have difficulty completing the self-test described above or are confused about their findings. (It can be tricky to do with small children, but it works well for school-aged kids.) First, your child breathes into a bag to supply a baseline sample; then, he/she drinks a small amount of a lactose solution and breathes into a different bag; and finally, lab technicians measure the amounts of hydrogen and methane gas exhaled in both samples.

A normal hydrogen level is 10 parts per million (ppm), whereas levels of 20 ppm or more are commonly found in the breath of people with lactose intolerance. A normal methane level is 0–7 ppm, and an increase in methane of 12 ppm or more between the two samples indicates lactose intolerance, even if the hydrogen level is normal. Measuring both hydrogen and methane considerably decreases the likelihood of a false result. The few false positive results of this test are generally caused by eating high-fiber foods beforehand, exposure to cigarette smoke, or sleeping during testing. False negative results occur 5 percent of the time and are commonly due to antibiotic, enema, or laxative use.

Sensitivity/Allergy Tests

As detailed in Chapter 11, sensitivity or allergy to foods and/or other substances contributes to many digestive and other health problems.

Elimination/Provocation Test for Food Sensitivity/Allergy

Elimination/provocation testing for foods is a two-stage process: an elimination diet and then a series of provocation "challenges" with the suspected offenders. Because you must radically change your child's diet in order to discover the foods to which he/she is reactive, this test requires determination and commitment. Often, the foods we are sensitive to are the ones we love the most, so your child may have to do without some of his/her favorites for awhile. Elimination/provocation testing is explained in detail in Chapter 11.

Blood Tests for Sensitivity/Allergy

True allergies are immunoglobulin E (IgE) antibody reactions that can cause anaphylactic shock, asthma, hives, itching, throat closing, and the like. Most doctors are familiar with IgE testing for allergies, and your child may already have had blood tests or scratch-tests for a limited number of foods plus pets, dust, and pollens. Your child's doctor may not know about (or believe in) testing for other antibodies such as immunoglobulins G, M, and A, but this is very useful for uncovering delayed hypersensitivity reactions. The tests are not 100-percent accurate but do provide good guidance about which foods may be most troublesome. Although many food sensitivities may be unmasked by the elimination/provocation challenge described above, others may remain hidden because delayed sensitivity reactions are more difficult to track; for example, your child may eat or be exposed to something troublesome today, but not show symptoms for seventy-two hours or more.

Many labs offer only IgG testing, but others offer IgE testing as well. The ELISA-ACT (available for children four years of age and older) assesses IgG, IgA, and IgM antibodies to foods and to common environmental chemicals and metals. In addition to a detailed read-out documenting your child's reactions with ratings from normal to severe, most labs also provide lists of foods that may be hidden sources of the offenders as well as a menu for a rotation diet and other educational materials to aid in the healing process.

Intestinal Permeability Test

As detailed in Chapter 12, intestinal permeability, or leaky gut syndrome, contributes to many digestive and other health problems. The mannitol-lactulose test has become the recognized standard for assessing intestinal permeability.

Mannitol and lactulose, two types of water-soluble sugar molecules that our cells cannot metabolize or use, are absorbed into the bloodstream at different rates due to their differing sizes and weights. Mannitol is easily absorbed by people with a healthy gut, whereas lactulose has such a large molecular size that it is only slightly absorbed by a healthy gut. Therefore, when a healthy child drinks a mannitol-lactulose solution, his/her urine test shows a high level of mannitol and a low level of lactulose. Different results, however, signify a health problem. High levels of both sugars, for example, indicate a leaky gut. Low levels of both sugars indicate general malabsorption of all nutrients. And low mannitol with high lactulose has been found in people with celiac disease, Crohn's disease, and ulcerative colitis.

Your doctor can provide a mannitol-lactulose test kit. After giving a random urine sample, your child drinks a mannitol-lactulose mixture and gives additional urine samples for six hours. The samples are then sent to the lab for analysis. This test is often done in conjunction with a CDSA or a parasite screening.

Indican Test

The indican test, or Obermeyer test, looks for the presence of a certain chemical in your child's urine. The level of indican (a type of indole) in urine gives information about how well your child metabolizes protein. Children with poor digestive function, malabsorption, dysbiosis, and gluten problems often putrefy foods. Indican testing uncovers this putrifaction. Indican testing is an inexpensive, noninvasive way to screen children for faulty digestion. The test doesn't identify where the problem begins, but it can be used to indicate whether digestion is an issue and monitor how well the treatment plan is working.

Provoked Urine Test for Toxic Metals

Many children retain high levels of toxic metals in their bodies. As detailed in Chapter 2, children are at higher risk for metal toxicity than adults are. Symptoms of metal toxicity in children may include anemia, behavioral and personality changes, colic, deafness, delays in growth and development, incoordination, irritability, learning problems, leg cramping, muscle weakness, neurological problems, poor memory, stomach-aches, tremors, vision changes, and more. Children with autism usually show metal toxicity. (I suspect that children with eosinophilic esophagitis/gastritis may also have metal toxicity issues, although this has not yet been studied.)

Blood testing only assesses your child's current exposure to heavy metals, whereas provoked urine testing assesses the deposition of metals in his/her bone and other tissues. For this fairly inexpensive test, your physician provides a small amount of a chelation drug such as DMPS, DMSA, EDTA, or penicillamine; you administer the drug and collect a urine sample from your child; and then you send the sample to the lab, where it will be measured for heavy metals and often for nutritional minerals as well.

Amino Acids Test

Testing urine or blood for amino acids can help detect inborn errors of metabolism in your child. It is most useful when your child's problems have not been lifelong or chronic. Amino acid testing is especially important for children who have learning, attention, behavioral, or neurological problems. It can also help determine whether your child is eating enough protein.

Amino acids link to form protein molecules. Protein, the primary component of muscles, neurotransmitters, many hormones, and all of our enzymes, is used in each cell in our bodies. From the eight (or nine) essential amino acids that we must obtain from our food, our bodies can normally manufacture the rest of the forty amino acids. Picture this process like a stream with waterfalls: The stream forms a pool, and then there is a small waterfall, then another pool, and so on. In some children, the upstream pools get huge, but nothing flows downstream, because these children are unable to manufacture the downstream amino acids. In a case like this, taking supplemental amino acids can dramatically change your child's overall health picture.

For this test, you simply collect your child's urine for twenty-four hours and send a sample of what you have collected to the lab for analysis.

Organic Acids Test

Organic acids are produced by metabolism throughout the body and by intestinal microbes. High levels of organic acids in urine can indicate metabolic problems, hormone irregularities, and dysbiosis. They can also be indicative of issues with detoxification pathways, inherited enzyme deficiencies, and drug effects. An organic acids test is a single, simple urine test that can be used to assess a large variety of nutritional and immunological factors including the metabolism of fatty acids, neurotransmitters, and carbohydrates, as well as oxidative damage, energy production, detoxification status, B-complex status, dysbiosis, methylation ability, and inflammatory reactions.

Quantitative Fluid Analysis

The philosophy of "biological terrain" argues that a healthy organism is more resistant to illness and disease. Quantitative fluid analysis, an update of biological terrain analysis, is used to evaluate the body's overall cellular health through three measurements each of blood, urine, and saliva. The measurements are pH (indicating acid/alkaline balance), oxidation-reduction potential (indicating oxidative stress), and resistivity (indicating availability of minerals to the cells). Quantitative fluid analysis provides a measurement of your child's overall resilience, and it can also be used to monitor how well supplementation, exercise, and other natural treatments are working to bring pH, oxidation-reduction potential, and resistivity into balance.

Electrical Acupuncture Voltage Test

Based upon supportive research, the electrical acupuncture voltage (EAV) test is widely used in Europe. In the right hands, an EAV test is a fast, noninvasive screening method that can pick up medical issues, emotional trauma, and problems from vaccinations. Your child holds a negatively charged rod in one hand, the practitioner places a positively charged pointer on a variety of designated acupuncture points on the child's skin, and a meter measures the electrical activity of the skin between the points. An EAV test can determine which organs are strong or weak, which foods help or hurt, and which nutrients are needed or are in excess. Many skilled professionals use this test to diagnose conditions and determine appropriate therapies. Be sure to go to someone who has a lot of expertise.

Heidelberg Capsule Test

As detailed in Chapter 3, hydrochloric acid (HCl), normally produced by the parietal cells of the stomach, is necessary for the initial stage of protein digestion and the absorption of vitamin B_{12} and many minerals. Common symptoms of low stomach acidity include belching or a burning sensation immediately after meals, bloating, a feeling that food just sits in the stomach without further digestion, and an inability to eat more than small amounts at any one sitting. Inadequate HCl levels have been associated with asthma, diabetes, eczema, gallbladder disease, hives, juvenile arthritis, lupus erythematosus, rosacea, underactive and overactive thyroid conditions, vitiligo, and weak adrenal glands.

The Heidelberg capsule test is a simple, accurate, and sensitive technique that uses radiotelemetry to determine how much HCl the stomach produces. Your child swallows an encapsulated radiotransmitter (about the size of a B-complex vitamin) that measures the stomach's resting pH and also its pH when administered baking soda, which is very alkaline. By observing how quickly the stomach returns to an acidic condition after the baking soda challenges, the physician can determine whether or not your child's stomach produces adequate HCl. Unfortunately, this test is not widely available.

Vitamin D Test

Children with autism, celiac disease, cystic fibrosis, diabetes, and inflammatory bowel disease have all shown an increased need for vitamin D. This test can easily be ordered by your physician to determine whether your child has adequate vitamin D levels. This test can be run through any medical laboratory. Typically, the test that is run is called 25-hydroxy vitamin D.

We naturally make vitamin D in our skin from sunlight. People who live in northern climates may not get enough vitamin D; children who spend their time indoors may also not make enough vitamin D. Vitamin D can also be taken as a supplement, by itself, in a multiple vitamin, or as a component of cod liver oil.

LABORATORIES TO CONTACT FOR TESTING

The diagnostic tests described above are not the ordinary tests that are readily found in your local medical lab or hospital; in fact, many of them were originally performed only by one or another of the laboratories listed below. Although your child's physician may be unfamiliar with some or many of the tests, don't be deterred from asking for any tests that you feel may be appropriate for your child. The doctor can call these labs for complete information packages, test kits, and assistance with interpretation of test results.

Diagnos-Techs, Inc., Clinical and Research Laboratory
6620 South 192nd Place J
Kent, WA 98032
800-878-3787, 425-251-0596
www.diagnostechs.com
Many tests including adrenal stress profile, DHE-4, male and female salivary hormones, parasitology, candida, Helicobacter pylori, *digestion efficiency, secretory IgA, gastric pH, and liver function.*

Doctor's Data, Inc. and Reference Laboratory
P.O. Box 111
West Chicago, IL 60186
800-323-2784, 630-377-8139
www.doctorsdata.com
Many tests including hair minerals, blood minerals, complete urinary and blood amino acids, mercapturic acid, D-glucaric acid, functional folic acid, methylmalonic acid (vitamin B_{12} status), and diet analysis.

ELISA-ACT Biotechnologies
14 Pidgeon Hill Drive, Suite 300
Sterling, VA 20165
800-553-5472, 703-450-2980, fax
    703-450-2981
www.ELISAACT.com—information
    about the laboratory
www.ELISAACT.org—information
    about functional immunology

Comprehensive food and environmental blood testing through the ELISA-ACT, which measures reactions to more than 300 foods, environmental chemicals, preservatives, mercury, and three major classes of yeasts. Comprehensive guides for physicians and patients provide lifestyle support related to the lab results.

Genova Diagnostics
63 Zillicoa Street
Asheville, NC 28801
800-522-4762
www.gdx.net

Many tests including CDSA2.0, lactose, small bowel overgrowth, liver detoxification profiles, intestinal permeability, Helicobacter pylori, *vitamin status, hair minerals, male and female hormones, DHE4/cortisol, secretory IgA, essential fatty acids, bone resorption, and homocysteine.*

Great Plains Laboratory
11813 West 77th
Lenexa, KS 66214
913-341-8949
www.greatplainslaboratory.com
Specializes in testing for children with autism and other learning disabilities.

ImmunoLaboratories, Inc.
1620 West Oakland Park
    Boulevard
Fort Lauderdale, FL 33311
305-486-4500, 800-231-9197,
    fax 305-739-6563
www.immunolabs.com
IgE, IgG4, and IgG1 food sensitivity assays.

Immunosciences Lab, Inc.
8693 Wilshire Boulevard,
    Suite 200
Beverly Hills, CA 90211
800-950-4686
www.immuno-sci-lab.com
Tests to detect immunological injury and environmental and genetic disposition include comprehensive immune function, lymphocyte and natural killer cell activity, immunotoxicology, silicone-related immune panels, chronic fatigue panels, gastrointestinal evaluation, viral/ parasite/candida/bacterial antibodies, and secretory IgA.

**Meridian Valley Clinical
    Laboratory**
801 SW 16th, Suite 126
Renton, WA 98055
425-271-8689
www.meridianvalleylab.com
A wide variety of tests including DHE4/cortisol, IgG and IgE food sensitivities/allergies, essential amino acids, adrenal steroids, parasitology, CDSA, essential fatty acids, and fractionated estrogens.

Meta Metrix Medical Laboratory

4855 Peachtree Industrial Boulevard, Suite 201

Norcross, GA 30092

800-221-4640, 770-441-2237, fax 770-441-2237

www.metametrix.com

A wide variety of tests including amino acids, fatty acids, lipid peroxides, anti-oxidant vitamin status, minerals in blood, urine, and hair, whole blood reduced carnitine, organic acids, glutathione, ATP, IgG and IgE food sensitivities/allergies, inhalant allergy, functional liver detoxification, intestinal permeability, plasma homocysteine, cysteine, total glutathione, and bone resorption.

Pacific Toxicology Laboratories

9348 De Soto Avenue

Chatsworth, CA 91311

800-328-6942

www.pactox.com

Tests for environmental pollutants and contaminants include panels for solvents and metabolites, pesticides, herbicides, polychlorinated and polybrominated biphenyls, PCBs, and heavy metals, as well as OSHA compliance panels.

SpectraCell Laboratories, Inc.

7051 Portwest Drive, Suite 100

Houston, TX 77024-8026

800-227-5227, 713-621-3101

www.spectracell.com

Functional vitamin, mineral, and antioxidant panels and comprehensive functional cardiovascular profiles.

US BioTek Laboratories, Inc.

13500 Linden Avenue North

Seattle, WA 98133

206-365-1256

www.usbiotek.com

Tests for organic acids, food allergies, and salivary hormones.

APPENDIX B

Healing Nutrients, Herbs, and Supplements

This appendix is a quick reference guide to the natural remedies mentioned throughout the book. Each has its own unique characteristics and nearly all of the remedies can be used in a wide variety of ways. *Note:* This guide highlights only the remedies of most interest in the context of this book and your child's digestive well-being. Many excellent books and websites can provide more detailed information (as a starting point, see the References and Resources sections). Enjoy!

ACACIA (*Acacia senegal;* also called Gum Arabic)

Demulcent, kidney-protective herb that soothes intestinal lining.

Helpful in inflammatory bowel disease, diarrhea, and dysentery.

Available as capsules, tea, gum, and syrup; gum usually dissolved in water with honey or sugar.

ADRENAL GLANDULARS

Adrenal gland extracts that build adrenal resilience.

Support adrenals in asthma and all allergic conditions.

Note: Look for an organic source.

Caution: Best taken before lunch time. Taken later in the day, adrenal glandulars can make your child "wired" and unable to sleep.

AGRIMONY (*Agrimonia eupatoria;* also called Stickwood and Cocklebur)

Astringent, tonic, muscle-toning herb.

In inflammatory bowel disease, reduces diarrhea.

Also used in skin and liver conditions.

ALKALIZING DIET

Dietary protocol intended to balance body's pH (see Chapter 7 for details).

Balanced internal pH is important for enhanced cellular function, optimal uptake of nutrients, optimal elimination of wastes, and disease prevention.

Helps rebalance gut flora, useful in all disease conditions including dysbiosis/candida infection.

In juvenile arthritis, conserves bone and reduces inflammation and pain.

In autism, promotes uptake of nutrients into cells and brain.

ALOE (*Aloe vera*)

Demulcent herb that soothes and heals membranes throughout the digestive tract.

Useful in irritable bowel disease and leaky gut syndrome.

Topical application of juice helps against baby's yeast infection/thrush.

Available as plant and juice; be sure juice is food-grade.

Recommended form is a fresh leaf from an aloe plant: peel skin off leaf, put insides with some water into a blender, blend into a gel, and drink as is or with juice.

AMERICAN CRANESBILL (*Geranium maculatum*)

Astringent, tonic herb.

Reduces diarrhea from inflammatory bowel disease and other causes.

For tea, steep 1 ounce dried herb in 1 pint water for 5–10 minutes.

ANISE/ANISEED (*Pimpinella anisum*)

Demulcent herb with sweet, pungent seeds.

Soothes digestive system.

Used for constipation/encopresis, flatulence/intestinal gas, and colic.

Available as tea or dried seeds.

For tea, use $\frac{1}{8}$ – $\frac{1}{4}$ teaspoon powdered seeds in 1 cup boiling water.

ANTIOXIDANTS

Substances that reduce oxidative damage throughout the body by scavenging free radicals.

In foods, highest levels are found in colored beans (like black or red) and fruits and vegetables.

Examples include vitamins C and E, beta-carotene and other carotenoids, coenzyme Q_{10}, glutathione/glutathione peroxidase, grapeseed extract/pycnogenol, lipoic acid, milk thistle, N-acetyl cysteine, selenium, sulfur-containing amino acids, super-oxide dismutase, and zinc.

Useful in any chronic or inflammatory disease: asthma, cystic fibrosis, diabetes, Down's syndrome, inflammatory bowel diseases, irritable bowel syndrome, and more.

APPLE-CIDER VINEGAR

Alkalizing food (see inset on page 68 for details) used historically in arthritis.

Contains many essential enzymes and minerals as well as malic acid.

Promotes digestion and numerous other bodily functions.

ASTRAGALUS (*Astragalus membranaceus*)

Immune-boosting herb widely used in Chinese medicine to strengthen lungs over time.

In asthma, used as a lung-strengthening tonic.

Available as capsules or tincture.

BARBERRY (*Berberis vulgaris*; also called Oregon Grape Root)

Herb containing antifungal substance berberine.

Used as a stomach aid and for diarrhea.

Often used as a preventive or therapy for candida overgrowth.

Available as capsules.

Caution: Should not be taken by anyone who is pregnant or breast-feeding, or who has high blood pressure or heart disease.

BASIL (*Ocimum basilicum*)

Digestion-enhancing herb.

Helpful against flatulence/intestinal gas.

Varieties called Holy Basil and Hairy Basil have been found helpful with type II diabetes.

Available fresh and dried.

Note: For diabetes, only use fresh herb.

For tea, steep 1 teaspoon herb in 1 cup water.

BAYBERRY (*Myrica cerifera*)

Astringent, stimulant, digestion-enhancing herb.

Helpful against flatulence/intestinal gas.

Used in inflammatory bowel disease to help stop bleeding and tone tissues.

For tea, steep 1 teaspoon herb in 1 cup water.

B-COMPLEX VITAMINS

Nutrient group important for energy production, stress management, and nervous system function.

Improve mouth ulcers/canker sores in people with B-complex deficiency.

In attention deficit disorders, helpful with energy, behavior, mood, and cognition.

Useful for children with autism and neurological or energy-deficiency illnesses.

May be included in supplements for blood glucose control in diabetes.

BETAINE HCl

Form of hydrochloric acid.

Aids protein digestion, defends against food poisoning and parasites, and permits duodenal absorption of minerals (calcium, magnesium, zinc, copper, iron, and potassium).

Can help with malabsorption or indigestion after eating a protein-containing meal.

May relieve eosinophilic esophagitis symptoms in children with an alkaline esophageal environment.

Caution: When taken unnecessarily, HCl causes a burning sensation in the stomach. If this occurs, stop administering or taking it.

BIOTIN

B-complex vitamin that helps body use glucose more efficiently and balance blood sugar levels.

Best food sources are egg yolk (cooked), liver, poultry, fish, legumes, and nutritional yeast.

Among nutrients used to help control candida overgrowth.

May be included in supplements for blood glucose control in diabetes.

Caution: Avidin, a protein in raw eggs, binds biotin, so don't eat many (or any) raw eggs.

BITTER MELON (*Momordica charantia*)

Bitter squash eaten widely in Philippines.

Research on use in controlling blood sugar regulation in type II diabetes is very promising.

Often included in supplements for blood glucose control in diabetes.

Available as capsules and tablets; also eaten as a food in vegetable dishes, soups, and stews.

BLACK SEED (*Nigella sativa;* also called Black Cumin)

Herb with flavorful seeds (used, for example, in string cheese).

Commonly used in Ayurvedic medicine; Mohammed said that it could cure any ill except death.

Used to treat parasitic infections, dispel worms, normalize blood sugar levels, and soothe bronchitis and coughs.

BLACK WALNUT (*Juglans nigra*)

Food nut that is an excellent source of iodine (important to thyroid function).

Traditionally used for ringworm, athlete's foot, and cracks in palms and feet.

Juice of unripe, green hulls of black walnuts is considered antiparasitic and antifungal.

Black walnut husk is a common ingredient in antiparasitic products.

BOLDO (*Peumus boldus;* also called Molina)

Gallbladder- and liver-supportive, detoxifying herb from Chilean mountains.

Commonly used in antiparasitic products.

Available as capsules, tablets, and liquid extract.

BORAGE (*Borago officinalis*)

Lovely garden plant with blue, star-shaped flowers.

Herbalists have said, "A garden without borage is like a man without courage."

Acts as an anti-inflammatory by shifting production of arachadonic acid to production of less-inflammatory prostaglandins.

Borage oil is high in gamma-linolenic acid (GLA); GLA research focuses on use against pain such as in arthritis and menstruation.

See also Gamma-linolenic Acid.

BOSWELLIA (*Boswellia serrata;* also called Indian Frankincense)

Anti-inflammatory herb used in Ayurvedic medicine for inflammatory bowel disease, osteoarthritis, rheumatoid arthritis, and general pain and inflammation.

Active ingredient is considered to be boswellic acid.

Unlike over-the-counter pain medications, does not irritate stomach.

Note: Taken long-term to protect against inflammation and prevent pain, rather than for immediate pain relief, although topical cream seems to be effective quickly.

Available as tablets, capsules, and topical cream.

Note: Look for a product standardized to a 60% concentration of boswellic acid.

BROMELAIN

Proteolytic enzyme derived from green stems of pineapple plant.

Enhances protein digestion, and also has anti-inflammatory and analgesic properties.

Helpful against arthritis pain, healing bruises and sprains, inflammation in respiratory infections, and cough.

Available as pills and capsules.

Note: As a digestive aid, to be taken with protein-containing meals. For use against pain and inflammation, must be taken between meals on an empty stomach.

BURDOCK ROOT (*Arctium lappa*)

Common weed in temperate climates (and the burs on your pants legs).

Supports liver function and detoxification, and considered a blood purifier.

Used for eczema and psoriasis.

Available as tincture; root can also be used to make a decoction.

For decoction, simmer 3 teaspoons root in 3 cups water for 15–20 minutes.

BUTTERBUR (*Petasites hybridus*)

Anti-inflammatory herb long used in Europe for such diverse problems as plague, cough, asthma, and skin wounds.

In migraine, can reduce frequency and severity of attacks (major side effect is burping).

Research also supports use in hay fever and allergy prevention and for fever reduction.

Caution: Should not be used by pregnant or breast-feeding women. In its natural state, butterbur contains liver toxins and is potentially cancer-causing; patented product Petadolex has removed these toxins.

BUTTERNUT (*Juglans cinera*; also called White Walnut)

Tree (relative of black walnut) with liver-supportive bark used as a mild laxative.

Bark is also commonly found in anti-parasitic products.

See also Black Walnut.

CABBAGE JUICE

Cancer-protective vegetable juice with high glutamine content.

Traditionally used to treat stomach ulcers, ulcerative colitis, and Crohn's disease.

Also available as powder.

CALCIUM

Alkalizing, bone-building mineral that also functions in muscle and nervous system activity.

Often deficient in children with ulcerative colitis or Crohn's disease.

Used along with magnesium for cramping, anxiety, and muscle tension.

Author's note: I recommend calcium and magnesium supplements for all children to support development of bones, muscles, and nerves, and for help with growing pains.

Note: Always combine with magnesium (magnesium dose is typically half of calcium or equal).

CALENDULA (*Calendula officinalis*; also called Pot Marigold)

Common garden flower and gentle antiseptic herb.

Topical application promotes wound healing and soothes diaper rash, irritated skin, cuts, and scrapes.

Tea relieves ulcers, stomach cramps, diarrhea, and nausea/vomiting.

Available as ointment, cream, and tincture; can also be juiced; flowers can be made into tea.

For tea, steep 1–2 teaspoons fresh or dried flowers in $\frac{1}{2}$ cup water for 10 minutes.

CAPRYLIC ACID

Coconut-derived fatty acid used to treat candida overgrowth.

Often an ingredient in antifungal products.

Author's note: Can irritate stomach and digestive tract, so I rarely use it with clients.

Caution: Do not give to a child with ulcerative colitis or Crohn's disease.

CAPSICUM

Derivative of cayenne pepper that blocks formation of inflammatory substances such as leukotrienes, arachadonic acid, and substance P.

Used topically to relieve pain (may produce a burning sensation when first applied).

In arthritis, cayenne cream has been well studied for temporary pain relief.

Available as cream.

CARAWAY SEED (*Carum carvi*)

Carminative seed commonly found in rye bread.

Stimulates appetite, settles stomach, and relieves nausea and flatulence/intestinal gas.

Can also relieve menstrual and other cramps.

Best as a tea.

Tea is helpful for colic.

CARDAMOM (*Elettaria cardamomum*)

Flavorful spice widely used in Indian cuisine, breads, desserts, baked fruit, and chai tea.

Stimulates appetite and relieves flatulence/intestinal gas.

Available as whole seeds (can be chewed) and powder.

For tea, use ¼ teaspoon powder per 1 cup boiling water.

For decoction, boil 2 teaspoons seeds in 1 cup water, cover, steep 10 minutes, and strain.

CARNITINE

Amino-acid-like nutrient that is protective of all muscles including heart.

Allows cells' mitochondria to use fats for energy and increases weight loss.

Red meats are best food source of carnitine; vegetarians are often carnitine-deficient.

Low blood carnitine levels have been found in children and teenagers with type I diabetes.

In attention deficit disorders, improves learning abilities and behavior.

In cystic fibrosis and diabetes, used along with taurine to improve fat metabolism.

May be taken alone or included in supplements for blood glucose control.

Available as tablets and capsules.

See also Taurine.

CARNOSINE

Compound of amino acids histidine and alanine.

In attention deficit disorders, improves learning abilities and behavior.

In autism, recent study of carnosine plus zinc showed significantly improved behavior and language comprehension.

Often packaged along with zinc and vitamin E.

See also Zinc and Vitamin E.

CATNIP (*Nepeta cataria;* also called Catmint)

Calming herb favored by felines.

Helpful against upset stomach, indigestion, flatulence/intestinal gas, menstrual cramps.

In colic, tea or tea-infused bathwater calms baby; tea also calms digestion of breast-feeding mother and passes through breast-milk to baby.

For tea, use 1 teaspoon herb in 1 cup boiled water.

CELERY

Alkalizing, cholagogic, digestion-stimulating vegetable, eaten raw and cooked.

CELERY SEED

Edible, digestion-enhancing seed used as seasoning or in tea.

Reduces flatulence/intestinal gas.

CHAMOMILE (*Matricaria chamomilla*)

Calming, antispasmodic herb used for tummy-aches by such notables as Peter Rabbit.

In irritable bowel syndrome and inflammatory bowel disease, relieves and expels intestinal gas, strengthens and tones stomach, and soothes pain.

In colic, tea or tea-infused bathwater calms baby; tea also calms digestion of breast-feeding mother and passes through breast-milk to baby.

Freeze tea into ice-cubes for teething.

Best as a tea or in bathwater.

CHARCOAL, ACTIVATED

Toxin- and gas-absorbing substance.

Relieves flatulence/intestinal gas.

Rated "safe and effective" by FDA for treatment of acute poisoning.

Also used in testing bowel transit time (turns stool black).

CHICKWEED (*Stellaria media*)

Soothing herb and edible weed with mild laxative effects.

In inflammatory bowel disease, soothes intestinal lining.

Available as capsules and tea, and fresh in your yard (it's commonly found in lawns); eat steamed or raw.

CHLOROPHYLL

The green chlopoplasts within plants ("energy factories").

Soothes and heals mucous membranes in mouth.

Helps prevent flatulence/intestinal gas.

For mouth ulcers/cankers, used as gargle or applied directly to sores.

Available as tablets and liquid.

CHROMIUM

Essential mineral that helps regulate blood sugar levels and has been shown to help reduce insulin resistance.

Nutritional yeast, an excellent chromium source, tastes great on popcorn, tofu, and vegetables.

Useful in both types of diabetes, hypoglycemia, and other insulin-resistant conditions.

Often included in supplements for blood glucose control in diabetes.

Caution: Increase your child's dosage slowly, especially if he/she is taking medication or insulin, as blood sugar levels can drop suddenly.

CLOVE (*Syzygium aromaticum*)

Fragrant, digestion-enhancing spice used to numb gums during teething and as an antiparasitic agent.

Available dried whole and as powder and oil.

For tea, steep ½ teaspoon whole cloves in 1 cup boiled water until cooled.

Caution: Don't use clove oil undiluted, as it can irritate tender gum tissue.

COBALAMINE
(also called Vitamin B$_{12}$)

B-complex vitamin essential for red blood cell formation, nervous system function, and energy production.

Deficiency leads to anemia, nerve damage, feeling tired and depressed, and poor memory.

Helpful in children with anemia,

asthma, chronic fatigue syndrome, fatigue, migraine, and more.

Not well absorbed orally, so best used in sublingual form or nasal sprays; recommended forms are methylcobalamine and hydroxycobalamine.

Note: Your pediatrician may recommend B_{12} injections.

COD LIVER OIL

Anti-inflammatory fish oil high in omega-3 fatty acids, vitamin A, and vitamin D.

Helpful in ulcerative colitis, Crohn's disease, and general pain and inflammation.

In cystic fibrosis, benefits include better growth, reduced bronchial inflammation, lowered IgG antibody levels, and fewer days of antibiotic treatment for infections.

Used in combination with other oils for constipation/encopresis.

Found helpful in autism by Mary Megson, M.D.

Available as liquid and capsules.

See also Omega-3 Fatty Acids, Vitamin A, and Vitamin D.

COENZYME Q$_{10}$ (CoQ$_{10}$)

Antioxidant nutrient used by cells' mitochondria to produce energy.

May be included in supplements for blood glucose control in diabetes.

Available as capsules, tablets, and chewable pills.

COLEUS FORSKOHLI (also called Forskolin)

Bronchodilating Ayurvedic herb.

Forskolin, an active ingredient marketed as a separate product.

Thought to stimulate cyclic AMP production, which may be impaired in children with asthma.

In asthma, often inhaled as a pressurized aerosol powder for bronchodilation.

Caution: Use under the care of a physician. Should not be taken by anyone on blood thinners.

COLOSTRUM

Cow's (or mother's) first milk after baby's birth.

Very high content of protective antibodies, gives a boost to immune system.

Used in arthritis and to help prevent colds and flu.

Available as capsules.

COMFREY (*Symphytum officianale*; also called Knitbone and Boneheal)

Soothing and gallbladder-supportive herb used to alleviate diarrhea and as a tea for colds and flu.

In inflammatory bowel disease, soothes intestinal lining.

Leaves can be used as a compress or poultice to relieve arthritis pain.

Available as capsules and tea.

Caution: Contains a liver-toxic alkaloid shown to cause liver cancer; however, comfrey leaves have been safely used for centuries as a tea and poultice. Avoid comfrey root.

COPPER

Essential trace mineral.

Traditionally worn as bracelets to relieve arthritis pain (copper is gradually dissolved by sweat and absorbed by skin).

People with rheumatoid arthritis often have marginal copper levels.

Available in bracelets and multivitamin-mineral supplements; a physician may also temporarily prescribe supplemental copper salicylate or sebacate until your child's copper level normalizes.

CORIANDER (*Coriandrum sativum*)

Delicious, edible seed of cilantro plant.

Enhances digestion, increases secretion of stomach acids, and reduces flatulence/intestinal gas.

For tea, use ¼ teaspoon in 1 cup boiling water.

COROSOLIC ACID

Extract of *Lagerstroemia speciosa* leaves.

Used to decrease blood glucose levels in type II diabetes.

Author's note: I have seen great benefits of supplemental corosolic acid in people with diabetes.

CURCUMIN

Antioxidant, anti-inflammatory bioflavonoid derived from turmeric.

Used in arthritis and cystic fibrosis, to prevent cancer, and to normalize blood pressure and cholesterol.

Concentrated, so it can be taken in smaller doses than turmeric.

See also Turmeric.

CURING PILLS (also called Kang Ning Wan)

Patented Chinese remedy for nausea, vomiting, and upset stomach.

Also used to treat diarrhea, motion sickness, chills, fever, and morning sickness.

DAIKON RADISH

Mildly flavored, gallbladder-supportive,

digestion-enhancing vegetable commonly used in Japanese cuisine.

Can be quite helpful in diet of children with cystic fibrosis.

DANDELION (*Taraxicum officinalis*)

Liver- and gallbladder-supportive, cholagogic herb and nutritious edible weed.

Root is used as tonic medicine and leaves are eaten as food.

Available as tea, tincture, capsules, and fresh in your yard (it's found in most lawns).

DEVIL'S CLAW (*Harpagophytum procumbens*)

Pain-killing, anti-inflammatory South African herb.

Historically used in irritable bowel syndrome and to stimulate digestion.

Commonly used to reduce pain and inflammation in arthritis.

Available as tea, tincture, capsules, and liquid extract.

DIGESTIVE ENZYMES

As adjunct to body's own pancreatic and other digestive enzymes, support/enhance digestion by breaking down foods more completely (see Chapters 3 and 4 for details).

See also Bromelain.

DILL (*Anethum graveolens*)

Delicious kitchen herb.

Weak tea or tea-infused bathwater can calm a colicky baby; tea also calms digestion of breast-feeding mother and passes through breast-milk to baby.

For tea, use 1–2 teaspoons of fresh parsley in 1 cup boiled water.

DIMETHYLAMINOETHANOL (DMAE)

Brain substance that improves synthesis of acetylcholine (a prominent neuro-transmitter).

Food sources include anchovies and sardines.

Used in attention deficit disorders.

DL-PHENYLALANINE (DLPA)

Amino acid that appears to inhibit breakdown of endorphins (body's natural pain relievers).

Used to treat pain, depression, rheumatoid arthritis, osteoarthritis, low-back pain, and migraine.

Note: "D" is naturally found form and "T" is its synthetic mirror; taking them in combination slows their release.

ECHINACEA (*Echinacea purpurea, E. angustifolia;* also called Purple Coneflower)

Immune-boosting herb believed to have antimicrobial properties.

After appendectomy, taken along with goldenseal for several days to prevent wound infection.

In inflammatory bowel disease, helps prevent infection.

Available as capsules, tablets, tincture, and tea.

ELDERBERRY (*Sambucus canadensis, S. nigra*)

Tasty berry of a large shrub.

Shortens duration and severity of flu and colds.

Available as syrup.

ELIMINATION/PROVOCATION DIET

Dietary protocol intended to help you discover your child's food sensitivities/allergies (see Chapter 11 for details).

EVENING PRIMROSE OIL

Anti-inflammatory oil high in gamma-linolenic acid (GLA); less concentrated than borage oil.

Helpful in arthritis and for other pain or inflammation.

See also Borage and Gamma-linolenic Acid.

FENNEL (*Foeniculum vulgare*)

Antispasmodic, digestion-enhancing, licorice-flavored herb.

Drinking tea or chewing sweet, pungent seeds relieves flatulence/intestinal gas.

Also used in constipation/encopresis as a gentle laxative.

Tea or tea-infused bathwater can calm a colicky baby; tea also calms digestion of breast-feeding mother and passes through breast-milk to baby.

For tea, steep 1 tablespoon crushed seeds in 1 cup boiled water for 5–10 minutes.

FEVERFEW (*Tanacetum parthenium*)

Anti-inflammatory herb historically used to aid digestion and for fever.

Soothing in inflammatory bowel disease.

In migraine, results of studies in preventing and minimizing severity are mixed.

Taken on a daily basis as a preventive measure rather than as a medication.

Available as fresh (works best) or dried leaves, tincture (approximates fresh leaves), and freeze-dried form; plant is easily grown for eating a few fresh leaves daily.

Note: If your child isn't relieved by one form, try another; fresh and dried differ, as do batches.

FIBER

Natural dietary substance that helps normalize gut bacteria, promote regular bowel movements, and slow release of glucose into bloodstream (see Chapter 8 for details).

Helpful in conditions including constipation/encopresis, diarrhea, and irritable bowel syndrome.

High-fiber diet is also useful in type II diabetes.

Caution: Increase dietary fiber slowly to avoid causing a lot of gas and discomfort (our flora "go wild" with sudden increase in fiber, and resulting fermentation produces gas).

FISH OIL

See Cod Liver Oil and Omega-3 Fatty Acids.

FOLIC ACID (also called Folate and Folinic Acid)

Cancer-protective B-complex vitamin that helps repair and maintain epithelial cells throughout digestive system and lungs and protects mucous membranes.

Helpful in leaky gut syndrome and asthma.

In children with type I diabetes, daily supplementation may protect blood vessels from damage (essential for preventing long-term complications such as eye, heart, and kidney disease).

Often low in people with inflammatory bowel disease (IBD); Asulfadine, a drug commonly used for IBD, depletes folic acid.

Author's note: In my clinical experience, I have found that a combination of glutamine and folic acid can rapidly reduce inflammation and irritation in active bowel disease. I recommend Folixor's 10-milligram sublingual tablets from Emerson Ecologics (see Resources).

See also Glutamine.

GAMMA-LINOLENIC ACID (GLA)

Essential fatty acid effective against pain and inflammation.

Food sources include whole grains, nuts, and seeds.

Also found in supplements such as borage oil, evening primrose oil, and black currant oil.

Reduces pain and stiffness in arthritis of all types.

See also Borage and Evening Primrose Oil.

GARLIC (*Allium sativum*)

Antibiotic, antifungal, antihelmintic, antispasmodic, cholagogic, and carminative food.

Historically used against pinworms.

An active component, allicin, is effective against amoebas and giardia.

Commonly used to treat candida overgrowth and thrush, also to treat and prevent colds and flu.

Eaten cooked or raw; also available as capsules and pills.

For sage-lemon-garlic tea, steep 2 tablespoons sage, half a lemon or more, 2 cloves chopped garlic, and honey to taste in 6 cups boiling water for 5 minutes. Tasty and can help reduce fever.

Author's note: I used a small, sugar-coated garlic pill made by Kwai to teach my children how to swallow pills while simultaneously protecting them from colds and flu.

GENTIAN ROOT (*Gentiana lutea*)

Liver- and gallbladder-supportive herb that stimulates gastric juices and appetite and tones intestinal muscles.

Commonly used for digestive disorders including flatulence/intestinal gas and stomachache.

Available as tea, tincture, capsules, and tablets; for children, tea is gentlest.

For tea, simmer 1 teaspoon whole root in 1 cup water 10–20 minutes, or pour 1 cup boiling water over ¼ teaspoon powder.

Caution: Should not be used by anyone with a stomach ulcer, active inflammatory bowel disease, or sores anywhere in gastrointestinal tract.

GENTIAN VIOLET

Purple tincture used against candida for decades in human and veterinary medicine.

Effective against thrush, diaper rash, and other yeast infections.

Available as 1% solution.

Caution: Stains baby, diapers, and parents.

GINGER (*Zingiber officinale*)

Pungent root commonly used in cooking.

Ayurvedic remedy for pain and swelling in rheumatoid arthritis and osteoarthritis.

Contains sugar-digesting and fat-digesting enzymes.

Prevents and eases nausea and dispels flatulence/intestinal gas.

Grated ginger added to foods is helpful for children with digestive problems.

Tea can temporarily relieve heartburn (gastroesophageal reflux disease); used regularly, ginger can help diminish heartburn over time.

In irritable bowel syndrome, helps relieve gas pains.

Available as fresh, pickled, dried, or candied root, powder, tea, and capsules.

For tea, steep a few thin slices fresh root, or ½ teaspoon powder or dried root, in 1 cup boiling water.

GINKGO (*Ginkgo biloba*)

Antioxidant, circulation-promoting, memory-enhancing herb (leaf of ginkgo tree).

Used to improve lung function and asthma, and also in children with attention deficit hyperactivity disorder.

Available as capsules and tablets.

GINSENG (*Panax ginseng,* also called American or Asian Ginseng)

Adaptogenic root that balances body's systems.

Used in Chinese medicine for a wide variety of ailments.

Increases beneficial gut bacteria *in vitro.*

Used with ginkgo in attention deficit disorder (some children experienced side effects).

Available as root, tea, tincture, and capsules; tea is gentle and easy for children's use.

See also Ginkgo and Siberian Ginseng.

GLUTAMINE

Amino acid used by small intestine for energy, maintenance, and repair.

Protects mucous membranes in lungs and digestive tract, reduces risk of infection, promotes muscle building and weight gain, and prevents muscle wasting.

Speeds healing after appendix removal.

Used to stop diarrhea in Crohn's disease, irritable bowel syndrome, leaky gut, stomach ulcer, and ulcerative colitis, and after gastric re-sectioning surgery.

Might be helpful in celiac disease, but this has not yet been studied.

Available as capsules and powder.

Caution: Too high a dose may cause constipation.

GOLDENSEAL (*Hydrastic canadensis*)

Antiseptic, astringent, laxative, tonic, antiparasitic herb that soothes mucous membranes.

Used historically for infections of gastrointestinal tract and lungs.

Active component, berberine sulfate, is effective against amoebas and giardia.

Effective against candida.

For mouth ulcers/canker sores, taken internally or dabbed directly on sores.

Available as tea, tincture, or tablets.

Note: Goldenseal is getting rare and is quite expensive.

GRAPEFRUIT-SEED EXTRACT

Antiparasitic, antibiotic, antifungal extract effective against candida infections and thrush; safe for babies and breast-feeding mothers.

A few drops diluted in a cup of water can be used topically on diaper rash.

Available as capsules and liquid (tastes very bitter).

GRAPESEED EXTRACT (also called Pycnogenol)

Powerful, gentle antioxidant containing active ingredient pycnogenol (also found in pine bark).

Many parents believe it to be helpful in attention deficit disorders.

Available as capsules and tablets, and in combination products.

GREEN TEA (*Camellia sinensis*)

Powerful antioxidant, cancer-preventive herb.

Its polyphenols increase beneficial intestinal bacteria and decrease clostridia.

Thought to have positive effects against serum cholesterol, tumors, and ulcers.

Available as tea, extract, tablets, and capsules.

GYMNEMA (*Gymnema sylvestre*)

Antidiabetic herb that enhances insulin's effect.

In India, leaves have been chewed for centuries to lower blood sugar levels.

In type I diabetes, controls blood glucose levels, lowers hemoglobin A1C levels, and lowers medication needs.

In type II diabetes, stimulates insulin production.

May be included in supplements for blood glucose control in diabetes.

HONEY

Delicious, nutritious natural sweetener. Natural prebiotic food.

In nausea/vomiting, 1 teaspoon (raw) helps settle stomach.

Caution: Do not give to babies younger than one year old (linked to infant botulism).

HOPS (*Humulus lupulus*)

Calming herb used traditionally for relaxation and to promote sleep.

Tea-infused bathwater can calm a colicky baby.

HORSERADISH

Gallbladder-supportive root used as a condiment.

Can be helpful in cystic fibrosis.

IRON

Mineral used by hemoglobin in red blood cells to carry oxygen throughout body.

Iron deficiency is called anemia.

People with inflammatory bowel disease are often iron-deficient.

Available as capsules or tablets.
    Caution: Keep out of reach of children.

JERUSALEM OAK (*Chenopodium anthelminticum; also called American Wormseed*)

Herb used in folk medicine throughout the Americas to expel roundworms, hookworms, and tapeworms, especially useful for children; more studies needed to confirm historical usage.

JOY GARDNER'S FLU CAPS

Anti-flu preparation of cayenne pepper, slippery elm, cinnamon, and goldenseal (see Chapter 25 for details).

LAVENDER (*Lavendula* species)

Fragrant, calming herb.

Tea-infused bathwater can calm a colicky baby.

LEMON BALM (*Melissa officinalis*)

Fragrant, calming, digestion-enhancing

herb used to reduce fever and relieve flatulence/intestinal gas.

Tea or tea-infused bathwater can calm a colicky baby; tea also calms digestion of breast-feeding mother and passes through breast-milk to baby.

LICORICE (*Glycyrrhiza glabra*)

Sweet, demulcent herb that soothes inflamed mucous membranes in esophagus and gastrointestinal tract.

Helpful in healing leaky gut.

Reduces nausea, vomiting, constipation, and encopresis.

Inhibits growth of *Helicobacter pylori* (bacteria that causes most stomach ulcers).

May be useful as adrenal support in asthma.

Available as tea, root, capsules, and chewable tablets; tea is safe for babies, root for older children (they'll like chewing on it).

Note: Most licorice candy contains no actual licorice, but Panda and some gourmet brands do.

Caution: Too much licorice may raise blood pressure. Deglycyrrhized (DGL) root is preferable, unless child has low blood pressure.

LINDEN FLOWER (*Tilia* species)

Calming herb used for sleep problems, colds, and flu.

Tea-infused bathwater can calm a colicky baby.

For tea, pour 1 cup boiling water over 1 teaspoon linden flowers and steep 5–10 minutes.

LIPOIC ACID (also called Alpha-Lipoic Acid)

Antioxidant nutrient.

In diabetes, protects liver function and may help control blood sugar levels.

Available as capsules and tablets.

LOBELIA (*Lobelia inflata;* also called Indian Tobacco)

Antispasmodic herb that helps adrenal glands produce hormones that relax bronchial muscles.

Helpful in asthma.

Recommended by herbalist Dr. John Christopher for gastroesophageal reflux disease and hiatal hernia when used externally.

Available as powder, tincture, and solid extract.

Caution: Too much lobelia causes vomiting.

MAGNESIUM

Alkalizing, muscle- and nerve-relaxing mineral with more than 300 uses in our bodies.

Children with inflammatory bowel disease or migraine are often magnesium-deficient.

People with diabetes or insulin resistance also have an increased need for magnesium.

In constipation/encopresis and irritable bowel syndrome, helpful for normalizing peristalsis.

Bronchodilating in asthma, and reduces severity and frequency of asthma attacks.

Reduces frequency of migraine, can help relieve growing pains.

Also used in attention deficit hyperactivity disorder.

Caution: Too much magnesium causes diarrhea.

Note: Some people have difficulty absorbing magnesium. If your child needs large amounts of magnesium, increase absorption by also giving a teaspoon of choline citrate (Perque brand; see Resources) per each 200 mg of magnesium.

MARJORAM (*Origanum vulgare*)

Antispasmodic, calming, digestion-enhancing herb and common seasoning.

Reduces flatulence/intestinal gas.

For tea, steep 1 teaspoon dried or 2 teaspoons fresh herb in 1 cup boiling water.

MARSHMALLOW (*Althaea officinalis*)

Demulcent, emollient herb that soothes mucous membranes in gastrointestinal tract and lungs.

In inflammatory bowel disease, soothes intestinal lining.

Available as capsules and tea.

MEDIUM-CHAIN TRIGLYCERIDES (MCTs) AND OTHER OILS

Healthful, helpful fats that stimulate digestion and bile production.

Food sources of MCTs such as linoleic acid include nuts, seeds, and whole grains.

In cystic fibrosis, supplementing with MCT oil and linoleic-acid-rich foods and oils can normalize fatty acid levels.

METHYLSULFONYLMETHANE (MSM)

Sulfur-rich antioxidant compound that reduces pain and inflammation.

Helps build cartilage and collagen.

Commonly used in arthritis.

Available as powder and capsules.

Note: For best absorption, should be taken with an equal amount of vitamin C.

MEYER'S COCKTAIL

Intravenous combination of magnesium, calcium, and vitamins B_5, B_6, B_{12}, and C.

Administered in a physician's office.

Used in asthma as well as other conditions not noted in this book.

Author's note: In asthma, I'd try this with an older child or with a smaller child whose asthma is severe.

MINERAL SALTS

Bicarbonates of calcium, magnesium, and/or potassium (for example, Alka-Seltzer Gold).

Can help buffer food sensitivity reactions.

In a tub of warm water, $1/2$ cup baking soda and $1/2$ cup Epsom salts alkalize, gently detoxify, relax, and cleanse (soak for at least 15 minutes); particularly useful in psoriasis and eczema.

See also Calcium and Magnesium.

MULLEIN (*Verbascum thapsus*)

Antispasmodic, demulcent, antibiotic, emollient, and expectorant herb.

In inflammatory bowel disease, soothes intestinal lining.

In asthma, cough, bronchitis, and lung disease, strengthens lung tissues.

Mullein oil (often combined with garlic) is used topically for ear infections (two or three drops in affected ear two or three times daily).

Available as capsules, tea, and oil.

For tea, pour 1 cup boiling water over 1 teaspoon dried leaf.

MUSTARD SEED (*Brassica nigra, B. hirta;* also called Black or White Mustard Seed)

Pungent, gallbladder-supportive, digestion-stimulating seeds used in cooking and condiments.

Prepared mustard is helpful in cystic fibrosis.

MYRRH (*Commiphora myrrha*)

Antiseptic, astringent, carminative, stomach-supportive herb.

Temporarily soothes canker sores, cough, and asthma.

Available as tea, powder, and tincture.

For tea, steep 1 teaspoon powdered myrrh in 2 cups water for 5 minutes and strain.

N-ACETYL CYSTEINE (NAC)

Antioxidant nutrient that protects lung function and helps chelate heavy metals.

Available as capsules.

NICOTINAMIDE (also called Niacin and Vitamin B_3)

B-complex nutrient thought to prevent free-radical toxicity.

In newly diagnosed type I diabetes, can slow progression of disease, put some children into remission, improve glucose control, and preserve some beta cell function.

OMEGA-3 FATTY ACIDS

Healthful fats eicosapentaenoic acid (EPA) and docosahexaenoic acid (DHA) found in all of our cells, especially critical for eyes, brain, nervous system, heart, and glands (see Chapter 8 for details).

Although many of us can manufacture DHA from other fats, some people lack enzymes and nutrients (vitamin B₆ and magnesium) necessary for this conversion.

Fish richest in EPA and DHA are salmon, halibut, tuna, mackerel, trout, sardines, eel, and herring. Marine algae and sea vegetables also offer significant amounts.

Beneficial in inflammatory and other conditions including Crohn's disease, ulcerative colitis, arthritis, psoriasis, eczema, migraine, asthma, cystic fibrosis, lupus, autism, attention deficit disorders, cancer, and more.

Caution: Fish oils increase blood-clotting time, and should not be taken by anyone who has hemophilia or who regularly takes anticoagulant medicines or aspirin.

See also Cod Liver Oil.

OREGANO (*Oreganum vulgare*)

Digestion-enhancing cooking herb.

Constituent carcavol has antibiotic and antifungal properties.

Taken internally for colds, flu, and fever, and to relieve flatulence/intestinal gas.

Oil of oregano is commonly used to treat candida overgrowth.

Also used externally for asthma, bronchitis, and arthritis.

Available as fresh or dried herb, tea, and oil.

OSCILLOCOCCINUM

Widely used homeopathic flu remedy.

Reported to decrease flu symptoms in twenty-four to thirty-six hours in about half of those who take it.

Available as sublingual pellets.

PANTOTHENIC ACID (also called Vitamin B₅)

B-complex nutrient that helps energy production and supports adrenal glands.

Used in asthma and allergies and to help heal leaky gut.

PARSLEY (*Carum petroselinum*)

Flavorful, diuretic, digestion-stimulating, gallbladder-supportive herb used as seasoning and garnish.

Relieves flatulence/intestinal gas and menstrual cramping.

Helpful as part of diet for children with cystic fibrosis.

Available fresh or dried.

PASSIONFLOWER (*Passiflora incarnata*)

Calming herb helpful in relaxation, sleep promotion, and irritable bowel syndrome.

Available as fresh or dried herb, capsules, and tincture often found with hops, valerian, and skullcap.

For tea, pour 1 cup boiling water over 1 teaspoon dried or 1 tablespoon fresh flowers.

PEPPERMINT (*Mentha piperita*)

Digestion-enhancing and muscle-relaxing herb.

Tea relieves flatulence/intestinal gas.

Peppermint oil is widely used in Great Britain as a muscle relaxant for irritable bowel syndrome spasms.

Note: Enteric-coated capsules can be taken between meals when your child is in spasm; one or two capsules daily can also be used preventively.

PLANTAIN (*Plantago major, P. lanceolata*)

Demulcent herb and edible weed.

As a poultice, used for toothaches and wound healing.

In inflammatory bowel disease, soothes intestinal lining.

Available as capsules, tea, and fresh in your yard (it's found in most lawns).

PROBIOTICS

Beneficial bacteria living in our intestines, lungs, and other mucous membranes as an important component of our immune and digestive systems, manufacturing vitamins, increasing nutrient absorption, and protecting mucous membranes (see Chapter 5 for details).

Taken after antibiotic use to re-establish gut ecology.

Effective against dysbiosis and candida infection.

Also helpful in asthma, attention deficit disorder, autism, colic, constipation, diabetes, diarrhea, encopresis, flatulence/intestinal gas, inflammatory bowel disease, irritable bowel syndrome, nausea, vomiting, and nearly every other disease.

Available as capsules and powder; also found in cultured and fermented foods and supplements.

Note: Powder can be mixed in cool or cold beverage (hot drinks kill the flora); probiotics will pass from breast-feeding mother to baby in breast-milk.

PROPOLIS (also called Bee Propolis)

Antibiotic and antifungal resin collected from trees and buds by bees (used to repair their hives).

In asthma, may decrease number and severity of night-time attacks, improve pulmonary function, and decrease levels of inflammatory cytokines.

Available as capsules, tincture, and resin.

Caution: People allergic to bee products should *not* use bee propolis.

PRUNE JUICE

Laxative beverage helpful in constipation and encopresis.

Note: Taken before bedtime, $1/3$ cup prune juice diluted in $2/3$ cup water can have a laxative effect by morning.

PSYLLIUM-SEED HUSKS

Good source of natural fiber, best known as fiber in Metamucil.

Helpful in constipation, diarrhea, and irritable bowel syndrome.

Pycnogenol. See Grape Seed Extract.

PYRIDOXINE (also called Vitamin B$_6$)

B-complex vitamin essential to health of nervous system, eyes, skin, mouth, liver, and brain.

Important for energy production and water balance, maintains muscle tone in digestive tract.

Used in diabetes, arthritis, depression, asthma, inflammatory bowel disease, autism, attention deficit disorder, and carpel tunnel syndrome.

Carl Pfeiffer, M.D., used B$_6$ for schizophrenia.

Caution: Too much B$_6$ can cause too much dreaming/REM sleep. If this occurs, reduce dosage.

Caution: Daily doses of 250 milligrams or more can produce reversible nervous system problems.

QUERCETIN

Anti-inflammatory bioflavonoid with antihistamine effects.

Food sources include apples, onions, and black tea.

Helpful in any illness with inflammation (virtually all).

Shown useful in arthritis, asthma, inflammatory bowel disease, food sensitivity/allergy, gout, hay-fever, heartburn, leaky gut syndrome, and migraine, as well as heart disease prevention and cancer prevention and treatment.

Possible help in eosinophilic esophagitis and eosinophilic gastritis not yet studied.

Available as capsules and tablets.

Recommended forms are quercetin dehydrate and quercetin chalcone.

RIBOFLAVIN (also called Vitamin B$_2$)

B-complex nutrient involved in energy production, brain's cellular communication, and health of the eyes and skin.

Daily supplementation can reduce frequency and severity of migraine.

Available as capsules and tablets.

ROSEMARY (*Rosmarinus officinalis*)

Antispasmodic, digestion-enhancing, calming, diaphoretic, astringent herb.

In irritable bowel syndrome, helps relieve and expel gas, strengthen and tone stomach, and soothe pain.

Available as fresh or dried herb, capsules, tincture, and tea.

S-ADENOSYLMETHIONINE (SAMe)

Naturally occurring amino acid found in every living cell.

Shown to be as potent an anti-inflammatory agent as indomethacin and other NSAIDs, but with fewer negative side effects.

Used for depression and arthritis.

Note: Should be taken with a good multivitamin that contains B-complex vitamins.

Note: This product is expensive because it is difficult to stabilize.

SEACURE

Fish-protein product containing peptides, amines, and omega-3 fatty acids.

Helpful in resolving leaky gut, inflammatory bowel disease, and irritable bowel syndrome.

SELENIUM

Antioxidant mineral that is protective against viral infection.

People with inflammatory bowel disease are often selenium-depleted.

Best-absorbed form is selenomethionine.

SIBERIAN GINSENG
(*Eleutherococcus senticosus*)

Adaptogenic herb that balances body systems, especially supportive to adrenal glands.

Used in asthma and allergy and to increase endurance.

Available as tincture, capsules, tablets, and tea.

SKULLCAP (*Scutellaria lateriflora*)

Calming herb used as a nervine for centuries.

Helpful in irritable bowel syndrome and for improving sleep quality.

Available as root, tincture, tea, and capsules; tea works well for children.

Often found with passionflower, hops, and valerian root.

For tea, simmer 1 teaspoon root in 1 cup water for 10 minutes and strain.

SLIPPERY ELM (*Ulmus fulva*)

Tree with demulcent, emollient, and nutritious inner bark that soothes mucous membranes in throat, esophagus, and stomach.

Used for heartburn/gastroesophageal reflux disease, nausea, sore throat, vomiting, and ulcer.

Available as tea, bark (can be chewed), and lozenges.

For tea, simmer 1 teaspoon bark in 2 cups water for 20 minutes and strain.

SPEARMINT (*Mentha viridis*)

Digestion-enhancing, muscle-relaxing herb.

Tea relieves flatulence/intestinal gas.

For tea, pour 1 cup boiling water over 1 teaspoon dry or 1 tablespoon fresh leaves.

Available fresh, dried, and in teabags.

SPECIFIC CARBOHYDRATE DIET

Dietary protocol very helpful for people with Crohn's disease or ulcerative colitis, outlined in Elaine Gottschall's book *Breaking the Vicious Cycle* (see Chapter 17 for details; see also www.scdiet.org).

SUPEROXIDE DISMUTASE (SOD)

Antioxidant enzyme containing manganese, zinc, or copper.

Relieves arthritis pain in human and veterinary medicine.

Available as sublingual pellets and wheatgrass extract.

See also Wheatgrass.

TAURINE

Liver- and gallbladder-protective amino acid that helps regulate bile flow.

Along with carnitine, used in cystic fibrosis to help with fat metabolism and heart function.

See also Carnitine.

TETRANDINE (*Stephania tetranda*)

Extract of Chinese medicinal herb Han-Fang Chi.

Historically used as an immune system suppressant and anti-inflammatory agent.

In arthritis, used in combination with *Tripterygium wilfordii* for greater effectiveness.

Caution: Potential toxic effects on liver and kidneys.

See also *Tripterygium wilfordii*.

THIAMINE (also called Vitamin B$_1$)

B-complex nutrient important for energy production, cellular communication, and nervous system.

Protective of pancreatic beta cells in children with type I diabetes.

THYME (*Thymus vulgaris*)

Digestion-enhancing herb used fresh or dried as seasoning or tea.

Can relieve flatulence/intestinal gas.

Thyme oil is used in remedies for candidiasis.

TRAUMEEL S

Homeopathic remedy (by Heel) of fourteen herbs and minerals.

Administered as a subcutaneous injection (ask your doctor).

In asthma, can improve symptoms significantly and reduce medication use and infection frequency.

Being studied as a mouthwash for effect against oral cancer.

TRIPTERYGIUM WILFORDII

Traditional Chinese medicinal herb with anti-inflammatory effects.

Used in adult rheumatoid arthritis, with fewer side effects than conventional medications.

Often used in combination with tetrandine for greater effectiveness.

See also Tetrandine.

TURMERIC (Curcuma longa)

Anti-inflammatory spice that gives flavor and yellow color to mustard and curry.

Used in Ayurvedic and Hawaiian medicine to reduce pain and swelling.

Contains bioflavonoids; an active ingredient, curcumin, is a known anti-inflammatory.

In arthritis, relieves pain and joint stiffness and reduces need for medication.

May also be used as a poultice on sprains.

Available as powder, capsules, or fresh root; powdered turneric can be used in food and juice; grown in warm areas as a lovely flowering plant.

Note: Highly effective when used fresh. Blend a 3-inch piece with 1–2 cups water and drink daily, and use in stir-frying and other cooking.

See also Curcumin.

UMEBOSHI PLUM

Salted, alkalizing, pickled plums used in Japanese cuisine.

Stimulates bile production and HCl and digestive juices in the stomach.

Helpful against nausea and flu symptoms.

In cystic fibrosis, promotes fat absorption.

Available whole and as paste; can be eaten straight (typically one or two daily, more for flu), made into tea, and used to flavor salad dressing.

Author's note: I saw a friend with the flu eat seven or eight umeboshi plums and feel completely fine within an hour.

VALERIAN (Valeriana officinalis)

Calming, antispasmodic herb commonly used to promote sleep and reduce anxiety and tension.

In irritable bowel syndrome and inflammatory bowel disease, relieves flatulence/intestinal gas, soothes pain, and relaxes and tones stomach muscles.

Available as capsules, tincture, and tea. Often found with passionflower, skullcap, and hops.

Note: Smells awful, but works really well.

VANADIUM

Essential mineral in animals; in humans, mimics effect of insulin.

We ingest 15–30 micrograms daily in food, but its role in our health is still being studied.

In type I and type II diabetes, significantly lowers blood sugar and can reduce need for oral medications and insulin.

Often included in supplements for blood glucose control in diabetes.

Safest source is vanadyl ascorbate.

VITAMIN A

Fat-soluble vitamin used throughout our bodies for health of respiratory, digestive, and genito-urinary system, as well as eyes and skin.

Often deficient in people with inflammatory bowel disease.

Used in leaky gut syndrome, asthma, and autism.

See also Cod Liver Oil.

VITAMIN B₆

See Pyridoxine.

VITAMIN B₁₂

See Cobalamine.

VITAMIN C (also called Ascorbate and Ascorbic Acid)

Antioxidant, antiviral, antimicrobial, anti-allergy, and anti-inflammatory vitamin.

Reduces bruising, protects blood vessels, and helps flush toxins and metals from body.

Ascorbate form can help balance pH.

Low in people with inflammatory bowel disease.

Taken preventively to reduce risk of infection, colds, and flu.

In arthritis, promotes formation of collagen and connective tissue.

In constipation and encopresis, softens stools.

Also used for leaky gut, allergy, and asthma.

Available as chewable pills, tablets, capsules, and powder.

Note: Can be taken in large amounts. When tissues are saturated, diarrhea occurs.

VITAMIN D

Fat-soluble vitamin present in virtually all of our cells and essential in calcium absorption, bone health, and cancer prevention.

Produced in body in response to sunlight, so it's important to spend at least half an hour a day outdoors (in summer, body stores vitamin D for future).

Helpful in autism, celiac disease, cystic fibrosis, diabetes, and inflammatory bowel disease.

Increased dietary vitamin D for type I diabetic mothers during pregnancy can reduce child's risk of type I diabetes.

Caution: If your child is taking doses higher than 1,000 international units, have his/her blood level of vitamin D checked.

VITAMIN E

Antioxidant nutrient.

Often deficient in people with inflammatory bowel disease.

May be included in supplements for blood glucose control in diabetes.

After appendectomy, promotes healing of surgical wound.

WATERCRESS

Slightly bitter, liver- and gallbladder-supportive, digestion-stimulating green, eaten cooked or in salads or sandwiches.

Can be helpful dietary addition in cystic fibrosis.

WHEATGRASS

Plant rich in chlorophyll and antioxidants.

In inflammatory bowel disease, can reduce rectal bleeding and disease severity.

Available as juice and powder.

See also Superoxide Dismutase.

WHEY PROTEIN (also called Whey Concentrate)

High-quality, easily digestible protein found in watery part of milk separated during cheese-making or in watery part of separated yogurt.

Rich in immunoprotective antibodies.

Tasty, quick, and easy addition to beverages or food, provides extra calories and protein.

Helpful in leaky gut syndrome.

In children with cystic fibrosis, can significantly increase levels of glutathione (important and much-needed antioxidant in this condition).

See also Glutathione.

WORMWOOD (*Artemisia annua;* also called Artemisia)

Herb used traditionally in China and Europe and commonly found in antiparasitic products.

Caution: Safe as tea or powder capsule, but pure wormwood oil is poisonous.

YOGURT/KEFIR/BUTTERMILK

Cultured dairy products containing beneficial probiotics that help normalize bowels (see Chapter 5).

Helpful against conditions including constipation, diarrhea, and encopresis.

YUCCA (*Yucca shidigera, Y. filamentosa*)

Anti-inflammatory, digestion-enhancing plant.

Commonly eaten by southwestern Native Americans to alleviate arthritis symptoms and improve digestion.

Improves triglyceride and cholesterol levels and helps lower blood pressure.

Shown to have benefits in arthritis.

Available as food and tablets.

ZINC

Antioxidant mineral essential for growth, wound healing, immune system function, healthy gut mucosa, and health of hair, skin, nails, and all of our cells.

Protects against viral infection.

Helpful in attention deficit disorders, autism, canker sores/mouth ulcers, diarrhea, inflammatory bowel disease, and post-surgical wound healing.

Note: You can easily self-test your child for zinc deficiency (see Chapter 20).

Caution: Too much zinc causes nausea.

References

Introduction

American Medical Association. "Migraines in children." *Medem* 1998. Available at www.medem.com/MedLB/article_detaillb.cfm?article_ID=ZZZIAZF99CC&sub_cat=56 7.

Galland L. *The Four Pillars of Healing.* New York: Random House, 1997.

Garrison M. "A systematic review of treatments for infant colic." *Pediatrics* 2000;106(1 pt 2):184–190.

Kluger J, Song S. "Young and bipolar." *Time* 2002;Aug 19.

MD Consult. "Atopic dermatitis." *MD Consult* 2002.

Orenstein S. "Gastroesophageal reflux disease in children." *Gastroent Clin* 1999;28.

Rubin G. "Constipation in children." *Clin Evid* 2003;9:350–355.

Spergel J, Pawlowski NA. "Food allergy: Mechanisms, diagnosis, and management in children." *Ped Clin N Am* 2002;49:73–96.

Surgeon General of the United States. "The surgeon general's call to action to prevent and decrease overweight and obesity in children and adolescents." U.S. Department of Health and Human Services 2003. Available at www.surgeongeneral.gov/topics/obesity/calltoaction/fact_adolescents.htm.

Whittington CJ, Kendall T, et al. "Selective serotonin reuptake inhibitors in childhood depression: Systematic review of published versus unpublished data." *Lancet* 2004;363(9418):1341–1345.

Chapter 1

Champagne CM, Ryan DH, Bray A. "Fast-food consumption among US adults and children: Dietary and nutrient intake profile." *J Am Diet Assoc* 2003;103(10):1332–1338.

Dietz WH. "Health consequences of obesity in youth." *Pediatrics* 1998;101:518–525.

Guthrie JF, Lin B, Frazao E. "Role of food prepared away from home in the American diet, 1977–78 versus 1994–96: Changes and consequences." *J Nutr Educ Behav* 2002;34(3):140–150.

King J. "Nutrition and your health: Dietary guidelines for Americans." *Dietary Guidelines Scientific Committee, USDA* 2005;Washington, D.C.

Lin BH, Frazao E, Guthrie J. "American children's diets not making the grade." *FoodReview* 2001;24(2). Available at www.ers.usda.gov/publications/FoodReview/May2001/FRV24I2b.pdf.

Nicklas TA, McQuarrie A, et al. "Efficiency of breakfast consumption patterns of ninth graders: Nutrient-to-cost comparisons." *J Am Diet Assoc* 2002;102(2):226–233.

Nielsen SJ, Popkin BM. "Patterns and trends in food portion sizes, 1977–1988." *JAMA* 2003;289(4):450–453.

Nielsen SJ, Siega-Riz AM, Popkin BM. "Trends in food locations and sources among adolescents and young adults." *Prev Med* 2002;35(2):107–113.

St-Onge MP, Keller KL, Heymsfield SB. "Changes in childhood food consumption patterns: A cause for concern in light of increasing body weights." *Am J Clin Nutr* 2003; 78(6):1068–1073.

Chapter 2

American Academy of Otolaryngology. "Secondhand smoke and children." Available at www.entnet.org/healthinfo/tobacco/secondhand_smoke.cfm.

Cosmetic Ingredient Review Panel. "Skin deep." FDA Office of Cosmetics and Colors 2003. Available at www.ewg.org/reports/skindeep/report/executive_summary.php.

The Cure Zone. Available at www.curezone.com/foods/microwave_oven_risk.html.

Environmental Working Group. "Skin deep, a safety assessment of ingredients in personal care products." 2005. Available at www.ewg.org/reports/skindeep.

Environmental Working Group. "Body burden—the pollution in newborns." July 14, 2005.

Hertel HU, Blanc B. *Nexus Mag*, U2 #25 April–May, 1995. www.ewg.org/reports/body-burdenz/execsumm.php

Lee L. "Health effects of microwave radiation—microwave ovens." Available at www.vaccinetruth.org/microwave.htm.

Mohan S, Tiller M, et al. "Mercury exposure of mothers and newborns in Surinam: A pilot study." *Clin Toxicol* 2005;43(2):101–104.

Nash R. "Mercury." Anti-aging Conference and Expo, Oct 28–31, 2004, Las Vegas, NV.

National Wildlife Federation. *Clean the Rain, Clean the Lakes II Report for New England.* 2001.

Needleman H, Schell A, et al. "The long-term effects of exposure to low doses of lead in childhood." *NEJM* 1990;322:83–88.

Oveson L, Jakobsen J, Leth T. "The effect of microwave heating on vitamins B_1 and E, and linoleic and linolenic acids, and immunoglobulins in human milk." *Int J Food Sci Nutr* 1996;47(5):427–436.

Porter JW. "Mercury emissions from China exceed USA." *The Virginian-Pilot* Aug 10 1998.

Wayne A, Newell L. "Radiation ovens: The proven dangers of microwave ovens." Available at www.lawgiver.org.

Wolfe SM. *Health Letter* 1989;5(7):1–5.

U.S. Centers for Disease Control. "National report on human exposure to environmental chemicals: Results lead." 2001. Available at www.cdc.gov/exposurereport.

U.S. Centers for Disease Control. "Second national report on human exposure to environmental chemicals." Jan 2003. Available at www.cdc.gov/exposurereport/2nd/pdf/ner summary.pdf.

U.S. Environmental Protection Agency. "Indoor air-smoke-free homes." Available at www.epa.gov/cgi-bin/epaprintonly.cgi.

Vahter M, Akesson A, et al. "Longitudinal study of methylmercury and inorganic mercury in blood and urine of pregnant and lactating women, as well as in umbilical cord blood." *Environ Res* 2000;84(2):186–194.

Chapter 3

Bland J. *20-Day Rejuvenation Diet Program.* Los Angeles, CA: Keats Publishing, 1997.

Gershon MD. *The Second Brain.* New York, NY: Harper Collins Publishers, 1998.

Robbins J. *May All Be Fed.* New York, NY: William Morrow & Co., 1992.

Thompson T. "Approach to gastrointestinal immune dysfunction and related health problems." Lecture, Fourth International Functional Medicine Meeting, Aspen, CO, 1997.

Chapter 4

Bender DA. *Introduction to Nutrition and Metabolism, Third Edition.* London, UK: Taylor and Francis Publishing, 2002.

Brody T. *Nutritional Biochemistry, Second Edition.* San Diego, CA: Academic Press, 1999.

Fuller D. *The Healing Power of Enzymes.* New York, NY: Forbes, 1998.

Lenhninger AL, Nelson DL, Cox MM. *Principles of Biochemistry.* New York, NY: Worth Publishing, 1993.

Lipski E. *How to Be Healthier with Enzymes.* Asheville, NC: Innovative Healing Press, 2005.

Mamadou M. *Oral Enzymes: Facts and Concepts.* Houston, TX: Transformation Enzyme Corporation, 1999.

Pizzorno JE, Murray MT. *Textbook of Natural Medicine, Second Edition,* Volumes 1 and 2. London, UK: Churchill Livingstone, 1999.

Segala M, editor. *Life Extension Foundation's Disease Prevention and Treatment, Third Edition.* Hollywood, FL: Life Extension Media, 2000.

Chapter 5

Alam NH, Ashraf H. "Treatment of infectious diarrhea in children." *Paediatr Drugs* 2003;5(3):151–165.

Biffi A, Coradini D, et al. "Antiproliferative effect of fermented milk on the growth of a human breast cancer cell line." *Nutr Cancer* 1997;28(1):93–99.

Bland J, Liska DA, et al. *Clinical Nutrition: A Functional Approach.* Gig Harbor, WA: Functional Medicine Institute, 1999.

Campieri C, Campieri M, et al. "Reduction of oxaluria after an oral course of lactic acid bacteria at high concentration." *Kidney Int* 2001;60(3):1097–1105.

Carper J. *Food Pharmacy.* New York, NY: Bantam Books, 1988.

Casas IA, Edens FW, Dobrogosz WJ. "*Lactobacillus reuteri:* An effective probiotic for poultry and other animals." In S Salminen, A von Wright, editors. *Lactic Acid Bacteria: Microbiology and Functional Aspects, Second Edition.* New York, NY: Marcel Dekker, Inc., 1998.

Chaitow L, Trenev N. *Probiotics.* London, UK: Thorsons Publications, 1990.

ConsumerLab. "Product review: probiotic supplements and foods (including *Lactobacillus acidophilus* and bifidobacterium)." Available at www.consumerlab.com/results/probiotics.asp.

Czerucka D, Roux L, Rampal P. "*Saccharomyces boulardii* inhibits secretagogue-mediated adenosine 3',5'-cyclic monophosphate induction in intestinal cells." *Gastroenterology* 1994;106(1):65–72.

"Florastor." Available at www.florastor.com/ProductInformation.asp.

Galland L. *Dysbiosis and Disease.* Audiotape. Asheville, NC: Great Smokies Diagnostic Lab and HealthComm International, 1993.

Great Smokies Diagnostic Lab and HealthComm International. *Solving the Digestive Puzzle.* Conference manual, San Francisco, CA, May 1995.

Gibson GR, Roberfroid MB. "Dietary modulation of the human colonic microbiota: Introducing the concept of probiotics." *J Nutr* 1995;125(6):1401–1412.

Gibson GR, Wang X. "Regulatory effects of *Bifidobacteria* on the growth of other colonic bacteria." *J Appl Bacteriol* 1994;77:412–420.

Guandalini S, Pensabene L, et al. "*Lactobacillus GG* administered in oral rehydration solution to children with acute diarrhea: A multicenter European trial." *J Pediatr Gastroenterol Nutr* 2000;30(1):54–60.

Kalliomäki M, Isolauri E. "Role of intestinal flora in the development of allergy." *Curr Opin Allergy Clin Immunol* 2003;3(1):15–20.

Kajiwara S, Gandhi H, Ustunol Z. "Effect of honey on the growth of and acid production by human intestinal *Bifidobacterium* spp.: An *in vitro* comparison with commercial oligosaccharides and inulin." *J Food Prot* 2002;65(1):214–218.

Kimmey MB, Elmer GW, et al. "Prevention of further recurrences of *Clostridium difficile* colitis with *Saccharomyces boulardii*." *Dig Dis Sci* 1990;35(7):897–901.

Kirjavainen PV, Salminen SJ, et al. "Probiotic bacteria in the management of atopic disease: Underscoring the importance of viability." *J Pediatr Gastroenterol Nutr* 2003;36(2):223–227.

Lipski, E. "Wondrous Bacteria," paper for course on evolution, Union Institute, 2000.

Macfarlane G, Cummings JH. "Probiotics and prebiotics: Can regulating the activities of intestinal bacteria benefit health?" *Br Med J* 1999;318:999–1003.

Mitsuuoka T. "Intestinal flora and aging." *Nutr Rev* 1992;50(12):438–446.

Pessi T, Sutas Y, et al. "Interleukin-10 generation in atopic children following oral *Lactobacillus rhamnosus GG*." *Clin Exp Allergy* 2000;30(12):1804–1808.

Plein K, Hotz J. "Therapeutic effects of *Saccharomyces boulardii* on mild residual symptoms in a stable phase of Crohn's disease with special respect to chronic diarrhea: A pilot study." *Gastroenterology* 1993;31(2):129–134.

Plummer N, Quilt P, Crockett C. "Fructooligosaccharides (FOS) and other prebiotics." *Townsend Lett Doctors Patients,* June 2003. Available at www.findarticles.com.

Reid G. "Probiotic agents to protect the urogenital tract against infection." *Am J Clin Nutr* 2001;73(suppl):437S–443S.

Reid G, Bruce AW. "Selection of *Lactobacillus* strains for urogenital probiotic applications." *J Infect Dis* 2001;183(suppl 1):S77–S80.

Rio ME, Zago Beatriz L, et al. "The nutritional status change the effectiveness of a dietary supplement of lactic bacteria on the emerging of respiratory tract diseases in children." *Arch Latinoam Nutr* 2002;52(1):29–34.

Roberfoid MB. "Prebiotics and synbiotics: concepts and nutritional properties." *Br J Nutr* 1998;80(4 suppl):S197–S202.

Rosenfeldt V, Benfeldt E, et al. "Effect of probiotic *Lactobacillus* strains in children with atopic dermatitis." *J Allergy Clin Immunol* 2003;111(2):389–395.

Saavedra JM, Abi-Hanna A, et al. "Long-term consumption of infant formulas containing live probiotic bacteria: Tolerance and safety." *Am J Clin Nutr* 2004;79(2):261–267.

Saran S, Gopalan S, et al. "Use of fermented foods to combat stunting and failure to thrive." *Nutrition* 2002;18(5):393–396.

Sazawal S, Dhingra U, et al. "Efficacy of milk fortified with a probiotic *Bifidobacterium lactis* (DR-10TM) and prebiotic galacto-oligosaccharides in prevention of morbidity and on nutritional status." *Asia Pac J Clin Nutr* 2004;13(suppl):S28.

Schrezenmeir J, Heller K, et al. "Benefits of oral supplementation with and without synbiotics in young children with acute bacterial infections" *Clin Pediatr* 2004;43(3): 239–249.

Sehnert K. "The garden within." *Health World Mag* 1989;9.

Sekine K, Ohta J, et al. "Analysis of antitumor properties of effector cells stimulated with a cell wall preparation (WPG) of *Bifidobacterium infantis*." *Biol Pharm Bull* 1995;18(1):148–153.

Sellars RL. "Acidophilus product." *Therapeutic Properties of Fermented Milks*. London, UK: Elsevier Applied Science, 1991.

Seppo L, Tauhiainen J, et al. "A fermented milk high in bioactive peptides has a blood pressure-lowering effect in hypertensive subjects." *Am J Clin Nutr* 2003;77(2):326–330.

Sghir A, Chow JM, Mackie RI. "Continuous culture selection of *Bifidobacteria* and *Lactobacilli* from human fecal samples using fructooligosaccharide as a selective substrate." *J Appl Microbiol* 1994;84(4):769–777.

Van Niel CW, Feudtner C, et al. "*Lactobacillus* therapy for acute infectious diarrhea in children: A meta-analysis." *Pediatrics* 2002;109(4):678–684.

Chapter 6

Begley S. "The end of antibiotics." *Newsweek* 1994;Mar 28:46–51.

Bjarnason I, Haylla J, et al. "Side effects of non-steroidal anti-inflammatory drugs on the small and large intestine in humans." *Gastroenterology* 1993;104(6):1832–1847.

Bland J. *Preventive Medicine Update*. Audiotape. Gig Harbor, WA: HealthComm, 1994.

Chaitow L, Trenev N. *Probiotics*. London, UK: Thorsons Publications, 1990.

Crook W. *The Yeast Connection and Women's Health*. Jackson, TN: Woman's Health Connection Inc., 2003.

Garrett L. *The Coming Plague*. New York, NY: Farrar, Straus, Giroux, 1994.

Koelz HR. "Ulcer prevention during anti-rheumatism therapy and in intensive medicine." *Schweizerische Rundschau fur Medizin Praxis* 1994;3(25–26):768–771.

Loosli AR. "Reversing sports-related iron and zinc deficiencies." *Physician Sportsmed* 1993;21(6):70–78.

MacKay D. "Can CAM therapies help reduce antibiotic resistance?" *Altern Med Rev* 2003;8(1):28–42.

McBride J. "Nutrient deficiency unleashes Jekyll-Hyde virus." *Ag Res* 1994;42(8): 14–16.

Mitsuoka T. "Intestinal flora and aging." *Nutr Rev* 1992;50(12):438–446.

Tippett K, Goldman JD. "Diets more healthful, but still fall short of dietary guidelines." *Food Rev* 1994;17(1):8–14.

Trowbridge J, Walker M. *The Yeast Syndrome*. New York, NY: Bantam Books, 1986.

Chapter 7

Aihara H. *Acid and Alkaline*. Oroville, CA: George Ohsawa Macrobiotic Foundation, 1986.

Brown SE, Jaffe R. "Acid-alkaline balance and its effect on bone health." *Intl J Integ Med* 2000;2(6).

Jaffe R. *Guided Health: A Constant Professional Reference*. Sterling, VA: Health Studies Collegium, 1993.

Jaffe R, Brown S, et al. *The Alkaline Way: Your Health Restoration*. Sterling, VA: ELISA-ACT Biotechnologies, 2004.

First Morning Urine pH after Rest and *Food and Chemical Effects on Acid/Alkaline Body Chemical Balance*. Sterling, VA: ELISA-ACT Biotechnologies, 2004.

Quilin P, Quilin N. *Beating Cancer with Nutrition*. Tulsa, OK: Nutrition Times Press, Inc., 1994.

Wiley R. *BioBalance*. Tacoma, WA: Life Sciences Press, 1989.

Chapter 8

Batmanghelidj F. *Your Body's Many Cries for Water.* Falls Church, VA: Global Health, 1992.

Carbonaro M, Mattera M, et al. "Modulation of antioxidant compounds in organic vs. conventional fruit." *J Ag Food Chem* 2002;50(19):5458–5462.

Carper J. *The Food Pharmacy.* New York: Bantam Books, 1989.

Constant J, Jaffe R. "The role of eggs, margarines and fish oils in the nutritional management of coronary artery disease and strokes." *Keio J Med* 2004;53(3):131–136.

Dallongeville J, Yarnell J, et al. "Fish consumption is associated with lower heart rates." *Circulation* 2004;109(9):e155–e156.

Donadio JV, Grande JP. "The role of fish oil/omega-3 fatty acids in the treatment of IgA nephropathy." *Semin Nephrol* 2004;24(3):225–243.

Donovan P, Jaffe R. *Guided Health: A Constant Professional Reference.* Reston, VA: Health Studies Collegium, 1993.

Eades MR, Eades MD. *Protein Power: The High-Protein/Low-Carbohydrate Way to Lose Weight, Feel Fit, and Boost Your Health—in Just Weeks!* New York: Bantam Books, 1997.

Jude S, Roger S, et al. "Dietary long-chain omega-3 fatty acids of marine origin: A comparison of their protective effects on coronary heart disease and breast cancers." *Prog Biophys Mol Biol* July 2005.

Kromhout D. "N-3 fatty acids and coronary heart disease: Epidemiology from Eskimos to Western populations." *J Intern Med Suppl* 1989;731:47–51.

Lappe FM. *Diet for a Small Planet.* New York: Ballantine Books, 1991.

MacKay D. "Can CAM therapies help reduce antibiotic resistance?" *Altern Med Rev* 2003;8(1):28–42.

Robbins J. *Diet for a New America.* Walpole, NH: Stillpoint Publishing, 1987.

Robbins J. *May All Be Fed.* Walpole, NH: Stillpoint Publishing, 1987.

Shauss A. "Dietary fish oil consumption and fish oil supplementation." In Pizzorno J and Murray M, editors, *A Textbook for Natural Medicine.* New York 1991, pp. 1–7.

Shnayerson M, Plotkin M. *The Killers Within: The Deadly Rise of Drug-Resistant Bacteria.* Boston: Little, Brown and Co., 2002.

Simopoulos AP. "The traditional diet of Greece and cancer." *Eur J Cancer Prev* 2004;13(3):219–230.

Young G, Conquer J. "Omega-3 fatty acids and neuropsychiatric disorders." *Reprod Nutr Dev* 2005;45(1):1–28.

Chapter 9

Dabrowski K, Lee KJ, et al. "Gossypol isomers bind specifically to blood plasma proteins and spermatozoa of rainbow trout fed diets containing cottonseed meal." *Biochim Biophys Acta* 2001;1525(1–2):37–42.

Kalla NR, Vasudev M. "Studies on the male antifertility agent gossypol acetic acid: *In vitro* studies on the effect of gossypol acetic acid on human spermatozoa." *IRCS J Med Sci* 1980;8(6):375–376.

Qiu J, Levin LR, et al. "Different pathways of cell killing by gossypol enantiomers." *Exp Biol Med* 2002;227(6):398–401.

Tso WW, Lee CS. "Cottonseed—a source of vaginal contraceptive (author's translation)." *Contracept Fertil Sex* 1982;10(7–8):465–468.

Chapter 10

Griffin KW, Botvin GJ, et al. "Parenting practices as predictors of substance use, delinquency, and aggression among urban minority youth: Moderating effects of family structure and gender." *Psychol Addict Behav* 2000;14(2):174–184.

International and American Association of Clinical Nutritionists. *Nutritional Advancements in Pediatric and Adolescent Care.* Conference proceedings, New Orleans, LA, 2004.

Johnsen CR. *Moms, Babies, and Breastfeeding.* Springfield, MA: 1st Books Publishing, 2003.

Mayoclinic.com. "Infant feeding and nutrition: Your newborn's needs." Nov 2004. Available at www.cnn.com/HEALTH/library/PR/00057.html.

Rapp D. *Is This Your Child?* New York, NY: Quill/William Morrow, 1991.

Satter E. *Child of Mine: Feeding with Love and Good Sense.* Palo Alto, CA: Bull Publishing Co., 1983.

Sears W. *The Family Nutrition Book: Everything You Need to Know about Feeding Your Children—From Birth through Adolescence.* New York, NY: Little, Brown, 1999.

University of Rhode Island Cooperative Extension. "Feeding the infant." *Expanded Food and Nutrition Program.* Available at www.uri.edu/ce/efnep/Infant percent20Feeding percent20p.1.htm.

Chapter 11

Bland J. *Applying New Essentials in Nutritional Medicine.* Gig Harbor, WA: Health Comm, 1995.

Bland J. *New Perspectives in Nutritional Therapies.* Gig Harbor, WA: Health Comm, 1996.

Caress SM, Steinemann AC. "Prevalence of multiple chemical sensitivities: A population-based study in the southeastern United States." *Am J Pub Health* 2004;94(5): 746–747.

Casmir G. "Anaphylaxis and food allergy in children: A major problem in public health." *Bull Mem Acad R Med Belg* 2004;159(7–9):425–433.

Golos N. *If This Is Tuesday, It Must Be Chicken.* New Canaan, CT: Keats Publishing, 1983.

International and American Association of Clinical Nutritionists. *Nutritional Advancements in Pediatric and Adolescent Care.* Conference proceedings, New Orleans, LA, 2004.

Kreutzer R, Neutra RR, Lashuay N. "Prevalence of people reporting sensitivities to chemicals in a population-based survey." *Am J Epidemiol* 1999;150:1–12.

Randolph T, Moss R. *An Alternative Approach to Allergies: The New Field of Clinical Ecology Unravels the Environmental Causes of Mental and Physical Ills.* New York, NY: Perennial Publishing, 1990.

Rapp D. *Is This Your Child?* New York, NY: Quill/William Morrow, 1991.

Chapter 12

Bahna SL. "Unusual presentations of food allergy." *Ann Allergy Asthma Immunol* 2001;86:414–420.

D'Adamo P. *Eat Right for Your Type.* New York, NY: Putnam Publishing Group, 1997.

Dagci H, Ustun S, et al. "Protozoon infections and intestinal permeability." *Acta Tropica* 2002;81:1–5.

Diebel LN, Liberati DM, et al. "Enterocyte apoptosis and barrier function are modulated by SIgA after exposure to bacteria and hypoxia/reoxygenation." *Surgery* 2003;134(4):574–580.

ELISA-ACT Handbook. Reston, VA: Serammune Physicians Lab, 1994.

Galland L. *Solving the Digestive Puzzle.* Great Smokies Diagnostic Lab and HealthComm International conference manual, San Francisco, CA, May 1995.

Guide to Health. Fort Lauderdale, FL: ImmunoLaboratories, Inc., 1994.

"Gut hyperpermeability." *Serammune Physicians Lab Newsletter* 1992 Jan;2(1).

Hang CH, Shi JX, et al. "Alterations of intestinal mucosa structure and barrier function following traumatic brain injury in rats." *World J Gastroenterol* 2003;9(12):2776–2781.

Holden W, Orchard T, Wordsworth P. "Enteropathic arthritis." *Rheum Dis Clin North Am* 2003;29(3):513–530, viii.

Hollander D. "Intestinal permeability, leaky gut, and intestinal disorders." *Curr Gastroenterol Rep* 1999;1(5):410–416.

Jaffe R, DeVane J, et al. *The Alkaline Way: Your Health Restoration.* Reston, VA: ELISA-ACT Biotechnologies LLC, 2004.

Kashavarzian A, Choudhary S, et al. "Preventing gut leakiness by oats supplementation ameliorates alcohol-induced liver damage in rats." *J Pharm Exp Therap* 2001;229(2): 442–448.

"The leaky gut." *Great Smokies Digest* 1990 summer;4.

Lipski E. *Leaky Gut Syndrome.* Los Angeles, CA: Keats Publishing, 1998.

Marks D, Marks L. "Food allergy: Manifestations, evaluation and management." *Postgrad Med* 1993;93(2):191–201.

Ren H, Musch MW, et al. "Short-chain fatty acids induce intestinal epithelial heat shock protein 25 expression in rats and IEC 18 cells." *Gastroenterology* 2001;121:631–639.

Ryan CM, Yarmush ML, et al. "Increased gut permeability early after burns correlates with the extent of burn injury." *Crit Care Med* 1992;20(11):1508–1512.

Schmitz H, Barmeyer C, et al. "Altered tight junction structure contributes to the impaired epithelial barrier function in ulcerative colitis." *Gastroenterology* 1999;116(2):301–309.

Sturniolo GC, Fries W, et al. "Effect of zinc supplementation on intestinal permeability in experimental colitis." *J Lab Clin Med* 2002;138(5):311–315.

Suenaert P, Bulteel V, et al. "Anti-tumor necrosis factor treatment restores the gut barrier in Crohn's disease." *Am J Gastroenterol* 2002;97(8):2000–2004.

Swanson M. *Comprehensive Digestive Stool Analysis and Intestinal Permeability.* Audiotape. Asheville, NC: Great Smokies Diagnostic Lab, 1993.

Trenev N. "Probiotics." Lecture, California State Chapter Meeting of the International and American Association of Clinical Nutritionists, Los Angeles, CA, April 1994.

Weber P, Brune T, et al. "Gastrointestinal symptoms and permeability in patients with juvenile idiopathic arthritis." *Clin Exp Rheumatol* 2003;21(5):657–662.

Chapter 13

Cradle-Cap and Eczema

Bateman B, Warner JO, et al. "The effects of a double blind, placebo controlled, artificial food colourings and benzoate preservative challenge on hyperactivity in a general population sample of preschool children." *Arch Dis Child* 2004;89(6):506–511.

Breuer K, Heratizadeh A, et al. "Late eczematous reactions to food in children with atopic dermatitis." *Clin Exp Allergy* 2004;34(5):817–824.

Burks WA, James J, et al. "Atopic dermatitis and food hypersensitivity reactions." *J Ped* 1998;132:132–136.

Horrobin DF. "Essential fatty acid metabolism and its modification in atopic eczema." *Am J Clin Nutr* 2000;71(1 suppl):367S–372S.

Kalimo K. "Yeast allergy in adult atopic dermatitis." *Immunological Pharmacological Aspects* 1991;4:164–167.

Khoo J, Shek L, et al. "Pattern of sensitization to common environmental allergens amongst atopic Singapore children in the first 3 years of life." *Asian Pac J Allergy Immunol* 2001;19(4):225–229.

Oliwiecki S, Burton JL, et al. "Levels of essential and other fatty acids in plasma and red cell phospholipids from normal controls and patients with atopic eczema." *Acta Derm Venereol* 1990;71:224–228.

Patzelt-Wenczler R, Ponce-Poschl E. "Proof of efficacy of Kamillosan® cream in atopic eczema." *Eur J Med Res* 2000;5(4):171–175.

Rosenfeldt V, Benfeldt E, et al. "Effect of probiotic *Lactobacillus* strains in children with atopic dermatitis." *J Allergy Clin Immunol* 2003;111(2):389–395.

Saeedi M, Morteza-Semnani K, Ghoreishi MR. "The treatment of atopic dermatitis with licorice gel." *J Dermatolog Treat* 2003;14(3):153–157.

Sampson HA. "The immunopathogenic role of food hypersensitivity in atopic dermatitis." *Acta Derm Venereol Suppl* 1992;176:34–37.

Sazanova NE, Varnacheva LN, et al. "Immunological aspects of food intolerance in children during first years of life." *Pediatriia* 1992;(3):14–18.

Soyland E, Lea T, et al. "Dietary supplementation with very long chain omega-3 fatty acids in patients with atopic dermatitis." *Br J Dermatol* 1994;130:757–764.

Tan BB, Weald D, et al. "Double-blind controlled trial of effect of housedust-mite allergen avoidance on atopic dermatitis." *Lancet* 1996;347:15–18.

Turjanmaa K. "'Atopy patch tests' in the diagnosis of delayed food hypersensitivity." *Allerg Immunol* 2002;34(3):95–97.

Werbach W. *Healing with Nutrition.* New York, NY: Harper Collins, 1993.

Projectile Vomiting

Hauben M, Amsden GW. "The association of erythromycin and infantile hypertrophic pyloric stenosis: Causal or coincidental?" *Drug Safety* 2002;25(13):929–942.

Rosenman MB, Mahon BE, et al. "Oral erythromycin prophylaxis vs. watchful waiting in caring for newborns exposed to *Chlamydia trachomatis.*" *Arch Pediatr Adolesc Med* 2003;157(6):565–571.

Sorensen HT, Skriver MV, et al. "Risk of infantile hypertrophic pyloric stenosis after maternal postnatal use of macrolides." *Scand J Infect Dis* 2003;35(2):104–106.

Ventura A, Pineschi A, et al. "Cow's milk intolerance and abdominal surgery: A puzzling connection." *Helv Paediatr Acta* 1986;41(6):487–494.

Ear Infection

American Academy of Pediatrics, American Academy of Physicians, et al. *Clinical Practice Guideline: Diagnosis and Management of Acute Otitis Media.* March 2004.

"Larch arabinogalactan." *Altern Med Rev* 2000;5(5):463–466.

MacKay D. "Can CAM therapies help reduce antibiotic resistance?" *Altern Med Rev* 2003;8(1):28–42.

"Otitis media with effusion." *Pediatrics* 2004;113(5):1412–1429.

Sarrell EM, Mandelberg A, et al. "Efficacy of naturopathic extracts in the management of ear pain associated with acute otitis media." *Arch Pediatr Adolesc Med* 2001;155(7): 796–799.

Schmidt M. *Childhood Ear Infections.* Berkeley, CA: North Atlantic Books, 1990.

Hirschsprung's Disease

Urao M, Fujimoto T, et al. "Does probiotics administration decrease serum endotoxin levels in infants?" *J Pediatr Surg* 1999;34(2):273–276.

Chapter 14

Canker Sores/Mouth Ulcers

Malstrom M, Salo OP, Fyhrquist F. "Immunogenetic markers and immune response in patients with recurrent oral ulceration." *Int J Oral Surg* 1983;12(1):23–30.

Nolan A, McIntosh WB, et al. "Recurrent apthous ulceration: Vitamin B_1, B_2, and B_6 status and response to replacement therapy." *J Oral Pathol Med* 1991;20(8):389–391.

O'Farrelly C, O'Mahoney C, et al. "Gliadin antibodies identify gluten-sensitive oral ulceration in the absence of villous atrophy." *J Oral Pathol Med* 1991;20(10):476–478.

Palopoli J, Waxman J. "Recurrent apthous stomatitis and vitamin B_{12} deficiency." *South Med J* 1990;83(4):475–477.

Porter SR, Scully C, Flint S. "Hematologic status in recurrent apthous stomatitis compared with other oral disease." *Med Oral Pathol* 1988;66(1):41–44.

Walker DM, Dolbie AE, et al. "Effect of gluten-free diet on recurrent apthous ulceration." *Br J Dermatol* 1980;103(1):111.

Wang SW, Li HK, et al. "The trace element zinc and apthosis: The determination of plasma zinc and the treatment of apthosis with zinc." *Rev Stomatol Chirur Maxillo-Faciale* 1986;87(5):339–343.

Wray D. "Gluten-sensitive recurrent arthritis stomatitis." *Dig Dis Sci* 1981;26(8): 737–740.

Eosinophilic Esophagitis and Eosinophilic Gastroenteritis

Feuer J. "Study in the *New England Journal of Medicine* identifies rapidly rising disorder." Cincinnati Children's Hospital Medical Center press release, Cincinnati, OH, 2004.

Liacouras CA, Ruchelli E. "Eosinophilic esophagitis." *Curr Opin Pediatr* 2004;16(5): 560–566.

Lim JR, Gupta SK, et al. "White specks in the esophageal mucosa: An endoscopic manifestation of non-reflux eosinophilic esophagitis in children." *Gastrointest Endosc* 2004;59(7):835–838.

Sant'Anna AM, Rolland S, et al. "Eosinophilic esophagitis in children: Symptoms, histology and pH probe results." *J Pediatr Gastroenterol Nutr* 2004;39(4):373–377.

Gastroesophageal Reflux and/or Hiatal Hernia

Boyle JT. "Acid secretion from birth to adulthood." *J Pediatr Gastroenterol Nutr* 2003; 37(suppl 1):S12–S16.

Fukai T, Marumo A, et al. "Anti-*Helicobacter pylori* flavonoids from licorice extract." *Life Sci* 2002;71(12):1449–1463.

Levine A, Milo T, et al. "Influence of *Helicobacter pylori* eradication on gastroesophageal reflux symptoms and epigastric pain in children and adolescents." *Pediatrics* 2004; 113:54–58.

Nelson SP, Chen EH, et al. "Prevalence of symptoms of gastroesophageal reflux during childhood: A pediatric practice-based survey. Pediatric Practice Research Group." *Arch Pediatr Adolesc Med* 2000;154(2):150–154.

Nielsen RG, Bindslev-Jensen C, et al. "Severe gastroesophageal reflux disease and cow milk hypersensitivity in infants and children: Disease association and evaluation of a new challenge procedure." *J Pediatr Gastroenterol Nutr* 2004;39(4):383–391.

Chapter 15

Celiac Diseases/Sprue/Gluten Intolerance

Catassi C, Ratsch IM, et al. "Celiac diseases in the year 2000: Exploring the iceburg." *Lancet* 1994;343:200–203.

Fasano A. "Celiac disease: How to handle a clinical chameleon." *N Engl J Med* 2003; 348:25.

Fasano A, Not T, et al. "Zonulin, a newly discovered modulator of intestinal permeability, and its expression in coeliac disease." *Lancet* 2001;358(9294):1729–1730.

Hollen E, Hogberg L, et al. "Antibodies to oat prolamines (avenins) in children with coeliac disease." *Scand J Gastroenterol* 2003;38(7):742–746.

Johnston SD, McMillan SA, et al. "A comparison of antibodies to tissue transglutaminase with conventional serological tests in the diagnosis of coeliac disease." *Eur J Gastroenterol Hepatol* 2003;15(9):1001–1004.

Kapur G, Patwari AK, et al. "Iron supplementation in children with celiac disease." *Indian J Pediatr* 2003;70(12):955–958.

Karnam US, Felder LR, Raskin JB. "Prevalence of occult celiac disease in patients with iron-deficiency anemia: A prospective study." *South Med J* 2004;97(1):30–34.

Lazzari R, Collina A, et al. "Sideropenic anemia and celiac disease." *Ped Med Chir* 1994;16(6):549–550.

Lundin KE, Nilsen EM, et al. "Oats induced villous atrophy in coeliac disease." *Gut* 2003;52(11):1649–1652.

Nielson D. "Gluten-sensitive enteropathy (celiac disease): more common than you think", *Amer. Family Physician* Dec 15, 2002, http://www.aafp.org/afp/20021215/2259.html.

O'Bryan T. "Neurological & cognitive complications of wheat sensitivity," IAACN Scientific Symposium, New Orleans, LA August 2004; Medline Plus, http://www.nlm.nih.gov/medlineplus/ency/article/000233.htm and WrongDiagnosis.com http://www.wrongdiagnosis.com/c/celiac_disease/symptoms.htm.

Prokopova L. "Celiac disease—a severe disease." *Vnitr Lek* 2003;49(6):474–481.

Storsrud S, Hulthen LR, Lenner RA. "Beneficial effects of oats in the gluten-free diet of adults with special reference to nutrient status, symptoms, and subjective experiences." *Br J Nutr* 2003;90(1):101–107.

Thompson T. "Oats and the gluten-free diet." *J Am Diet Assoc* 2003;103(3):376–379.

WrongDiagnosis.com; http://www.wrongdiagnosis.com/c/celiac_disease/symptoms.htm.

Flatulence/Intestinal Gas

Platel K, Srinivasan K. "Influence of dietary spices and their active principles on pancreatic digestive enzymes in albino rats." *Nahrung* 2000;44(1):42–46.

Parasitic Infection

Markell EK, Udkow MP. "*Blastocystic hominis:* Pathogen or fellow traveler?" *Am J Trop Med Hyg* 1986;35(5):1023–1026.

Phillipson JD, Wright CW. "Medicinal plants in tropical medicine: Medicinal plants against protozoal diseases." *Trans Royal Soc Trop Med Hyg* 1991;85:18–21.

Sky PR. "Of parasites and pollens." *Discover* 1993 Sep;14(9):56–62.

Chapter 16

Diarrhea

Alam NH, Ashraf H. "Treatment of infectious diarrhea in children." *Paediatr Drugs* 2003;5(3):151–165.

Bolin TD, Davis AE, Duncombe VM. "A prospective study of persistent diarrhea." *Aus/NZ J Med* 1982;12(1):22–26.

Wilson JM. "Hand washing reduces diarrhea episodes: A study in Lombok, Indonesia." *Trans Royal Soc Trop Med Hyg* 1991;85:819–821.

Constipation

Benninga MA, Buller HA, et al. "Biofeedback training in chronic constipation." *Arch Dis Child* 1993;68:126–129.

Bleijenberg G, Kuijpers HC. "Biofeedback treatment of constipation: A comparison of two methods." *Am J Gastroenterol* 1994;89(7):1021–1026.

Constipation Fact Sheet. Publication no. 92-2754. Washington, DC: National Institutes of Health, National Institute of Diabetes and Digestive and Kidney Diseases, 1992.

Iwai N, Iwata G, et al. "Is a new biofeedback therapy effective for fecal incontinence in patients who have anorectal malformations?" *J Ped Surg* 1997;32(11):1626–1629.

Loening-Baucke V. "Prevalence, symptoms and outcome of constipation in infants and toddlers." *J Pediatr* 2005;146(3):359–363.

Lundblad B, Hellstrom AL. "Perceptions of school toilets as a cause for irregular toilet habits among schoolchildren aged 6 to 16 years." *J Sch Health* 2005;75(4):125–128.

McRorie JW, Daggy BP, et al. "Psyllium is superior to docusate sodium for treatment of chronic constipation." *Aliment Pharmacol Ther* 1998;12:491–497.

Chapter 17

Inflammatory Bowel Disease

Ammon HP. "Boswellic acids (components of frankincense) as the active principle in treatment of chronic inflammatory diseases." *Wien Med Wochenschr* 2002;152(15–16): 373–378.

Aslan A, Triadafilopoulos G. "Fish oil fatty acid supplementation and active ulcerative colitis: A double-blind, placebo-controlled crossover study." *Am J Gastroenterol* 1992; 87(4):432–433.

Babbs CF. "Oxygen radicals in ulcerative colitis." *Free Rad Biol Med* 1992;13(2): 169–181.

Ben-Arye E, Goldin E, et al. "Wheat grass juice in the treatment of active distal ulcerative colitis: A randomized double-blind placebo-controlled trial." *Scand J Gastroenterol* 2002;37(4):444–449.

Biasco G, Zannoni U, et al. "Folic acid supplementation and cell kinetics of rectal mucosa in patients with ulcerative colitis." *Cancer Epidem Biomarkers Prev* 1997;6: 469–471.

Borrelli O, Bascietto C, et al. "Infliximab heals intestinal inflammatory lesions and restores growth in children with Crohn's disease." *Dig Liver Dis* 2004;36(5):342–347.

Borody TJ, Warren EF, et al. "Treatment of ulcerative colitis using fecal bacteriotherapy." *J Clin Gastroenterol* 2003;37(1):42–47.

Candy S, Borok G, et al. "The value of an elimination diet in the management of patients with ulcerative colitis." *S Afr Med J* 1995;83(11):1176–1179.

Chen W, Li D, et al. "High prevalence of *Mycoplasma pneumoniae* in intestinal mucosal biopsies from patients with inflammatory bowel disease and controls." *Dig Dis Sci* 2001;46(11):2529–2535.

"Crohn's disease linked to measles." *Med Trib* 1993; May 13:10.

Davis RL, Bohlke K. "Measles vaccination and inflammatory bowel disease: Controversy laid to rest?" *Drug Safety* 2001;24(13):939–946.

De Ridder L, Escher JC, et al. "Infliximab therapy in 30 patients with refractory pediatric Crohn disease with and without fistulas in The Netherlands." *J Pediatr Gastroenterol Nutr* 2004;39(1):46–52.

Dieleman LA, Heizer WD. "Nutritional issues in inflammatory bowel disease." *Gastroenterol Clin North Am* 1998;27(2):435–451.

Fernandez-Banares F, Cabre E, et al. "Enteral nutrition as a primary therapy in Crohn's disease." *Gut* 1994;35(1suppl):S55–S59.

Floch MH. "Probiotics, irritable bowel syndrome, and inflammatory bowel disease." *Curr Treat Options Gastroenterol* 2003;6(4):283–288.

Gaby A, Wright J. "Ulcerative colitis." *Nutr Healing Newsletter* 1995;2(1).

Gil A. "Is eicosapentaenoic acid useful in the treatment of ulcerative colitis in children?" *J Pediatr Gastroenterol Nutr* 2003;37(5):536–537.

Gottschall E. *Food and the Gut Reaction.* Kirkton, Ontario: Kirkton Press, 1986.

Gross V, Arndt H, et al. "Free radicals and inflammatory bowel diseases: Pathophysiology and therapeutic implications." *Hepatogastroenterology* 1994;41:320–327.

Gryboski JD. "Ulcerative colitis in children 10 years old or younger." *J Ped Gastroenterol Nutr* 1993;17(1):24–31.

Gupta I, Parihar A, et al. "Effects of *Boswellia serrata* gum resin in patients with ulcerative colitis." *Eur J Med Res* 1997;2(1):37–43.

Hanauer SB. "Inflammatory bowel disease: Novel aspects of clinical genetics and potential for probiotic therapy." *Medscape* 2002. Available at www.medscape.com/ viewarticle/434522.

Hanauer SB, Peppercorn MA, Present DH. "Current concepts, new therapies in IBD." *Patient Care* 1992;26(13):79–102.

Head KA, Jurenka JS. "Inflammatory bowel disease part 1: Ulcerative colitis—pathophysiology and conventional and alternative treatment options." *Altern Med Rev* 2003;8(3):247–283.

Hotz J, Plein K. "Effectiveness of plantago seed husks in comparison with wheat bran on stool frequency and manifestations of irritable colon syndrome with constipation." *Medizin Klin* 1994;89(12):645–651.

Jian YT, Wang JD, et al. "Modulation of intestinal mucosal inflammatory factors by curcumin in rats with colitis." *Di Yi Jun Yi Da Xue Xue Bao* 2004;24(12):1353–1358.

Karlinger K, Gyorke T, et al. "The epidemiology and the pathogenesis of inflammatory bowel disease." *Eur J Radiol* 2000;35(3):154–167.

Kruis W, Fric P, et al. "Maintaining remission of ulcerative colitis with the probiotic *Escherichia coli* Nissle 1917 is as effective as with standard mesalazine." *Gut* 2004; 53(11):1617–1623.

Langmead L, Feakins RM, et al. "Randomized, double-blind, placebo-controlled trial of oral *Aloe vera* gel for active ulcerative colitis." *Aliment Pharmacol Ther* 2004;19(7): 739–747.

Langmead L, Makins RJ, et al. "Anti-inflammatory effects of *Aloe vera* gel in human colorectal mucosa *in vitro*." *Aliment Pharmacol Ther* 2004;19(5):521–527.

Lichtenstein GR, MacDermott RP. "Recent advances in the treatment of inflammatory bowel disease: The role of biologics and immunodulators." *Medscape* 2002. Available at www.medscape.com/viewarticle/434521.

Mylonaki M, Langmead L, et al. "Enteric infection in relapse of inflammatory bowel disease: Importance of microbiological examination of stool." *Eur J Gastroenterol Hepatol* 2004;16(8):775–778.

Nellist CC. "Elemental diet therapy a good option for Crohn's." *Fam Pract News* 1994;1:7.

Reinisch W, Nahavandi H, et al. "Extracorporeal photochemotherapy in patients with steroid-dependent Crohn's disease: A prospective pilot study." *Aliment Pharmacol Ther* 2001;15:1313–1322.

Robinson RJ, Krzywicki T, et al. "Effect of a low-impact exercise program on bone mineral density in Crohn's disease: A randomized controlled trial." *Gastroenterology* 1998; 115:36–41.

Roediger WEW. "Decreased sulfur amino acid intake in ulcerative colitis." *Lancet* 1998; 351:1555.

Salh B, Assi K, et al. "Curcumin attenuates DNB-induced murine colitis." *Am J Physiol Gastrointest Liver Physiol* 2003;285(1):G235–G243.

Satsangi J, Morecroft J, et al. "Genetics of inflammatory bowel disease: Scientific and clinical implications." *Best Pract Res Clin Gastroenterol* 2003;17(1):3–18.

Seigel J. "Inflammatory bowel disease: Another possible effect of the allergic diathesis." *Ann Allergy* 1981;47(2):92–94.

Shanahan F. "Host-flora interactions in inflammatory bowel disease." *Inflamm Bowel Dis* 2004 Feb;10(suppl 1):S16–S24.

Tamboli CP, Neut C, et al. "Dysbiosis in inflammatory bowel disease." *Gut* 2004; 53(1):1–4.

Thompson NP, Montgomery SM, et al. "Is measles vaccination a risk factor for inflammatory bowel disease?" *Lancet* 1995;345:1071–1074.

Ukil A, Maity S, et al. "Curcumin, the major component of food flavour turmeric, reduces mucosal injury in trinitrobenzene sulphonic acid-induced colitis." *Br J Pharmacol* 2003; 139(2):209–218.

Vierhapper H, Nowotny P, et al. "Prevalence of hypergastrinemia in patients with hyper- and hypothyroidism: Impact for calcitonin?" *Horm Res* 2002;57(3–4):85–89.

Irritable Bowel Syndrome

Baran E, Dupont C. "Modification of intestinal permeability during food provocation procedures in pediatric irritable bowel syndrome." *J Ped Gastroenterol Nutr* 1990;11:72–77.

Bazzocchi G, Gionchetti P, et al. "Intestinal microflora and oral bacteriotherapy in irritable bowel syndrome." *Dig Liver Dis* 2002;34(suppl 2):S48–S53.

Born P, Vierling T, et al. "Fructose malabsorption and irritable bowel syndrome." *Gastroenterology* 1991;101(5):1454.

Borok G. "Irritable bowel syndrome and diet." *Gastroenterol Forum* 1994;29.

Dunlop SP, Jenkins D, Spiller RC. "Distinctive clinical, psychological, and histological features of postinfective irritable bowel syndrome." *Am J Gastroenterol* 2003;98(7): 1578–1583.

Dunlop SP, Jenkins D, et al. "Relative importance of enterochromaffin cell hyperplasia, anxiety, and depression in postinfectious IBS." *Gastroenterology* 2003;125(6): 1651–1659.

Fernandez-Banares F, Esteve-Pardo M, et al. "Role of fructose-sorbitol malabsorption and irritable bowel syndrome." *Gastroenterology* 1991;101(5):1453–1454.

Floch MH. "Probiotics, irritable bowel syndrome, and inflammatory bowel disease." *Curr Treat Options Gastroenterol* 2003;6(4):283–288.

Francis CW, Whorwell PJ, et al. "Bran and irritable bowel syndrome: Time for reappraisal." *Lancet* 1994;334:339–340.

Gershon MD. "Serotonin and its implication for the management of irritable bowel syndrome." *Rev Gastroenterol Disord* 2003;3(suppl 2):S25–S34.

Hanaway P. "Irritable bowel syndrome: An integrated approach to 'gut feelings.'" *Integr Med* 2004;3(5):16–21.

Hotz J, Plein K. "Effectiveness of plantago seed husks in comparison with wheat bran on stool frequency and manifestations of irritable colon syndrome with constipation." *Medizin Klin* 1994;89(12):645–651.

Kim HJ, Camilleri M, et al. "A randomized controlled trial of a probiotic, VSL#3, on gut transit and symptoms in diarrhoea-predominant irritable bowel syndrome." *Aliment Pharmacol Ther* 2003;17(7):895–904.

Moukarzel AA, Lesicka H, et al. "Irritable bowel syndrome and nonspecific diarrhea in infancy and childhood—relationship with juice carbohydrate malabsorption." *Clin Pediatr* 2002;41(3):145–150.

Rumessen JJ. "Functional bowel disease: The role of fructose and sorbitol." *Gastroenterology* 1991;101:1452–1460.

Vernia P, et al. "Lactose intolerance and irritable bowel syndrome: Relative weight in inducing abdominal symptoms in high-prevalence area." *Gastroenterology* 1992;102(4 part 11):A5 3 0.

Vernia P, Di Camillo M, Marinaro V. "Lactose malabsorption, irritable bowel syndrome and self-reported milk intolerance." *Dig Liver Dis* 2001;33(3):234–239.

Vernia P, Marinaro V, et al. "Self-reported milk intolerance in irritable bowel syndrome: What should we believe?" *Clin Nutr* 2004;23(5):996–1000.

Vernia P, Ricciardi MR, et al. "Lactose malabsorption and irritable bowel syndrome. Effect of a long-term lactose-free diet." *Ital J Gastroenterol* 1995;27(3):117–121.

Chapter 18

Abrams SA, Lipnick RN, et al. "Calcium absorption and metabolism in children with juvenile rheumatoid arthritis assessed using stable isotopes." *J Rheumatol* 1993;20(7): 1196–1200.

Alpigiani MG, Ravera G, et al. "The use of n-3 fatty acids in chronic juvenile arthritis [article in Italian]." *Pediatr Med Chir* 1996;18(4):387–390.

Banerjee M, Tripathi LM, et al. "Modulation of inflammatory mediators by ibuprofen and curcumin treatment during chronic inflammation in rat." *Immunopharmacol Immunotoxicol* 2003;25(2):213–224.

Chang DM, Chang WY, et al. "The effects of traditional antirheumatic herbal medicines on immune response cells." *J Rheumatol* 1997;24(3):436–441.

Curtis CL, Hughes CE, et al. "N-3 fatty acids specifically modulate catabolic factors involved in articular cartilage degradation." *J Biol Chem* 2000;275(2):721–724.

Espersen GT, Grunnet N, et al. "Decreased interleukin-1 beta levels in plasma from rheumatoid arthritis patients after dietary supplementation with n-3 polyunsaturated fatty acids." *Clin Rheumatol* 1992;11(3):393–395.

Flynn M. "The effect of folate and cobalamine on osteoarthritis and hands." *J Am Coll Nutr* 1994;13(4):351–356.

Gaby AR. "Natural treatments for osteoarthritis." *Altern Med Rev* 1999;4(5):330–341.

Gotia S, Popovici I, et al. "Antioxidant enzyme levels in children with juvenile rheumatoid arthritis." *Rev Med Chir Soc Med Nat Iasi* 2001;105(3):499–503.

Hatakka K, Martio J, et al. "Effects of probiotic therapy on the activity and activation of mild rheumatoid arthritis—a pilot study." *Scand J Rheumatol* 2003;32(4):211–215.

Haugen M, Kjeldsen-Kragh J, et al. "Diet and disease symptoms in rheumatic diseases—results of a questionnaire-based survey." *Clin Rheumatol* 1991;10(4):401–407.

Helgeland M, Svendsen E, et al. "Dietary intake and serum concentrations of antioxidants in children with juvenile arthritis." *Clin Exp Rheumatol* 2000;18(5):637–641.

Henderson CJ, Cawkwell GD, et al. "Predictors of total body bone mineral density in non-corticosteroid-treated prepubertal children with juvenile rheumatoid arthritis." *Arthr Rheum* 1997;40(11):1967–1975.

Ho LJ. "Chinese herbs as immunomodulators and potential disease-modifying antirheumatic drugs in autoimmune disorders." *Curr Drug Metab* 2004;5(2):181–192.

Holden W, Orchard T, Wordsworth P. "Enteropathic arthritis." *Rheum Dis Clin North Am* 2003;29(3):513–530, viii.

Horrobin DF. "Essential fatty acid and prostaglandin metabolism in Sjogren's syndrome, systemic sclerosis and rheumatoid arthritis." *Scand J Rheumatol* 1986;61(suppl): S242–S245.

James MJ, Gibson RA, et al. "Dietary polyunsaturated fatty acids and inflammatory mediator production." *Am J Clin Nutr* 2000;71(1 suppl):343S–348S.

Kamaeva OI, Reznikov P, et al. "Antigliadin antibodies in the absence of celiac disease." *Klin Med* 1998;76(2):33–35.

Katargina LA, Starikova AV, et al. "Clinical and pathogenetic significance of *Proteus mirabilis* antibodies in uveitis associated with joint lesions in children and adolescents." *Vestn Oftalmol* 2002;118(3):28–30.

Katz JP, GR Lichtenstein. "Rheumatologic manifestations of gastrointestinal diseases." *Gastroenterol Clin North Am* 1998;27(3):533–562, v.

Kimmatkar N, Thawani V, et al. "Efficacy and tolerability of *Boswellia serrata* extract in treatment of osteoarthritis of knee—a randomized double blind placebo controlled trial." *Phytomedicine* 2003;10(1):3–7.

Kjeldsen-Kraugh J. "Dietary treatment of rheumatoid arthritis." *Scand J Rheumatol* 1996:63.

Leirisalo-Repo M. "Enteropathic arthritis, Whipple's disease, juvenile spondyloarthropathy, and uveitis." *Curr Opin Rheumatol* 1994;6(4):385–390.

Lepore L, Pennesi M, et al. "Anti-alpha-gliadin antibodies are not predictive of celiac disease in juvenile chronic arthritis." *Acta Paediatr* 1993;82(6–7):569–573.

Leventhal LJ, Boyce EG, et al. "Treatment of rheumatoid arthritis with gamma-linolenic acid." *Ann Intern Med* 1993;119(9):867–873.

Lozovksaia LS, Soboleva VD, et al. "Etiological connection between juvenile rheumatoid arthritis and the chronic form of coxsackie virus infection." *Vopr Virusol* 1996;41(3): 122–126.

Mamadou M. "Cellular injury, part 2: Inflammation control and oral enzymes." *Transformation Enzyme Corporation Newsletter* 2003 Nov;12:1–6.

Machtey I. "Vitamin E and arthritis/vitamin E and rheumatoid arthritis." *Arthr Rheum* 1991;34(9):1205.

Min SY, Hwang SY, et al. "Increase of cyclooxygenase-2 expression by interleukin 15 in rheumatoid synoviocytes." *J Rheumatol* 2004;31(5):875–883.

Mulberg AE, Linz C, et al. "Identification of nonsteroidal anti-inflammatory drug-induced gastroduodenal injury in children with juvenile rheumatoid arthritis." *J Pediatr* 1993; 122(4):647–649.

Murray KJ, Moroldo MB, et al. "Age-specific effects of juvenile rheumatoid arthritis-associated HLA alleles." *Arthr Rheum* 1999;42(9):1843–1853.

Nielsen GL, Faarvang KL, et al. "The effects of dietary supplementation with N-3 polyunsaturated fatty acids in patients with rheumatoid arthritis." *Eur J Clin Invest* 1992; 22:687–691.

Petty RE. "Viruses and childhood arthritis." *Ann Med* 1997;29(2):149–152.

Picco P, Gattorno M, et al. "Increased gut permeability in juvenile chronic arthritides. A multivariate analysis of the diagnostic parameters." *Clin Exp Rheumatol* 2000;18(6): 773–778.

Ramos VA, Ramos PA, et al. "Role of oxidative stress in the maintenance of inflammation in patients with juvenile rheumatoid arthritis." *J Pediatr* 2000;76(2):125–132.

Rister M, Bauermeister K. "Superoxide-dismutase and superoxide-radical-release in rheumatoid arthritis (author's translation)." *Klin Wochenschr* 1982;60(11):561–565.

Sato M, Miyazaki T, et al. "Quercetin, a bioflavonoid, inhibits the induction of interleukin-8 and monocyte chemoattractant protein-1 expression by tumor necrosis factor-alpha in cultured human synovial cells." *J Rheumatol* 1997;24(9):1680–1684.

Seignalet J. "Diet, fasting, and rheumatoid arthritis." *Lancet* 1993;339:68–69.

Silverio Amancio OM, Alves Chaud DM, et al. "Copper and zinc intake and serum levels in patients with juvenile rheumatoid arthritis." *Eur J Clin Nutr* 2003;57(5):706–712.

Sklodowska M, Gromadzinska J, et al. "Vitamin E, thiobarbituric acid reactive substance concentrations and superoxide dismutase activity in the blood of children with juvenile rheumatoid arthritis." *Clin Exp Rheumatol* 1996;14(4):433–439.

Smith N, Cox L, et al. "Antibody responses to gut bacteria in ankylosing spondylitis, rheumatoid arthritis, Crohn's disease, and ulcerative colitis." *Rheumatol Int* 1997;17(1): 11–16.

Srivastava KC, Mustafa T. "Ginger [*Zingiber officinale*] in rheumatism and musculoskeletal disorders." *Med Hypotheses* 1992;39(4):342–348.

Sukenik S, Giryes H, et al. "Treatment of psoriatic arthritis at the Dead Sea." *J Rheumatol* 1994;21(7):1305–1309.

Sundrarjun T, Komindr S, et al. "Effects of n-3 fatty acids on serum interleukin-6, tumour necrosis factor-alpha and soluble tumour necrosis factor receptor p55 in active rheumatoid arthritis." *J Int Med Res* 2004;32(5):443–454.

Tao X, Cush JJ, et al. "A phase I study of ethyl acetate extract of the Chinese antirheumatic herb *Tripterygium wilfordii* hook F in rheumatoid arthritis." *J Rheumatol* 2001; 28(10):2160–2167.

Trock DH, Bollet AJ, et al. "A double-blind trial of the clinical effects of pulsed electromagnetic fields in osteoarthritis." *J Rheumatol* 1993;20(3):456–460.

Vargova V, Vesely R, et al. "Will administration of omega-3 unsaturated fatty acids reduce the use of nonsteroidal antirheumatic agents in children with chronic juvenile arthritis?" *Cas Lek Cesk* 1998;137(21):651–653.

Venkatraman JT, Chu WC. "Effects of dietary omega-3 and omega-6 lipids and vitamin E on serum cytokines, lipid mediators and anti-DNA antibodies in a mouse model for rheumatoid arthritis." *J Am Coll Nutr* 1999;18(6):602–613.

Warady BD, Lindsley CB, et al. "Effects of nutritional supplementation on bone mineral status of children with rheumatic diseases receiving corticosteroid therapy." *J Rheumatol* 1994;21(3):530–535.

Weber P, Brune T, et al. "Gastrointestinal symptoms and permeability in patients with juvenile idiopathic arthritis." *Clin Exp Rheumatol* 2003;21(5):657–662.

Chapter 19

Anibarro B, Caballero T, et al. "Asthma with sulfite intolerance in children: A blocking study with cyanocobalamin." *J Allergy Clin Immunol* 1992;90(1):103–109.

Bahna SL. "Unusual presentations of food allergy." *Ann Allergy Asthma Immunol* 2001; 86:414–420.

CDC, National Center for Environmental Health, "Asthma's impact on children and adolescents." http://www.edc.gov/nceh/airpollution/asthma/children.htm

Gumowski P, Lech B, et al. "Chronic asthma and rhinitis due to *Candida albicans,* Epidermophyton, and Trichophyton." *Ann Allergy* 1987;59(1):48–51.

Kalliomaki M, Salminen S, et al. "Probiotics in primary prevention of atopic disease: A randomised placebo-controlled trial." *Lancet* 2001;357(9262):1076–1079.

Khayyal MT, el-Gazalaly MA, et al. "A clinical pharmacological study of the potential beneficial effects of a propolis food product as an adjuvant in asthmatic patients." *Fundam Clin Pharmacol* 2003;17(1):93–102.

Li MH, Zhang HL, et al. "Effects of ginkgo leave concentrated oral liquor in treating asthma." *Zhongguo Zhong Xi Yi Jie He Za Zhi* 1997;17(4):216–218.

Matusiewicz R. "The homeopathic treatment of corticosteroid-dependent asthma: A double-blind, placebo-controlled study." *Biomed Ther* 1997;15(4):117–122.

Mellis CM. "Is asthma prevention possible with dietary manipulation?" *Med J Aust* 2002;177(suppl):S78–S80.

Merchant JA, Naleway AL, et al. "Asthma and farm exposures in a cohort of rural Iowa children." *Environmental Health Perspectives.* 2005 Mar;113(3):350–356.

Ramachandran S, Shah A, et al. "Allergic bronchopulmonary aspergillosis and *Candida albicans* colonization of the respiratory tract in corticosteroid-dependent asthma." *Asian Pac J Allergy Immunol* 1990;8(2):123–126.

Rance F, Micheau P, et al. "Food allergy and asthma in children." *Rev Pneumol Clin* 2003;59(2 pt 1):109–113.

Schmidt WP. "Model of the epidemic of childhood atopy." *Med Sci Monit* 2004; 10(2): HY5–HY9.

Woods RK, Walters EH, et al. "Food and nutrient intakes and asthma risk in young adults." *Am J Clin Nutr* 2003;78(3):414–421.

Chapter 20

Bilici M, Yildirim F, et al. "Double-blind, placebo-controlled study of zinc sulfate in the treatment of attention deficit hyperactivity disorder." *Prog Neuropsychopharmacol Biol Psychiatry* 2004;28(1):181–190.

Bland J. "Nutrition and allergy-related disorders in toddlers and children." *New Perspectives in Nutritional Therapies.* Gig Harbor, WA: Institute for Functional Medicine, 1996.

Boris J, Mandel FS. "Foods and additives are common causes of the attention deficit hyperactive disorder in children." *Ann Allergy* 1994;72(5):462–468.

Bornstein RA, Baker GB, et al. "Plasma amino acids in attention deficit disorder." *Psychiatry Res* 1990;33(3):301–306.

Carter CM, Urbanowicz M, et al. "Effects of a few food diet in attention deficit disorder." *Arch Disor Chil* 1993;69(5):564–568.

Hagerman RJ, Falkenstein AR. "An association between recurrent otitis media in infancy and later hyperactivity." *Clin Pediatr* 1987;26(5):253–257.

Harding KL, Judah RD, et al. "Outcome-based comparison of Ritalin versus food-supplement treated children with AD/HD." *Altern Med Rev* 2003;8(3):319–330.

Kidd PM. "Attention deficit/hyperactivity disorder (ADHD) in children: Rationale for its integrative management." *Altern Med Rev* 2000;5(5):402–428.

Kozielec T, Starobrat-Hermelin B. "Assessment of magnesium levels in children with attention deficit hyperactivity disorder (ADHD)." *Mag Res* 1997;10(2):143–148.

Lyon M, Cline J. "The effect of an oligoantigenic diet with or without a prescribed medical food product on the behavior and physiological parameters of children with attention deficit hyperactivity disorder." *Proceedings of the Sixth International Symposium on Functional Medicine.* Gig Harbor, WA: Institute for Functional Medicine, 1999.

Lyon MR, Cline JC, et al. "Effect of the herbal extract combination *Panax quinquefolium* and *Ginkgo biloba* on attention-deficit hyperactivity disorder: A pilot study." *J Psychiatry Neurosci* 2001;26(3):221–228.

"Magnesium reduces hyperactivity." *Autism Res Rev Int* 1998;12(2):4.

Newmark SC. "ADHD and food sensitivity." *Altern Ther Health Med* 2002;8(3):18, reply 18.

Pelsser LM, Buitelaar JK. "Favourable effect of a standard elimination diet on the behavior of young children with attention deficit hyperactivity disorder (ADHD): A pilot study." *Ned Tijdschr Geneeskd* 2002;146(52):2543–2547.

Richardson AJ, Montgomery P. "The Oxford-Durham study: A randomized, controlled trial of dietary supplementation with fatty acids in children with developmental coordination disorder." *Pediatrics* 2005;115(5):1360–1366.

Richardson AJ, Puri BK. "A randomized double-blind, placebo-controlled study of the effects of supplementation with highly unsaturated fatty acids on ADHD-related symptoms in children with specific learning difficulties." *Neuropsychopharmacol Biol Psychiatry* 2002;26:233–239.

Rowe KS. "Synthetic food colourings and 'hyperactivity': A double-blind crossover study." *Aust Paediatr J* 1988;24(2):143–147.

Scahill L, deGraft-Johnson A. "Food allergies, asthma, and attention deficit hyperactivity disorder." *J Child Adolesc Psychiatr Nurs* 1997;10(2):36–40.

Schnoll R, Burshteyn D, et al. "Nutrition in the treatment of attention-deficit hyperactivity disorder: A neglected but important aspect." *Appl Psychophysiol Biofeedback* 2003; 28(1):63–75.

Schulte-Korne G, Deimel W, et al. "Effect of an oligo-antigen diet on the behavior of hyperkinetic children." *Z Kinder Jugendpsychiatr Psychother* 1996;24(3):176–183.

Starobrat-Hemerlin B. "The effect of deficiency of selected bioelements on hyperactivity in children with certain specified mental disorders." *Ann Acad Med Stetin* 1998;44: 297–314.

Starobrat-Hemerlin B, Kozielec R. "The effects of magnesium physiological supplementation on hyperactivity in children with attention deficit hyperactivity disorder (ADHD). Positive response to magnesium oral loading test." *Mag Res* 1997;10(2): 149–156.

Tuthill R. "Hair lead levels related to children's classroom attention-deficit disorder." *Arch Environ Health* 1996;51(3):214–220.

Uhlig T, Merkenschlager A, et al. "Topographic mapping of brain electrical activity in children with food-induced attention deficit hyperkinetic disorder." *Eur J Pediatr* 1997; 156(7):557–561.

Warner JO. "Food and behaviour." *Clin Exp Allergy* 1995;25(suppl 1):S23–S26.

Chapter 21

Read, read, and read! The information in this chapter is only the tip of the iceberg. Many wonderful books and articles can educate you on this important topic. The Autism Research Institute at www.autismwebsite.com/ari/ is a clearinghouse for autism literature and research, with a fabulous bookstore offering many resources on autism and Asperger's syndrome. Books from the Autism Research Institute include *Autism: Effective Biomedical Treatments* and *Biological Treatments for Autism and PDD* as well as *Treating Autism* (2003) and *Vaccines, Autism and Childhood Disorders* (2003). Additional good books are *What Your Doctor May Not Tell You about Childhood Vaccinations* (Warner Books, 2001); *Facing Autism* (WaterBrook Press, 2000); and *Unraveling the Mystery of Autism* (Broadway, 2002), *Thinking In Pictures: And Other Reports from My Life with Autism* (Vintage, 1995), and *Children with Starving Brains* (Bramble Books, 2003). See also Resources.

Autism Research Institute. "Magnesium reduces hyperactivity." *Autism Res Rev Int* 1998; 12:4.

Andrews N, Miller E, et al. "Thimerosal exposure in infants and developmental disorders: A retrospective cohort study in the United Kingdom does not support a causal association." *Pediatrics* 2004;114(3):584–591.

Bernard S, Enayati A, et al. "The role of mercury in the pathogenesis of autism." *Mol Psychiatry* 2002;7(suppl 2):S42–S43.

Bernard S, Enayati ABS, et al. *Autism: A Unique Type of Mercury Poisoning.* Cranford, NJ: ARC Research, 2000.

Blaxill MF, Redwood L, et al. "Thimerosal and autism? A plausible hypothesis that should not be dismissed." *Med Hypotheses* 2004;62(5):788–794.

Burton D. "The future challenges of autism: A survey of the ongoing initiatives in the federal government to address the epidemic." Hearing before the House Governmental

Reform Subcommittee on wellness and human rights representative Dan Burten, Chairman, Washington, D.C. November 20, 2003.

Chakrabarti S, Fombonne E. "Pervasive developmental disorders in preschool children." *JAMA* 2001;285(24):3093–3099.

Chez MG, Buchanan CP, et al. "Double-blind, placebo-controlled study of L-carnosine supplementation in children with autistic spectrum disorders." *J Child Neurol* 2002; 17(11):833–837.

"Children with autism." Report to the Chairman and Ranking Minority Member, Subcommittee on Human Rights and Wellness, Committee on Government Reform, U.S. House of Representatives, 2005. Available at www.gao.gov/new.items/d05220.pdf.

Geier DA, Geier MR. "A comparative evaluation of the effects of MMR immunization and mercury doses from thimerosal-containing childhood vaccines on the population prevalence of autism." *Med Sci Monit* 2004;10(3):PI33–PI39.

Geier DA, Geier MR. "An assessment of the impact of thimerosal on childhood neurodevelopmental disorders." *Pediatr Rehab* 2003;6(2):97–102.

Hessel L. "Mercury in vaccines." *Bull Acad Natl Med* 2003;187(8):1501–1510.

Holmes AS, Blaxill MF, et al. "Reduced levels of mercury in first baby haircuts of autistic children." *Int J Toxicol* 2003;22(4):277–285.

Meadows M. "IOM report: No link between vaccines and autism." *FDA Consum* 2004; 38(5):18–19.

Merrick J, Kandel I, et al. "Trends in autism." *Int J Adolesc Med Health* 2004;16(1): 75–78.

Nash R. *Clinical Methods for Identifying, Reducing and Eliminating Heavy Metal Toxicity: Integrative Medical Therapeutics for Anti-Aging.* Las Vegas, NV: Primedia, 2004.

Nelson KB, Bauman ML. "Thimerosal and autism?" *Pediatrics* 2003;111(3):674–679.

Newschaffer CJ, Falb MD, Gurney JG. "National autism prevalence trends from United States special education data." *Pediatrics* 2005;115(3):277–282.

Parker SK, Schwartz B, et al. "Thimerosal-containing vaccines and autistic spectrum disorder: A critical review of published original data." *Pediatrics* 2004;114(3):793–804.

Sandler RH, Feingold SM, et al. "Short-term benefit from oral vancomycin treatment of regressive-onset autism." *J Child Neurol* 2000;15:429–435.

Singh VK, Rivas WH. "Detection of antinuclear and antilaminin antibodies in autistic children who received thimerosal-containing vaccines." *J Biomed Sci* 2004;11(5): 607–610.

Stehr-Green P, Tull P, et al. "Autism and thimerosal-containing vaccines: Lack of consistent evidence for an association." *Am J Prev Med* 2003;25(2):101–106.

Verstraeten T, Davis RL, et al. "Safety of thimerosal-containing vaccines: A two-phased study of computerized health maintenance organization databases." *Pediatrics* 2003; 112(5):1039–1048.

Wakefield AJ. "Measles, mumps, and rubella vaccination and autism." *N Engl J Med* 2003;348(10):951–954.

Chapter 22

Alvarez S, Herrero C, Bru E, Perdigon G. "Effect of *Lactobacillus casei* and yogurt administration on prevention of *Pseudomonas aeruginosa* infection in young mice." *J Food Prot* 2001;64(11):1768-1774.

Campbell DC. "Vitamin A deficiency in cystic fibrosis resulting in xerophthalmia." *J Human Nutr Dietetics* 1998;11:529–532.

Carrasco S, Codoceo R, et al. "Effect of taurine supplements on growth, fat absorption and bile acid on cystic fibrosis." *Acta Univ Carol [Med]* 1990;36(1–4):152–156.

Charmathy LM, Reinstein LJ, et al. "Desensitization to pancreatic enzyme intolerance in a child with cystic fibrosis." *Pediatrics* 1998;102(1):13.

Cobanoglu N, Oczelik U, et al. "Antioxidant effect of carotene in cystic fibrosis and bronchiectasis: Clinical and laboratory parameters of a pilot study." *Acta Paediatr* 2002;91:793–798.

Croft NM, Marshall TG, Ferguson A. "Gut inflammation in children with cystic fibrosis on high-dose enzyme supplements." *Lancet* 1995;346(8985):1265–1267.

De Curtis M, Santamaria F, et al. "Effect of taurine supplementation on fat and energy absorption in cystic fibrosis." *Arch Dis Child* 1992;67(9):1082–1085.

Egan ME, Pearson M, et al. "Curcumin, a major constituent of turmeric, corrects cystic fibrosis defects." *Science* 2004;304(5670):600–602.

Eid NS, Shoemaker LR, Samierc TD. "Vitamin A and cystic fibrosis: Case report and review of the literature." *J Pediatric Gastroenterol Nutr* 1990;10(2):265–269.

Escobar H, Perdomo M, et al. "Intestinal permeability to 51Cr-EDTA and orocecal transit time and cystic fibrosis." *J Pediatr Gastroenterol Nutr* 1992;14(2):204–207.

Farrell PM, Bieri JF, et al. "The occurrence and effects of human vitamin E deficiency: A study in patients with cystic fibrosis." *J Clin Invest* 1977;60:233–241.

Kalivianakis M, Minich DM, et al. "Fat malabsorption in cystic fibrosis patients receiving enzyme replacement therapy is due to impaired intestinal uptake of long-chain fatty acids." *Am J Clin Nutr* 1999;69:127–134.

Kovesi TA, Lehotay DC, et al. "Plasma carnitine levels in cystic fibrosis." *J Pediatr Gastroenterol Nutr* 1994;19(4):421–424.

Krebs NF, Sontag M, et al. "Low plasma zinc concentrations in young infants with cystic fibrosis." *J Pediatr* 1998;133(6):761–764.

Lloyd-Still JD, Johnson SB, et al. "Essential fatty acid status and fluidity of plasma phospholipids in cystic fibrosis infants." *Am J Clin Nutr* 1991;(54):1029–1035.

Lloyd-Still JD, Powers C. "Carnitine metabolites in infants with cystic fibrosis." *Acta Univ Carol [Med]* 1990;36(1–4):78–80.

Lloyd-Still JD, Powers CA, et al. "Acetylcarnitine is low in cord blood and cystic fibrosis." *ACTA Pediatr Scand* 1990;(79):427–439.

Lloyd-Still JD, Powers CA, et al. "Carnitine metabolites in infants with cystic fibrosis: A prospective study." *Acta Paediatr* 1993;82(2):145–149.

Lucarelli S, Quattrucci S, et al. "Food allergy in cystic fibrosis." *Minerva Pediatr* 1994;46(12):543–548.

Mall M, Grubb BR, et al. "Increased airway epithelial NA+ absorption produces cystic fibrosis-like lung disease in mice." *Nat Med* 2004;10(5):452–454.

McCabe H. "Riboflavin deficiency in cystic fibrosis: Three case reports." *Nutr Dietet* 2000;14:365–370.

Ramsey BW, Farrell PM, Pencharz P. "Nutritional assessment and management in cystic fibrosis: A consensus report." *Am J Clin Nutr* 1992;(55):108–116.

Rashid M, Durie P, et al. "Prevalence of vitamin K deficiency in cystic fibrosis." *Am J Clin Nutr* 1999;70:378–382.

Skopnik H, Kusenbach G, et al. "Taurine supplementation in cystic fibrosis (CF): Effect on vitamin E absorption kinetics." *Klin Padiatr* 1991;203(1):28–32.

Smith LJ, Lacaille F, et al. "Taurine decreases fecal fatty acid and sterol excretion in cystic fibrosis. A randomized double-blind trial." *Am J Dis Child* 1991;145(12): 1401–1404.

Wood LG, Fitzgerald DA, et al. "Increased plasma fatty acid concentrations after respiratory exacerbations are associated with elevated oxidative stress in cystic fibrosis patients." *Am J Clin Nutr* 2002;75:668–675.

Wos H, Krauze M, et al. "Total carnitine level in infants with cystic fibrosis and deficit supplementation by means of pharmacologic preparations and diet. Introductory remarks." *Pediatr Pol* 1995;70(8):661–666.

Yoshimura T, Matsushima K, et al. "Purification of a human monocyte-derived neutrophil chemotactic factor that has peptide sequence similarity to other host defense cytokines." *Proc Natl Acad Sci USA* 1987;84(24):9233–9237.

Chapter 23

Al-Qadreh A, Voskaki I, et al. "Treatment of osteopenia in children with insulin-dependent diabetes mellitus: The effect of 1 alpha-hydroxyvitamin D3." *Eur J Pediatr* 1996; 155(1):15–17.

American Dietetic Association, Dietitians of Canada. "Position of the American Dietetic Association and Dietitians of Canada: Vegetarian diets." *Can J Diet Pract Res* 2003; 64(2):62–81.

American Diabetes Association. "Type 2 diabetes in children and adolescents." *Diabetes Care* 2000;23(3):381–389.

Annis AM, Caulder MS, et al. "Family history, diabetes, and other demographic and risk factors among participants of the National Health and Nutrition Examination Survey 1999–2002." *Prev Chronic Dis* 2005. Available at www.cdc.gov/pcd/issues/2005/apr/04_0131.htm.

Calero P, Ribes-Koninckx C, et al. "IgA antigliadin antibodies as a screening method for nonovert celiac disease in children with insulin-dependent diabetes mellitus." *J Pediatr Gastroenterol Nutr* 1996;23(1):29–33.

Cefalu WT, Hu FB. "Role of chromium in human health and in diabetes." *Diabetes Care* 2004;27(11):2741–2751.

Chen HL, Sheu WH, et al. "Konjac supplement alleviated hypercholesterolemia and hyperglycemia in type 2 diabetic subjects—a randomized double-blind trial." *J Am Coll Nutr* 2003;22(1):36–42.

Cicero AF, Derosa G, Gaddi A. "What do herbalists suggest to diabetic patients in order to improve glycemic control? Evaluation of scientific evidence and potential risks." *Acta Diabetol* 2004;41(3):91–98.

Crino A, Schiaffini R, et al. "A randomized trial of nicotinamide and vitamin E in children with recent onset type 1 diabetes (IMDIAB IX)." *Eur J Endocrinol* 2004;150(5): 719–724.

Dahlquist G, Savilhati E, Landin-Olsson M. "An increased level of antibodies to beta-lactoglobulin is a risk determinant for early-onset type 1 (insulin dependent) diabetes mellitus independent of islet cell antibodies and early introduction of cow's milk." *Diabetologia* 1992;35:980–984.

Damci T, Nuhoglu I, et al. "Increased intestinal permeability as a cause of fluctuating postprandial blood glucose levels in type 1 diabetic patients." *Eur J Clin Invest* 2003; 33(5):397–401.

De Block CE. "Diabetes mellitus type 1 and associated organ-specific autoimmunity." *Verh K Acad Geneeskd Belg* 2000;62(4):285–328.

Fasano A, Not T, et al. "Zonulin, a newly discovered modulator of intestinal permeability, and its expression in coeliac disease." *Lancet* 2001;358(9294):1729–1730.

Fronczak CM, Baron AE, et al. "*In utero* dietary exposures and risk of islet autoimmunity in children." *Diabetes Care* 2003;26(12):3237–3242.

Husmann MJ, Fuchs P, et al. "Extracellular magnesium depletion in pediatric patients with insulin-dependent diabetes mellitus." *Miner Electrolyte Metab* 1997;23(2):121–124.

Jaffe RM, Deuster PA, Reeser C. "Determining the role of food/environmental sensitivities in reducing risk factors in patients with NIDDM." Reston, VA: Health Studies Collegium, 2001.

Jaffe RM, Mani J, et al. "Tolerance loss in diabetes: Association with foreign antigen exposure." *Diabetic Medicine*.

Jenkins DJ, Kendall CW, et al. "Type 2 diabetes and the vegetarian diet." *Am J Clin Nutr* 2003;78(3 suppl):610S–616S.

Kohno T, Kobashiri Y, et al. "Antibodies to food antigens in Japanese patients with type 1 diabetes mellitus." *Diabetes Res Clin Pract* 2002;55(1):1–9.

Krawczuk-Rybak M, Peczynska J, Urban M. "Usefulness of antioxidant vitamin supplementation in children and adolescents with newly diagnosed diabetes mellitus type I." *Endokrynol Diabetol Chor Przemiany Materii Wieku Rozw* 1999;5(1):11–20.

Mamoulakis D, Galanakis E, et al. "Carnitine deficiency in children and adolescents with type 1 diabetes." *J Diabetes Complications* 2004;18(5):27.

Pena AS, Wiltshire E, et al. "Folic acid improves endothelial function in children and adolescents with type 1 diabetes." *J Pediatr* 2004;144(4):500–504.

Pozzilli P, Browne PD, Kolb H. "Meta-analysis of nicotinamide treatment in patients with recent-onset IDDM. The Nicotinamide Trialists." *Diabetes Care* 1996;19(12): 1357–1363.

Roffi M, Kanaka C, et al. "Hypermagnesiuria in children with newly diagnosed insulin-dependent diabetes mellitus." *Am J Nephrol* 1994;14(3):201–206.

Rohn RD, Pleban P, Jenkins LL. "Magnesium, zinc and copper in plasma and blood cellular components in children with IDDM." *Clin Chim Acta* 1993;215(1):21–28.

Saggese G, Federico G, et al. "Hypomagnesemia and the parathyroid hormone-vitamin D endocrine system in children with insulin-dependent diabetes mellitus: Effects of magnesium administration." *J Pediatr* 1991;118(2):220–225.

Sakurai H. "Therapeutic potential of vanadium in treating diabetes mellitus." *Clin Calcium* 2005;15(1):49–57.

Secondulfo M, Iafusco D, et al. "Ultrastructural mucosal alterations and increased intestinal permeability in non-celiac, type I diabetic patients." *Dig Liver Dis* 2004;36(1):35–45.

Shanmugasundaram ER, Rageswari G, et al. "Use of *Gymnema sylvestre* leaf extract in the control of blood glucose in insulin-dependent diabetes mellitus." *J Ethnopharmacol* 1990;30(3):281–294.

Srivastava AK, Mehdi MZ. "Insulino-mimetic and anti-diabetic effects of vanadium compounds." *Diabet Med* 2005;22(1):2–13.

Stene LC, Ulriksen J, et al. "Use of cod liver oil during pregnancy associated with lower risk of type I diabetes in the offspring." *Diabetologia* 2000;43(9):1093–1098.

Takaya J, Higashino H, et al. "Intracellular magnesium of platelets in children with diabetes and obesity." *Metabolism* 2003;52(4):468–471.

Tuvemo T, Ewald U, et al. "Serum magnesium and protein concentrations during the first five years of insulin-dependent diabetes in children." *Acta Paediatr Suppl* 1997;418:7–10.

Vaarala O. "The gut immune system and type 1 diabetes." *Ann NY Acad Sci* 2002;958:39–46.

Vaarala O, Klennetti P, et al. "Cellular immune response to cow's milk beta-lactoglobulin in patients with newly diagnosed IDDM." *Diabetes* 1996;45:178–182.

Valerio G, Franzese A, et al. "Long-term follow-up of diabetes in two patients with thiamine-responsive megaloblastic anemia syndrome." *Diabetes Care* 1998;21(1):38–41.

Visalli N, Cavallo MG, et al. "A multi-centre randomized trial of two different doses of nicotinamide in patients with recent-onset type 1 diabetes (the IMDIAB VI)." *Diabetes Metab Res Rev* 1999;15(3):181–185.

Vuksan V, Sievenpiper JL, et al. "Beneficial effects of viscous dietary fiber from Konjac-mannan in subjects with the insulin resistance syndrome: Results of a controlled metabolic trial." *Diabetes Care* 2000;23(1):9–14.

Wiltshire EJ, Gent R, et al. "Endothelial dysfunction relates to folate status in children and adolescents with type 1 diabetes." *Diabetes* 2002;51(7):2282–2286.

Yeh GY, Eisenberg DM, et al. "Systematic review of herbs and dietary supplements for glycemic control in diabetes." *Diabetes Care* 2003;26(4):1277–1294.

Zhao HX, Mold MD, et al. "Drinking water composition and childhood-onset type 1 diabetes mellitus in Devon and Cornwall, England." *Diabet Med* 2001;18(9):709–717.

Chapter 24

Al-Gazali LI, Padmanabhan R, et al. "Abnormal folate metabolism and genetic polymorphism of the folate pathway in a child with Down syndrome and neural tube defect." *Am J Med Genet* 2001;103(2):128–132.

Bade MA, Rammeloo EM, et al. "Symptoms of disease and food allergy in children with Down syndrome." *Ned Tijdschr Geneeskd* 1995;139(33):1680–1684.

Bonamico M, Mariani P, et al. "Prevalence and clinical picture of celiac disease in Italian Down syndrome patients: A multicenter study." *J Pediatr Gastroenterol Nutr* 2001; 33(2):139–143.

Book L, Hart A, et al. "Prevalence and clinical characteristics of celiac disease in Downs syndrome in a US study." *Am J Med Genet* 2001;98(1):70–74.

Bucci I, Napolitano G, et al. "Zinc sulfate supplementation improves thyroid function in hypozincemic Down children." *Biol Trace Elem Res* 1999;67(3):257–268.

Carnicer J, Farre C, et al. "Prevalence of coeliac disease in Down's syndrome." *Eur J Gastroenterol Hepatol* 2001;13(3):263–267.

Cogulu O, Ozkinay F, et al. "Celiac disease in children with Down syndrome: Importance of follow-up and serologic screening." *Pediatr Int* 2003;45(4):395–399.

Corsi MM, Ponti W, et al. "Proapoptotic activated T-cells in the blood of children with Down's syndrome: Relationship with dietary antigens and intestinal alterations." *Int J Tissue React* 2003;25(3):117–125.

Dinani S, Carpenter S. "Down's syndrome and thyroid disorder." *J Ment Defic Res* 1990;34(pt 2):187–193.

Fuchtenbusch M, Karges W, et al. "Antibodies to bovine serum albumin (BSA) in type 1 diabetes and other autoimmune disorders." *Exp Clin Endocrinol Diabetes* 1997; 105(2):86–91.

Goldacre MJ, Wotton CJ, et al. "Cancers and immune related diseases associated with Down's syndrome: A record linkage study." *Arch Dis Child* 2004;89(11):1014–1017.

Harrell RF, Capp RH, et al. "Can nutritional supplements help mentally retarded children? An exploratory study." *Proc Natl Acad Sci USA* 1981;78(1):574–578.

Kanavin OJ, Aaseth J, et al. "Thyroid hypofunction in Down's syndrome: Is it related to oxidative stress?" *Biol Trace Elem Res* 2000;78(1–3):35–42.

Kolek A, Vospelova J, et al. "Occurrence of coeliac disease in children with Down's syndrome in north Moravia, Czech Republic." *Eur J Pediatr* 2003;162(3):207–208.

Mackey J, Treem WR, et al. "Frequency of celiac disease in individuals with Down syndrome in the United States." *Clin Pediatr* 2001;40(5):249–252.

Napolitano G, Palka G, et al. "Is zinc deficiency a cause of subclinical hypothyroidism in Down syndrome?" *Ann Genet* 1990;33(1):9–15.

Oliveira AT, Longui CA, et al. "Evaluation of the hypothalamic-pituitary-thyroid axis in children with Down syndrome." *J Pediatr* 2002;78(4):295–300.

Pogribna M, Melnyk S, et al. "Homocysteine metabolism in children with Down syndrome: *In vitro* modulation." *Am J Hum Genet* 2001;69(1):88–95.

Pozzan GB, Rigon F, et al. "Thyroid function in patients with Down syndrome: Preliminary results from non-institutionalized patients in the Veneto region." *Am J Med Genet* 1990;7(suppl):S57–S58.

Reading CM. "Down's syndrome: Nutritional intervention." *Nutr Health* 1984;3(1–2): 91–111.

Reichelt KL, Lindback T, et al. "Increased levels of antibodies to food proteins in Down syndrome." *Acta Paediatr Jpn* 1994;36(5):489–492.

Rumbo M, Chirdo FG, et al. "Evaluation of coeliac disease serological markers in Down syndrome patients." *Dig Liver Dis* 2002;34(2):116–121.

Sanchez-Albisua I, Storm W, et al. "How frequent is coeliac disease in Down syndrome?" *Eur J Pediatr* 2002;161(12):683–684.

Sciberras C, Vella C, et al. "The prevalence of coeliac disease in Down's syndrome in Malta." *Ann Trop Paediatr* 2004;24(1):81–83.

Thiel RJ, Fowkes SW. "Down syndrome and epilepsy: A nutritional connection?" *Med Hypotheses* 2004;62(1):35–44.

Turkel H. *Medical Treatment of Down Syndrome and Genetic Diseases, Fourth Edition.* Southfield, MI: Ubiotica.

Tuysuz B, Beker DB. "Thyroid dysfunction in children with Down's syndrome." *Acta Paediatr* 2001;90(12):1389–1393.

Chapter 25

Barak V, Birkenfeld S, et al. "The effect of herbal remedies on the production of human inflammatory and anti-inflammatory cytokines." *Isr Med Assoc J* 2002;4(11 suppl): S919–S922.

Barak V, Halperin T, et al. "The effect of Sambucol, a black elderberry-based, natural product, on the production of human cytokines: I. Inflammatory cytokines." *Eur Cytokine Netw* 2001;12(2):290–296.

Centers for Disease Control. "Key facts about avian influenza (bird flu) and avian influenza A (H5N1) virus." Accessed May 24, 2005. Available at www.cdc.gov/flu/avian/gen-info/facts.htm.

Jaber R. "Respiratory and allergic diseases: From upper respiratory tract infections to asthma." *Prim Care* 2002;29(2):231–261.

Jefferson T, Rivetti D, et al. "Efficacy and effectiveness of influenza vaccines in elderly people: A systematic review." *Lancet* 2005:3566(9492):1165–1174.

Jefferson T, Smith S, et al. "Assessment of the efficacy and effectiveness of influenza vaccines in healthy children: Systematic review." *Lancet* 2005;365(9461): 773–780.

Konlee M. "A new triple combination therapy." *Posit Health News* 1998;17:12–14.

Zakay-Rones Z, Thom E, et al. "Randomized study of the efficacy and safety of oral elderberry extract in the treatment of influenza A and B virus infections." *J Int Med Res* 2004;32(2):132–140.

Chapter 26

Annequin D, Dumas C, et al. "Migraine and chronic headache in children." *Rev Neurol* 2000;156(suppl 4):4S68–4S74.

Anthony M. "Platelet superoxide dismutase in migraine and tension type headaches." *Cephalalgia* 1994;14:1818–1813.

Bates B. "Low-fat, high-carbohydrate diet averts migraines." *Family Practice News* 1996;1:16.

Bigal ME, Bordini CA, et al. "Intravenous magnesium sulphate in the acute treatment of migraine without aura and migraine with aura. A randomized, double-blind, placebo-controlled study." *Cephalalgia* 2002;22(5):345–353.

Black M. "Nicotinic acid and headache." *Cortlandt Forum* 1990:26–30.

Carter CM, Egger J, et al. "A dietary management of severe childhood migraine." *Hum Nutr Appl Nutr* 1985;39(4):294–303.

Cavanagh N. "Dietary treatment of childhood migraine." *Midwife Health Visit Community Nurse* 1986;22(8):279–231.

"Certain foods provoke migraine." *Nutr Rev* 1984;42(2):41–42.

Corbo J, Esses D, et al. "Randomized clinical trial of intravenous magnesium sulfate as an adjunctive medication for emergency department treatment of migraine headache." *Ann Emerg Med* 2001;38(6):621–627.

Dalton K, Dalton ME. "Food intake before migraine attacks in children." *J R Coll Gen Pract* 1979;29(208):662–665.

Danesch U, Rittinghausen R. "Safety of a patented special butterbur root extract for migraine prevention." *Headache* 2003;43(1):76–78.

Diener HC, Rahlfs VW, et al. "The first placebo-controlled trial of a special butterbur root extract for the prevention of migraine: Reanalysis of efficacy criteria." *Eur Neurol* 2004;51(2):89–97.

Egger J, Carter CM, et al. "Is migraine food allergy? A double-blind controlled trial of oligoantigenic diet treatment." *Lancet* 1983;2(8355):865–869.

Galli V, Ciccarone V, et al. "Hemicrania and food in the child." *Pediatr Med Chir* 1985;7(1):17–21.

Guariso G, Bertoli S, et al. "Migraine and food intolerance: A controlled study in pediatric patients." *Pediatr Med Chir* 1993;15(1):57–61.

Harel Z, Gascon G, et al. "Supplementation with omega-3 polyunsaturated fatty acids in the management of recurrent migraines in adolescents." *J Adolesc Health* 2002;31(2):154–161.

Hesse J, Mogelvang B, et al. "Acupuncture versus metoprolol in migraine prophylaxis: A randomized trial of trigger point inactivation." *J Intern Med* 1994;235:451–456.

Heuser G. "*Candida albicans* and migraine headaches: A possible link." *J Advancement Med* 1992;5(3):177–187.

Johnson ES, Kadam NP, et al. "Efficacy of feverfew as prophylactic treatment of migraine." *Br Med J* 1985;2291(6495):569–573.

Jones M. "Migraine headaches and food." *NOHA News* 1989;14(2).

Kabbouche MA, Powers SW, et al. "Carnitine palmityltransferase II (CPT2) deficiency and migraine headache: Two case reports." *Headache* 2003;43(5):490–495.

Kalin P. "The common butterbur (*Petasites hybridus*)—portrait of a medicinal herb." *Forsch Komplementarmed Klass Naturheilkd* 2003;10(suppl 1):S41–S44.

Lipton RB, Gobel H, et al. "*Petasites hybridus* root (butterbur) is an effective preventive treatment for migraine." *Neurology* 2004;63(12):2240–2244.

Lucarelli S, Lendvai D, et al. "Hemicrania and food allergy in children." *Minerva Pediatr* 1990;42(6):215–218.

Mazzotta G, Sarchielli P, et al. "Intracellular Mg++ concentration and electromyographical ischemic test in juvenile headache." *Cephalalgia* 1999;19(9):802–809.

Medina JL, Diamond S. "The role of diet in migraine." *Headache* 1978;18(1):31–34.

"Monograph. *Petasites hybridus*." *Altern Med Rev* 2001;6(2):207–209.

Mylek D. "Migraine as one of the symptoms of food allergy." *Pol Tyg Lek* 1992;47 (3–4):89–91.

National Institute of Neurological Disorders and Stroke, American Academy of Neurology. "21st century prevention and management of migraine headaches." *Clinical Courier* 2001;9. Available at www.ninds.nih.gov/doctors/OP129D_Clinical_ Courier_fa.pdf.

Palmero Becares ML. "Migraine, food and additives." *Med Clin* 1986;87(3):87–89.

Pfaffenrath V, Diener HC, et al. "The efficacy and safety of *Tanacetum parthenium* (feverfew) in migraine prophylaxis—a double-blind, multicentre, randomized placebo-controlled dose-response study." *Cephalalgia* 2002;22(7):523–532.

Pittler M, Ernst E. "Feverfew for preventing migraine." *Cochrane Database Syst Rev* 2004;1:CD002286.

Rios J, Passe MM. "Evidence-based use of botanicals, minerals, and vitamins in the prophylactic treatment of migraines." *J Am Acad Nurse Pract* 2004;16(6):251–256.

Robbins L. "Precipitating factors in migraine: A retrospective review of 494 patients." *Headache* 1994;34(4):214–216.

Russell G, Abu-Arafeh I, et al. "Abdominal migraine: Evidence for existence and treatment options." *Paediatr Drugs* 2002;4(1):1–8.

Schoenen J, Jacquy J, et al. "Effectiveness of high-dose riboflavin in migraine prophylaxis: A randomized controlled trial." *Neurology* 1998;50:466–470.

Schoenen J, Lenaerts M, Bastings E. "High-dose riboflavin as a prophylactic treatment of migraine: Results of an open pilot study." *Cephalagia* 1994;14:328–329.

Serratrice J, Disdier P, et al. "Migraine and coeliac disease." *Headache* 1998;38(8): 627–628.

Silberstein SD, Lipton RB. "Epidemiology of migraine." *Neuroepidemiology* 1993; 12(3):179–184.

Soriani S, Arnaldi C, et al. "Serum and red blood cell magnesium levels in juvenile migraine patients." *Headache* 1995;35(1):14–16.

Stewart WF, Schechter A, Rasmussen BK. "Migraine prevalence. A review of population-based studies." *Neurology* 1994;44(6 suppl 4):S17–S23.

Taubert K. "Magnesium in migraine. Results of a multicenter pilot study." *Portschreit Medizin* 1994;112(24):238–230.

Thiel R. "Natural interventions for migraine sufferers." *ANMA Monitor* 1998;2(3):5–9.

Thomas J, Tomb E, et al. "Migraine treatment by oral magnesium intake and correction of the irritation of buccofacial and cervical muscles as a side effect of mandibular imbalance." *Mag Res* 1994;7(2):123–127.

Wager W, Nootbaar-Wagner U. "Prophylactic treatment of migraine with gamma-linolenic and alpha-linolenic acids." *Cephalalgia* 1997;17:127–130.

Wang F, Van Den Eeden SK, et al. "Oral magnesium oxide prophylaxis of frequent migrainous headache in children: A randomized, double-blind, placebo-controlled trial." *Headache* 2003;43(6):601–610.

Zelnik N, Pacht A, et al. "Range of neurologic disorders in patients with celiac disease." *Pediatrics* 2004;113(6):1672–1676.

Appendix A

Application Guide: Bacterial Overgrowth of the Small Intestine. Asheville, NC: Great Smokies Diagnostic Laboratory, 1994.

Application Guide: Functional Liver Testing. Asheville, NC: Great Smokies Diagnostic Laboratory, 1994.

Bland J. *New Clinical Breakthroughs in the Management of Chronic Fatigue Syndrome, Intestinal Dysbiosis, Immune Dysregulation and Cellular Toxicity.* Gig Harbor, WA: Health Comm, 1992.

Brown S, Jaffe R. "Acid-alkaline balance and its effect on bone health." *Int J Integr Med* 2000;2:6.

Cusak MA, O'Mahony MS, Woodhouse K. "Giardia in older people." *Age Ageing* 2001;30:419–421.

Gittleman AL. *Guess What Came to Dinner?* Garden City Park, NY: Avery Publishing Group, 1993.

Jaffe R, Donovan P. *Your Health: A Professional User's Guide.* Sterling, VA: Health Studies Collegium, 1993.

Kirsch M. "Bacterial overgrowth." *Am J Gastroenterol* 1990;85(3):231–237.

Lab Manual. Asheville, NC: Great Smokies Diagnostic Laboratory, 1995.

Rider MS, Acterbert J, et al. "Effect of immune system imagery on secretory IgA." *Biofeedback Self-Reg* 1990;15(4):317–333.

GENERAL REFERENCES

Websites

About Natural Healing, www.healing.about.com

About Alternative Medicine, www.altmedicine.about.com

Centers for Disease Control, www.cdc.gov/ncidod/diseases

Clinical Pearls Database version 5.02, IT Services, Sacramento, CA, www.clinicalpearls.com

Pediatrician Alan Greene, M.D., www.drgreene.com

Family Doctor, www.familydoctor.org

Kids' Health for Parents, www.kidshealth.org

Mayo Clinic, www.mayoclinic.com

Medline Plus, www.nlm.nih.gov/medlineplus

National Digestive Diseases Clearinghouse, www.digestive.niddk.nih.gov

Books

Hoffman R. *Seven Weeks to a Settled Stomach.* New York, NY: Pocket Books, 1990.

Bove M. *An Encyclopedia of Natural Healing for Children and Infants.* New York, NY: Keats/McGraw Hill, 2001.

Gershon MD. *The Second Brain.* New York, NY: Harper Collins Publishers, 1998.

Gardner J. *The New Healing Yourself: Natural Remedies for Adults and Children.* Freedom, CA: Crossing Press, 1989.

Jaffe R, Brown S, et al. *The Alkaline Way: Your Health Restoration.* Sterling, VA: ELISA-ACT Biotechnologies, 2004.

Murray M, Pizzorno J. *Encyclopedia of Natural Medicine.* Rocklin, CA: Prima Publishing, 1991.

Shabert J. *The Ultimate Nutrient: Glutamine.* Garden City Park, NY: Avery Publishing Group, 1994.

Wright J. *Dr. Wright's Guide to Healing with Nutrition.* Emmaus, PA: Rodale Books, 1984.

Zand J, Roundtree R, Walton R. *Smart Medicine for a Healthier Child, Second Edition.* New York, NY: Avery, 2003.

Index